Praise for
Reconcilable Differences

"One virtue of the book is its utter realism.... Offers a slew of tools that couples can use to reconcile their differences without the help of a therapist."

—JANE BRODY, *The New York Times*

"When partners fight, they often push each other to change. But seeing conflicts from the other's perspective helps move the couple away from anger and blame. This invaluable book provides concrete strategies to do just that. With a deeper understanding of your partner's emotional vulnerabilities, you can build trust and intimacy, and maybe even bring about the changes that matter most to you."

—JANIS ABRAHMS SPRING, PHD, author of *After the Affair*

"No matter how many books you have read to improve your relationship, read this one, and follow the research-based principles it presents! The authors are internationally known scientists who have produced a book that all couples need to read. It's not the differences between you and your partner that matter, but how you handle them, and this book shows exactly how and why."

—HOWARD J. MARKMAN, PHD, coauthor of *Fighting for Your Marriage*

"This deceptively simple book can change lives. You and your partner will learn numerous ways to accept each other and achieve a new level of happiness and comfort in your relationship. The genius of the book is that these techniques are not difficult, and they can help put an end to perpetual conflict."

—PEPPER SCHWARTZ, PHD, coauthor of *The Normal Bar: The Surprising Secrets of Happy Couples and What They Reveal about Creating a New Normal in Your Relationship*

"It is often so difficult for quarreling couples to find a way through the thicket of blame, accusation, and resentment that ensnares them, but this splendid book illuminates some pathways out. The first edition was terrific, but this revision goes beyond it, bringing in new research, fresh ideas, and, as usual, practical solutions. All couples who find themselves enduring repeated conflicts—which is to say, nearly all couples—will benefit from this fine book."

—CAROL TAVRIS, PHD, coauthor of *Mistakes Were Made (but Not by Me)*

"There are lots of books for couples that make interesting reading, and some that provide specific, doable suggestions for improving your relationship, but just a handful—including this one—based on principles that have been scientifically shown to work. Any couple that wants to better understand and overcome problems in their relationship will find this book a great place to start."

—W. KIM HALFORD, PHD, School of Psychology, University of Queensland, Australia

"Gives several guides to building acceptance."

—*USA Today*

"Packed with data, wisdom, and common sense."

—POLLY DREW, *Milwaukee Journal Sentinel*

Reconcilable Differences

Reconcilable Differences

SECOND EDITION

Rebuild Your Relationship by Rediscovering the Partner You Love—without Losing Yourself

ANDREW CHRISTENSEN, PhD

BRIAN D. DOSS, PhD

NEIL S. JACOBSON, PhD

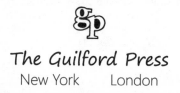

The Guilford Press

New York   London

10/6/14
LN
$15.95

© 2014 The Guilford Press
A Division of Guilford Publications, Inc.
72 Spring Street, New York, NY 10012
www.guilford.com

Printed in the United States of America

This book is printed on acid-free paper.

Last digit is print number: 9   8   7   6   5   4   3   2   1

Library of Congress Cataloging-in-Publication Data

Christensen, Andrew, 1946–
    Reconcilable differences : rebuild your relationship by rediscovering
the partner you love—without losing yourself / Andrew Christensen,
Brian D. Doss, and Neil S. Jacobson. — Second edition
        pages   cm
    Includes bibliographical references and index.
    ISBN 978-1-4625-0243-1 (pbk.) — ISBN 978-1-4625-1231-7 (hardcover)
    1. Couples.   2. Man–woman relationships.   3. Interpersonal
communication.   4. Interpersonal relations.   5. Conflict management.
    I. Doss, Brian David, 1975–   II. Jacobson, Neil S., 1949–1999   III. Title.
    HQ801.C4867 2014
    306.7—dc23

                                                          2013037587

During the production phase for the first edition of this book, Neil S. Jacobson died suddenly and unexpectedly. His death is an incalculable loss to his family and friends and to the three fields in which he was a leading scholar and researcher: marital therapy, domestic violence, and depression.

As his close collaborator and friend for years, I miss him greatly. This book is dedicated to his honor and memory.

—A. C.

Contents

Acknowledgments

There are those who influenced my ideas, those who helped me articulate them in this book, those who helped me implement these ideas with couples, and those who helped me live the reality of these ideas. All deserve acknowledgment.

Clearly my coauthors, Neil S. Jacobson and Brian D. Doss, have had the foremost influence on my ideas about couple therapy. Through years of productive discussion, joint writing projects, and joint supervision of our clinicians, the late Neil Jacobson and I developed and refined our approach to couple therapy. We each might have been able to develop this approach alone, but not nearly as well and not nearly as enjoyably. My former graduate student and now colleague and coauthor Brian Doss brought a keen interest in dissemination to our work and creativity in adapting integrative behavioral couple therapy (IBCT) to a larger audience. From his early research on what leads people to seek couple therapy to his current, monumental effort to translate IBCT into an online program accessible to all, he has demonstrated not only an ability to think big but also the energy and tenacity to follow through. Aside from Neil and Brian, other important influences on my thinking were Robert Weiss, a father of behavioral couple therapy and my first marital therapy supervisor; Gayla Margolin, with whom I conducted my first clinical study of marital therapy; the late Harold Kelley, an influential social psychologist with whom I worked early in my career; and Dan Wile, whose clinical writings, though coming from a dramatically different theoretical perspective, directly influenced my own work with couples. And, finally, the couples with whom I worked, either directly in my private practice or indirectly by watching hours of their therapy sessions on videotape, were a continued challenge to my thinking and a repeated reminder that the dirty and tender reality of conflict and love is always more complicated than our theories envision.

My editor at The Guilford Press, Christine Benton, was an enormous help in translating my ideas into ink. She understood what I was trying to say about acceptance in relationships, and she kept the rudder of this book clearly on that course through two editions. She helped me say what I wanted to say—which is all that anyone can ask of an editor. I also want to thank Melissa Fu and Betty Horng for their secretarial assistance with this book. They cheerfully worked on the manuscript as it went through its various drafts.

The therapists on our project, in both Los Angeles and Seattle, brought the ideas of our treatment approach to bear on the lives of our struggling couples. Alfredo Crespo, Shelly Harrell, Megan Sullaway, and Anthony Zamudio, in Los Angeles, and Peter Fehrenbach, Carol Henry, Christopher Martel, and Debra Wilk, in Seattle, are talented therapists who demonstrated the special skill of attending to the research demands of our project while providing quality care to each of their couples. I appreciate the competent efforts of Professor Bill George, who took over administration of the project at the University of Washington after Neil Jacobson's untimely death. The graduate students at UCLA and at the University of Washington, now all but one PhDs themselves, were remarkably able clinical assessors and researchers who ran the day-to-day operations of this large research project. Brian Baucom, Katherine Williams Baucom, Lisa Benson, Brian Doss, Kathleen Eldridge, Krista Gattis, Amanda Jensen, Janice Jones, Meghan McGinn, Felicia De La Garza Mercer, Mia Sevier, and Lorelei Simpson were graduate students on the project at UCLA; David Atkins, Sara Berns, Jean Yi, and Jennifer Wheeler were graduate students on the project at the University of Washington. In addition, the consummate methodological and statistical skills of David Atkins were essential to this project. Finally, I wish to acknowledge the competent project coordinators at UCLA, with whom I worked closely: Nancy Chen, Nikki Frousakis, Cindy Heng, Betty Horng, Melissa McElrea, Adam Rico, Marietta Watson, Mike Wong, and Wai-Ling Wu. They helped the project run smoothly and happily.

And, finally, I want to thank those who have helped me live my ideas of conflict, acceptance, and intimacy in a true learning laboratory of love, our home: my wife, Louise; our daughter, Lisa; and our son, Sean.

ANDREW CHRISTENSEN

I was honored to be asked to join the second edition of *Reconcilable Differences*. The first edition that Andy and Neil wrote was an outstanding example of their ability to bridge and integrate three areas of expertise: knowledge of the research literature on couple therapy, therapist skills honed while working with hundreds of distressed couples, and an ability to translate the concepts into a format that couples could apply on their own to their own relationships.

My contributions to the second edition are a result of the countless opportunities for mentoring and collaboration I've had over the years. My coauthor, Andy, was my PhD mentor and dissertation chair at UCLA; he more than anyone else has helped shape my ideas on couple distress and intervention. Just as important, he provides a shining example of how one can be successful both personally and professionally.

I've been lucky to have other important mentors in the couple field, including Doug Snyder, who was my colleague at Texas A&M for 5 years; Scott Stanley and Howard Markman, who have helped shape my ideas on prevention; and Julian Libet at the Charleston VA Medical Center, who helped me in my struggle to adapt my approaches to couple therapy with disadvantaged couples. I have also benefited immensely from my repeated collaborations with my colleagues Galena Rhoades and Lorelei Simpson, who provide me with both the challenge and the opportunity of new perspectives.

Some of the new ideas we've introduced in the second edition were forged and tested as part of our National Institutes of Health (NIH) grant to develop a web-based program for couples experiencing difficulties in their relationship (*www.OurRelationship.com*). So, I would like to thank NIH for their support of this work and the people who have made that project possible. In particular, Emily Georgia, Larisa Cicila, and Judith Biesen have played central roles in the design and implementation of the web-based program. Kelly Koerner, Cammy Bean, and Mark Harrison helped guide me in translating our therapy approach into a self-help format, and those lessons were critical in formulating many of the revisions in this edition. Our editors at Guilford, Christine Benton and Kitty Moore, were also extremely helpful in that regard. And Cherelle Carrington deserves a strong dose of appreciation for preparing the index for this book.

Finally, I would like to acknowledge the incalculable support that I've gotten from my wife, Mandy, and our two children, Abby and Matthew. While I could say a lot more than that, one of the most important lessons I've learned from them is the importance of separating my professional life from my personal life. So, I'll keep it simple here—thank you!

BRIAN D. DOSS

Preface

No matter how much we have in common with the one we love, each of us remains a unique human being. And no matter how much we love each other, the differences between us will eventually cause conflict. We feel hurt or ignored, resentful or angry, and our arguments often make the problem worse. Something's got to give, and we usually nominate our partner.

Sound familiar? If so, you're not alone. Trying to get your partner to change when strife seems to be pulling your relationship apart is human nature. It's easy to understand your own point of view; it's much harder to see where the one you love is coming from. That your relationship would improve drastically if only he or she would see things your way and make a few little alterations in behavior seems like an obvious conclusion.

As you undoubtedly know, however, trying to change another person, even one motivated by love and loyalty toward you, is a tall order. Eliciting change from your partner without demonstrating acceptance of his or her unique position is difficult, often impossible, as we have learned over decades of clinical practice and research in the field of couple therapy.

When Neil S. Jacobson and I met early in our careers, we were both proponents of the behavioral approach to couple therapy in which we had been trained. This type of therapy teaches couples communication and problem-solving skills so that partners can make positive changes in their behavior toward each other. In studies conducted in North America, Germany, Australia, and elsewhere, the behavioral approach proved superior in helping couples improve their degree of satisfaction and reduce the conflict in their relationship compared to getting no treatment at all. The efficacy of the behavioral approach is supported by more research than any other therapy for couples. Neil became a leading exponent of this type of couple therapy and produced some of the best research studies showing its effectiveness. However, his studies and those of others showed the limitations of this approach: a good third of couples did not respond to the treatment, and even among those who did respond positively, a substantial number relapsed in the years following treatment. From a scientific standpoint, the best available wasn't that good.

In 1991, when Neil invited me to speak at the University of Washington, we discovered that we had, separately and simultaneously, started to experiment with a different approach to couples in conflict. Though they were not identical, our interventions had one thing in common: the promotion of acceptance over change. We had developed ways in which partners could experience and accept the normal vulnerabilities that we all have and the very natural incompatibilities that crop up between two unique individuals. With this acceptance, something paradoxical often occurred: many of the needs and demands for change evaporated, and each partner became more amenable to making the changes that were truly important to the other.

We decided to combine forces in developing our new treatment and in seeking a grant that would allow us to test its effectiveness. In 1993 we obtained a 3-year grant from the National Institute of Mental Health to conduct a small pilot study comparing our treatment to traditional behavioral couple therapy (TBCT). As part of our pilot study, we trained five therapists in our new approach, which we called integrative behavioral couple therapy (IBCT), as well as in the traditional behavioral approach. Twenty-one distressed couples were randomly assigned to one of the two approaches and received up to 25 sessions of therapy. Based on extensive evaluations of these couples prior to treatment, immediately after treatment, and at follow-up periods, the couples in our integrative treatment performed substantially better than those in the traditional treatment, even though they, as expected, also showed improvement.

Encouraged by these results, we knew that only a larger study with a more diverse sample of couples and more extensive evaluation and follow-up would provide definitive evidence of the relative outcome of our new treatment, IBCT. In 1997 we received funding from the National Institute of Mental Health for a 5-year study of 134 couples, which to our knowledge is the largest and most extensive evaluation of couple therapy conducted to date. We selected couples in Los Angeles and Seattle who had serious and chronic marital discord; all were randomly assigned to one of the two treatments and received up to 26 sessions of couple therapy over about 8 months. Couples were followed for 2 years posttreatment.

In 1998, Brian Doss joined the project as a graduate student with me at UCLA. In 1999, just 2 years into the project, Neil suffered a sudden, major heart attack and died at age 50. A personal tragedy for all of those who knew and cared for him, it was also a major setback for our research. Fortunately, faculty and graduate students at the University of Washington as well as graduate students at UCLA stepped up to the challenge of working without Neil, and the project continued. We even obtained additional funding in 2003 to continue following couples for 5 years after the termination of therapy.

Despite being seriously and chronically distressed, couples in both treatments showed substantial improvement that was largely maintained through 2 years of follow-up, even though the study design prohibited any additional therapy from our project for these couples after treatment ended. During each of the 6-month assessments through these first 2 years of follow-up, couples who had received IBCT showed significantly greater maintenance of change than couples who had received TBCT. At the 2-year follow-up, 69% of the couples in IBCT and 60% of the couples in TBCT evidenced clinically significant improvement relative to their initial functioning. During years 3 to 5 of follow-up, couples showed some deterioration, and differences between the two treatments were erased. Yet 50% of couples still showed significant clinical improvement relative to their initial functioning at the final, 5-year follow-up. We concluded that with these seriously and chronically distressed couples, additional booster sessions were probably needed to maintain treatment gains and the superior outcome of IBCT. For more information about this research, including copies of some of our research papers, please see our website: *http://ibct.psych.ucla.edu.*

All couples who received our IBCT got the first edition of this book as a companion guide to their treatment. Although you are not getting one of the therapists we have trained along with the book, we believe that you can use this book to lessen conflict and increase intimacy in your relationship. Some of you may want to use the book as you seek professional assistance from a couple therapist (see Chapter 16). Others may find the book sufficient on its own.

After the completion of our study, we have engaged in two major efforts at dissemination. First, the U.S. Department of Veterans Affairs chose IBCT as one of the evidence-based treatments to make available to veteran couples in need. Since 2010, I have been heavily involved in training VA therapists and consultants. Second, Brian spearheaded an effort to adapt IBCT for online delivery. Now a professor at the University of Miami, Brian obtained funding from the National Institute of Child Health and Human Development to develop and test this online system. Since 2009, Brian and I have worked together with our separate graduate students to develop and test this program. Both of these projects forced us to rethink IBCT and develop ways to make it more accessible. We wanted to incorporate these developments into our book and thus decided to revise *Reconcilable Differences.*

This revised edition is different from the first edition in five important ways. First, we help readers define one core problem on which they will focus as they work through the book. Although couples often have a number of concerns, usually those concerns center around one or two themes. For example, one couple might constantly struggle with responsibilities (who should do what in terms of child care and housework and according to whose standards). Another couple might struggle with intimacy issues (how close should we be physically and emotionally). We believe it helps to focus in depth on one core issue. After success with this core issue, you can focus on other issues. Second, we provide a number of evidence-based questionnaires with instructions on scoring and interpretation so you may evaluate your relationship and proceed based on sound knowledge. Third, we have introduced an acronym, the DEEP analysis, to assist you in understanding your struggles. *D* stands for differences in personality and interests that may contribute to conflict. The first *E* stands for emotional sensitivities that may make the differences more difficult to handle. The second *E* stands for external stressors that may complicate resolution of the problem. And, finally, the *P* stands for patterns of communication. Couples interact about their difficulties as a way of resolving them, but often this communication not only does not solve the problem but actually makes it worse. Early in the book there are chapters devoted to each of these aspects of a DEEP analysis, with questionnaires to help readers assess and evaluate these areas. Fourth, we have shortened parts of the book and tried to streamline it and make it more readable. Finally, we have tried to be more inclusive with this edition. Although we suggested in the first edition that IBCT could work well with gay and lesbian couples, our examples focused exclusively on heterosexual couples. In this revision, we include examples from gay and lesbian couples as well. We believe these changes make the book much more usable in facilitating changes in your relationship.

If there is one thing we have discovered in our years of work with couples, it is that advice is easy to give, hard to take, and even harder to implement. Although this book is aimed at ushering you and your partner to an understanding of how couples interact, what causes conflict, and how you might lessen yours, it purposely avoids "sounds-good," "one-size-fits-all" advice. Instead, we guide you toward an understanding of your own unique relationship and suggest ways to foster acceptance. To bring our points home, we have filled the pages with illustrations of couples facing problems a lot like yours. As the primary author of this book, I have generated these examples from my own practice, my supervision of couple therapy, and my personal experience, but each is a constructed amalgam so as to protect the confidentiality of any real couple.

Because conflict is a window on the vulnerabilities and sensitivities of warring partners, it offers the promise of greater connection as well as the threat of alienation. We believe that by understanding your conflicts and emotionally accepting your positions in the conflict, the two of you can achieve genuine intimacy. You can, in the end, reconcile the differences that keep you apart.

ANDREW CHRISTENSEN
University of California, Los Angeles

PART I

The Conflicting Sides of Conflict

CHAPTER 1

Three Sides to Every Story

- Debra thinks Frank is emotionally bankrupt. Frank thinks Debra is insecure.
- Frank thinks Debra's on an endless emotional roller coaster. Debra thinks Frank hides his feelings.
- Debra wants to talk about what's bothering her. Frank wants to decompress by *not* talking about what's bothering him.
- Frank thinks Debra is relentless. Debra thinks Frank just doesn't care.

How did this couple end up feeling like adversaries when what brought them together a decade ago was love? As it turns out, there are three sides to every story. Let's hear each of them.

Debra's Story

How long can you be married to a stranger? Looks like I may be about to set a record of some kind.

After 8 years of marriage—10 years of being together—I still can't communicate with Frank. The problem is, he doesn't listen to me. He never shares his feelings with me, just turns off, withdraws. I hardly ever can figure out what's going on with him.

It's gotten to the point where I feel closer to my friend Joan, a woman I've been working with for just a year. At least I never have to wonder what she's thinking or feeling—she lets me know. Huh, communication—imagine that! I swear, I think Joan knows more about what's going on with me after a 5-minute coffee break than Frank does after an entire weekend together.

Frank and I are intimate in some ways, of course. I know his body very well, from years of stroking and exploring. And from his grunts and moans, I've figured out his sexual preferences pretty well. I could write a book about his personal habits: the obsessive way he flosses his teeth, the careful way he blow-dries his hair to cover his bald spot, the meticulous way he lines up his clothes in the closet.

But I sure don't know what he's thinking and feeling most of the time. He gets this look that's part tired, part concerned, part preoccupied. But when I ask him if anything's wrong, he says, "No." When I ask him what he's feeling, he says, "Tired." When I ask him what he's thinking about, he says, "Work." If I ask him *what* about work, he says, "Just some problems." All his answers seem perfunctory and dutiful, like he doesn't want to tell me but has to. He might as well say it right out: "I don't want to talk about this anymore." He'd rather watch a stupid show on television than connect with his own wife.

Sometimes I wonder if he even *has* any feelings other than fatigue. (Is that really a feeling?) He just plods through life, always taking care of business, preoccupied with getting his work done but never showing much excitement or pain. He says his style shows how emotionally stable he is. I say it just shows he's passive and bored.

In many ways I'm just the opposite: I have a lot of ups and downs. But most of the time I'm energetic, optimistic, spontaneous. Of course I get upset, angry, and frustrated sometimes. He says this shows I'm emotionally immature, that "I have a lot of growing up to do." I think it just shows I'm human. He's the one who's emotionally stunted.

I do share most of my thoughts and feelings with him: my problems at work, my reactions to my friends, my emotional highs and lows. His response? A sort of bland tolerance—sometimes interested, sometimes not, sometimes just going along out of habit, sometimes. . . . I really don't know. How can I, when he doesn't tell me what's going on with him? So I just ramble on, feeling more and more like I'm talking to myself. The chatterbox wife with the bored husband.

It wasn't like this at first. He was never very expressive, but he enjoyed listening to me. And he would tell me things about himself. In the beginning, even though the communication between us was never balanced, it was at least mutual. I thought he'd eventually get more comfortable with me and confide in me more, but he actually confides less now than when we first met!

His lack of communication bothers me most when we disagree about something. I want to discuss our differences and try to work out a solution. I expect conflict in a close relationship; I'm not threatened by it, and I want to deal with it openly. But Frank won't even discuss it. At the first sign of tension, he runs. He offers some feeble platitude like "Things will work themselves out."

I think the root of our problem is Frank's sensitivity to criticism. He can't stand any suggestion that he might have done something wrong, especially if I show that I'm angry about it. It's like he wants our relationship to be elevator "muzak"—so boring, nondescript, and utterly forgettable that it fades into the background. Well, guess what, Frank? This is real life! He's not perfect, I'm not perfect—we're different people with different needs. So of course we're going to get angry sometimes. That doesn't mean we don't love each other—in fact, it probably means we *do*. Yet whenever I get critical or angry, he acts as if I've violated some sacred law of nature. And then he gets even more critical and angry at me (for being critical and angry at him) than I was with him in the first place.

I remember one incident that kind of sums up the way I see Frank. We went out to dinner with a couple who had just moved to town. The husband was a friend of one of Frank's college roommates, and the evening started out great. They were a charming couple, and since we'd never met and they were new in town, we had a lot to talk about. As the evening wore on, I became more and more aware of how wonderful their life was. They seemed genuinely in love, even though they had been married longer than we have. No matter how much the man talked to us, he always kept in contact with his wife: touching her, making eye contact with her, or including her in the conversation. And he used "we" a lot to refer to them. Watching them made me realize how little Frank and I touch, how rarely we look at each other, and how separately we participate in a conversation. I wanted to put my hand on Frank's knee or hold his hand, just to have the appearance of being a couple. But I was afraid Frank wouldn't respond or, worse, would give me that look that says "Not now!" Sometimes I think he is embarrassed to be with me.

Anyway, I admit it. I was envious of this other couple. And to make matters worse, they had *money*. Of course, they were much too polite to mention it, but as they casually referred to the private schools their kids went to and the vacations they took, I realized they were not struggling to get by. After dinner, we went back to their place, and their house was incredible—not ostentatious, but tasteful, classy, and expensive, with some beautiful antique furniture and some oriental rugs that I was tempted to steal. We once looked for a house in their neighborhood, but we couldn't afford even the least expensive ones.

They seemed to have it all: loving family, beautiful home, leisure, luxury. What a contrast to Frank and me: struggling along, both working full-time jobs, trying to save money, sometimes barely managing to pay the bills. I wouldn't mind that so much, if only we worked at it *together*. But we're so distant. Even though we have similar goals in mind, it doesn't feel like we're on the same team.

When we got home, I started expressing those feelings. I wanted to reevaluate our life—as a way of getting closer. I don't like the materialistic side of myself; envying other people's wealth makes me feel shallow. I thought maybe we needed to adjust our priorities, not struggle so much for the almighty dollar. Maybe we couldn't be as wealthy as these people, but there was no reason we couldn't have the closeness and warmth they had.

As usual, Frank didn't want to talk about it. When he said he was tired and wanted to go to bed, I got angry. It was Friday night, and neither of us had to get up early the next day; the only thing keeping us from being together was his stubbornness. It made me mad. I was fed up with giving in to his need for sleep whenever I brought up an issue to discuss. I thought, why can't he stay awake just for me sometimes?

I wouldn't let him sleep. When he turned off the lights, I turned them back on. When he rolled over to go to sleep, I kept talking. When he put a pillow over his head, I talked louder. He told me I was a baby. I told him he was insensitive. It escalated from there and got ugly. No violence but lots of words that shouldn't have been said. He finally went to the guest bedroom, locked the door from the inside, and went to sleep.

The next morning we were both worn out and distant. He criticized me for being so irrational. Which was probably true. I do get irrational when I get desperate. But I think he uses that accusation as a way of justifying himself. It's sort of like "If you're irrational, then I can dismiss all your complaints and I am blameless." But I didn't make much of a protest. I just thought, what's the use?

Frank's Story

Debra never seems to be satisfied. I'm never doing enough, never giving enough, never loving enough, never sharing enough. You name it, I apparently don't do enough of it. There's a line from an old song that goes "Too much is not enough." That's Debra.

Or to put it another way, I sometimes think of the old Dylan song "Too Much of Nothing." Debra sometimes acts like everything I do to please her amounts to nothing. I get no credit for what I do for her.

Sometimes she gets me believing I really am a bad husband. I start feeling as though I've let her down, disappointed her, not met my obligations as a loving, supportive husband. But then I give myself a dose of reality. What have I done that's wrong? I'm an okay human being. People usually like me, respect me. I hold down a responsible job. I don't cheat on her or lie to her. I'm not a drunk or a gambler. I'm moderately attractive, and I'm a sensitive lover. I even make her laugh a lot. Yet I don't get an ounce of appreciation from her—just complaints that I'm not doing enough.

I think she must be insecure. She wants constant reassurance. I told her once in desperation, "Look. I love you. Until further notice to the contrary, you can assume that I still love you. I promise to inform you of any change in the status of these feelings. You don't need to keep checking." Maybe she's bored with her life and blames that on me. She's always looking for high drama and excitement in the relationship. It's really a soap-opera view of love, where everything has to be heavy and emotional. But marriage should be a place where I can retreat from the stresses and demands of my life, not an addition to them.

She's always asking me how I'm feeling. The truth is, sometimes I'm not feeling a damn thing—and that feels damn good! It's like she assumes I have all these emotions bottled up inside and I'm refusing to share my inner life with her. But that's not the way it is. Often I'm exhausted from work and just want to veg out—flip on the television, crash on the sofa, and suck on a beer. It doesn't matter what show is on—heck, I even like the commercials. I'm not there for intellectual stimulation or social chit-chat. Maybe one of these days I'll start growing vines from my ears, as Debra suggests. But to me it's relaxing. Now I ask you: Is what I'm doing morally wrong? Is it constitutionally forbidden? Is it a positive sign of decadence? To hear Debra, you'd certainly think so.

Don't get me wrong. I'm not always exhausted or stressed out. In fact, I think I pace myself rather well—especially compared to Debra. I organize my life so I'm prepared for the demands and stresses that go with my job and my home life. I'm not thrown by events the way Debra is. Her feelings are like a roller coaster: it's a fun ride sometimes, but you never know if there's a stomach-churning drop around the next turn. I can't live that way. A nice steady cruising speed is more my style.

But I don't put Debra down for being the way she is. I'm basically a tolerant person. People, including spouses, come in all shapes and sizes. They aren't tailored to fit your particular needs. So I don't take offense at little annoyances; I don't feel compelled to talk about every difference or dislike; I don't feel every potential area of disagreement has to be explored in detail. I just let things ride.

I expect my partner to do the same for me. But when Debra picks at me about every detail that doesn't fit with her idea of what's right, I do react strongly. My cool disappears, and I explode.

Debra accuses me of being an emotional pack rat, of storing bad feelings until an opportune time, but that's not true. I don't go around dwelling
on whatever injustices or irritations I've had to put up with. I don't hoard
them in secret until I can reveal them in some dramatic display. But when
I'm criticized for some small thing, I suddenly remember what I've suffered
without a word, and I get furious at the injustice of it.

I can handle most of my problems myself. I don't lay them on other
people, and I don't hold others responsible for solving my problems. Debra
can't seem to understand that there are certain things that I can only work
through alone.

I remember driving home with Debra after a night out with a couple
we had just met. The husband was a friend of my college roommate, Willie.
They were an attractive, impressive couple. He had come to town to manage
one of our commercial banks; she had joined one of our family law firms.
I was surprised that old goofball Willie, whom I had always thought of as
sort of shallow, had such interesting and classy friends.

On the way home I was wondering what kind of impression I'd made
on them. I was tired that evening and not at my best. Sometimes I can be
clever and funny in a small group, but not that night. Maybe I was trying
too hard. Sometimes I have high standards for myself and get down on
myself when I can't live up to them. But this other couple wasn't particularly clever either. Maybe we were all sizing each other up, like on a first
date. I never much liked first dates, always wanted to get past them to the
comfortable stage.

Debra interrupted my ruminations with a seemingly innocent question: "Did you notice how much in tune those two were with each other?"
Now, I know what's behind that kind of question—or at least where that
kind of question will lead. It always leads right back to us, specifically to
me. Eventually the point becomes "We aren't in tune with each other,"
which is code for "You're not in tune with me."

I dread these conversations that chew over what's wrong with us as a
couple, because the real question, which goes unstated in the civil conversations, but gets stated bluntly in the uncivil ones, is "What's wrong with
Frank?" So I tried to avoid an unnecessary fight by answering that they
were a nice couple.

But Debra pushed it. She insisted on evaluating them in comparison to
us. They had money and intimacy. We had neither. Maybe we couldn't be
wealthy, but we could at least be intimate. Why couldn't we be intimate?
Meaning: Why couldn't I be intimate? I tried to lighten up the conversation,
suggesting that maybe we lacked an intimacy gene. She was not amused.

When we got home, I tried to defuse the tension by saying I was tired and suggesting we go to bed. I *was* tired, and the last thing I wanted was to get into the same old fight all over again. But Debra was relentless. She argued that there was no reason we couldn't stay up and discuss this. I wanted to say that there was no point in discussing because it wouldn't be a discussion—it'd be a trial. But I didn't because that would be just another piece of evidence she would use to convict me.

I proceeded with my bedtime routine, giving her the most minimal of responses. If she won't respect my feelings, why should I respect hers? She talked at me while I put on my pajamas and brushed my teeth; she wouldn't even let me alone in the bathroom. When I finally got into bed and turned off the light, she turned it back on. I rolled over to go to sleep, but she kept talking. You'd think she'd have gotten the message when I put the pillow over my head—but no, she pulled it off. At that point I lost it. I told her she was a baby, a crazy person—I don't remember everything I said. Finally, in desperation, I went to the guest bedroom and locked the door. I was too upset to go to sleep right away, and I didn't sleep well at all.

In the morning, I was still angry at her. I told her she was irrational. For once, she didn't have much to say. The truth is, we were both exhausted.

The Third Side: An Objective Story

The differences that Frank and Debra find so upsetting in each other were there from the beginning. Debra was emotional and outgoing. She formed close ties to others and got emotional support and stimulation from these relationships. Her style was to speak her mind and be open about her feelings.

Frank, on the other hand, was private and shy. An only child, he had grown up an outsider, with few friends. He didn't like to socialize much and often felt uncomfortable in the presence of others. He sought security, not so much in the company of others, but in a stable, organized, rational life. You could always depend on Frank. His checkbook was always balanced, literally and figuratively. His life was a lesson in the avoidance of excess.

Frank and Debra had much in common: similar backgrounds, almost identical values, and some common interests in sports. They found each other physically attractive, and even the differences between them were a source of attraction. Frank's calm manner was a nice balance for Debra's moodiness, while her comfort in social situations allowed him to be private but still take part in the conversation. Frank's penchant for organization helped Debra live at a less frenetic pace, while her optimism and enthusiasm added energy to his plodding style.

Ideally, these differences would have brought them to a happy medium.

Frank might have learned to be more open about how he felt, while Debra might have become more comfortable with privacy and time alone. He might have developed a more zestful, spontaneous approach to life, while she might have learned to pace herself. He might have become more comfortable in social situations, while she might have learned to value the peace and quiet of solitude.

Because the contrasts between them at first seemed appealing, Frank and Debra appreciated them and were open to mutual influence and change early in their relationship. However, in time, their own needs and the inability of the other to satisfy them made those already existing differences larger. Frank's need for time alone conflicted with Debra's need for time together. The more he sought independence, the more she pressed for closeness. The more emotional she became, the more he "turned off."

These differences were difficult for them to manage because of enduring emotional sensitivities that each brought to the relationship. Debra experienced Frank's withdrawal as rejection of her, which at times it was. A difficult and painful period of adolescence, where she felt unattractive to any boy, probably contributed to her sensitivity to rejection. Because of this experience, Frank's frequent need for distance was especially difficult for her to accept, unless there was the buffering of closeness and intimacy beforehand. Frank's experience as an only child, carefully reared by protective parents who shielded him from any criticism, made him react strongly to it as an adult, particularly from a spouse, unless it was buffered by praise and appreciation. And Debra often leveled her criticisms sharply. These sensitivities provided the emotional fuel that often triggered conflict over their natural differences.

Stressful events often played a part in exacerbating the differences between them and triggering their sensitivities. When work was demanding for Frank and not going well—calling his competence into question— he especially needed time alone and was particularly sensitive to criticism. When her interpersonal relationships at work or with her family weren't going well, Debra especially needed quality time with Frank and was particularly sensitive to rejection. Thus, stress was a catalyst for triggering behaviors that were difficult and painful for the other, a pain intensified by those very stressors.

Their differences, emotional sensitivities, and stresses then became a source of argument—an intricate dance of criticism, defensiveness, withdrawal, and counterattack. They had danced this dance many times before, but neither was quite sure how to turn off the music. Given her greater comfort with communication, especially negative communication, Debra was more likely to start a conversation about their differences by expressing her needs or feelings, particularly when Frank had been distant. But Frank felt criticized by her statements—partly because they often *were* critical and partly because he was already sensitive to criticism and had become more so during the course of his relationship with Debra.

For example, Debra's comments about the other couple on the way home from their evening out seemed to Frank a statement about him—one carrying the strong implication that he wasn't as "in tune" with Debra as their new male friend was with his wife. It's hardly surprising that Frank took the comment as a criticism, since she has criticized him many times for not being sensitive to her. Debra has often complained, with some justification, that Frank is not attentive and involved enough with her. So, although her remark about the other couple was heard by Frank as a criticism of him, criticism was not what she had intended. In fact, her feeling at the time was more envy of their friends and a longing for the intimacy they seemed to have than a particular complaint about Frank. However, their past conflicts over intimacy and being "in tune" with each other, plus Frank's acquired sensitivity to Debra's criticism, led him to take her comment personally.

Because Frank feared an ugly argument with Debra, he sidestepped her comment. Sometimes diversions like this work for Frank because they bypass the conversation and avert an argument. However, sometimes—as on this occasion—his tactics frustrate Debra and contribute to the very conflict he is trying to prevent. The more he withdraws, the angrier she gets. What little conversation they have consists of mutual attacks and defensive maneuvers, and the dance goes on. So stuck are they in their respective roles that they fail to notice the feelings they have in common—on this particular evening, they were both envious of their new friends.

As Debra and Frank's problems have accumulated, each has developed a theory of how the other's difficulties are damaging the relationship. They each think the other is at fault, and thus they both selectively remember parts of their life, focusing on those parts that support their own points of view. For example, Debra thinks Frank is socially awkward and afraid of intimacy. He has few friends and no close friends. When she tries to talk to him about their own lack of closeness—such as after the night out with their new acquaintances—he avoids the discussion. This avoidance, in Debra's view, proves that his fear of intimacy, even with his own wife, is the source of their problems.

In contrast, Frank believes Debra's insecurity and immaturity are the source of their problems. He uses the same incident, but interpreted differently, to support his point of view. As he sees it, Debra got upset that night merely because their friends made more money and were more affectionate in public than he and Debra. Frank thinks they have problems because

Debra cannot accept herself and others (even her own husband) for what they are. He sees her emotionality as immaturity, her energetic tempo as exhausting, and her desire for closeness as weakness.

As they each carry around these theories about the other, they become entrenched in their positions and blinded to the various ways one *could* look at their problems. Debra ignores any evidence of Frank's social competence, such as his sense of humor, his kindness and consideration toward others, or his passionate lovemaking. Yet these positive qualities were reasons Debra was attracted to Frank. In parallel fashion, Frank overlooks obvious signs of Debra's psychological security, such as her persistence and optimism in the face of disappointment. Each expects the other to be inadequate, acts as if he or she is, and in so doing promotes the very characteristic that is so disliked. Debra, assuming Frank won't participate much in social encounters, provides little opportunity or incentive for him to speak and thus contributes to his shyness and social withdrawal. Frank, assuming Debra will get upset at any bad news, doesn't tell her things like his problems at work that he thinks will bother her. When she eventually finds out, she gets more upset than she would have had he told her in the first place. Plus now she is angry with him for concealing information from her.

Every couple starts out, like Frank and Debra, with a number of differences between them—differences that may nourish the relationship or damage it. When the differences are linked with emotional sensitivities, as they often are, or when stress exacerbates the differences, as it often does, the stage is set for conflict. Like Debra and Frank, the couple may argue. Each partner alternates between criticizing the other for being different and defending against the other's criticisms. Or, instead of outright argument, they may withdraw from each other, expressing their dissatisfaction through avoidance. Rather than solving the problems or minimizing the differences, these destructive cycles can maintain and even exaggerate the very differences that caused the problems in the first place. The end product of this vicious cycle is that the differences often seem irreconcilable.

The Purpose of This Book: Creating Acceptance and Change in Relationships

In the last 20 years, we have developed a new approach to couple therapy, called integrative behavioral couple therapy (IBCT), and done research on it. We have collected extensive data on its effectiveness. We completed two randomized clinical trials sponsored by the National Institute of Mental Health and, in the largest randomized trial of couple therapy ever conducted, showed that our approach can strengthen relationships and prevent divorce in most couples for at least 5 years (the last point we contacted couples). But we also know that therapy isn't for everyone, and we wanted to help people who are looking to improve or strengthen their relationship on their own—people just like you. That's why we wrote *Reconcilable Differences.* We took the best and most important parts of our proven couple therapy and designed them so that you could benefit from them on your own time, in your own home, without needing to talk to a therapist. Of course, talking to a therapist about topics in this book can also be very helpful, and, as we'll explore in the last section of this book, perhaps necessary in some cases.

Since the first edition of *Reconcilable Differences,* published over 10 years ago in 2000, we have learned much about how to disseminate IBCT, primarily through two large programs. First, this treatment was adopted by the U.S. Department of Veterans Affairs (VA) as one of its evidence-based psychological treatments, and as a result, we have spent a lot of time training VA therapists in the treatment. Second, we received a grant from the National Institute of Child Health and Human Development to adapt this treatment for an online intervention. As a result of both of these efforts, we have learned ways to describe the approach that make it easier to understand and follow. Human relationships are complex, and efforts to change them can be difficult. Our motivation in making the current revision of *Reconcilable Differences* was to include these simpler ways of teaching about relationships and how to improve them. As part of this effort to simplify, in this edition of the book we have you focus on one core issue in your relationship. By applying each of the concepts in the book to this core issue, we believe you will achieve a more profound understanding of yourself and your partner and have a better chance of improving your relationship.

The purpose of this book is to help you understand the conflicts you have with your partner and then to transform those conflicts into greater peace and intimacy. When you get embroiled in conflict with your partner, you both may blame the trouble on faults in the other. You each try to correct these faults by changing the other. But the other resists change, and so you get locked in a struggle that erodes your good feelings for each other. Each of you can feel stuck, not knowing how to cope with unwelcome differences in the other and resorting to blame, criticism, defensiveness, and withdrawal. These ways of coping serve only to hurt each other's feelings. Bruised and injured by your attempts to resolve your differences, you may feel that the chasm has become impossible to breach.

In this book we will show you a way out of this impasse: by accepting your partner. The natural inclination is to try to change your partner, but efforts directed solely at such change often make the conflict worse. When you genuinely accept your partner, you may achieve peace from the conflict and, paradoxically, change from your partner. Your partner probably wants to make you happy. When you are able to accept each other's experience, and often the behavior that results from that experience, you both may make spontaneous changes to accommodate to the other. Acceptance offers a route for you both to move toward a happier and closer union.

How can you achieve genuine acceptance? And how can acceptance transform conflicts into intimacy? Although they are painful, conflicts offer a window into the emotions of both of you: your disappointments, hopes, strengths, and weaknesses. If you can look at these conflicts not with the goal of blaming and fault finding but with the goal of understanding the strong emotions that drive each of you, you can learn more about yourself and your partner individually as well as how you interact. This understanding allows you to appreciate each other more completely and more honestly and can inspire compassion for each other's position. Through this understanding you also may gain some perspective that will lessen your conflicts, perhaps even enabling you to laugh at them at times. Understanding and compassion for each other and greater perspective on your conflicts may then lead you to an acceptance of each other's feelings and behavior, which in turn breaks your vicious cycles of argument, disagreement, and withdrawal—or at least allows you to recover from those cycles more quickly. At the very least, the process of analyzing and discussing your differences and conflicts in an atmosphere of acceptance will promote greater tolerance between you; in the best case, it can enhance the intimacy between you. Conflict offers not only the threat of alienation but also the possibility of intimacy.

Change is the brother of acceptance, but it is the younger brother. When acceptance comes first, it paves the way for change. When you and your partner experience greater acceptance from each other, your resistance to change often dissolves. You may be more open to adapting to each other and accommodating in ways that reduce conflict. You may be able to communicate more clearly and negotiate and problem-solve more effectively since you are no longer adversaries. In this book we will also discuss strategies for promoting change in relationships once greater acceptance has been achieved.

How the Book Is Organized

Our book is divided into five parts.

Part I, "The Conflicting Sides of Conflict," which you have already begun, describes common ways of interpreting arguments that just make these arguments worse. As part of this section, you will complete some questionnaires about your relationship to understand how it is functioning now. You will also have a chance to select a particular ongoing core conflict between you and your partner so that you can apply your growing understanding and skill to easing this struggle.

Part II, "A DEEP Understanding of Conflict: The Third Side of the Story," introduces a new way of understanding conflicts that can lead to their acceptance and resolution. *DEEP* is an acronym that stands for the four major factors that come into play in conflicts and hold the key to resolution through both acceptance and change: natural *d*ifferences between the two of you, *e*motional sensitivities in each of you, *e*xternal circumstances that create stress for each of you, and the *p*atterns of communication in which you get stuck as you try to resolve the conflict. You will be given plenty of illustrations from other couples and will be asked to apply this "DEEP understanding" model to the core conflict between you and your partner that you selected. By the time you have finished reading Part II, you will have an essential foundation for using the rest of the book.

Part III, "From Argument to Acceptance," shows the ways that you and your partner can foster acceptance of each other, focusing first on the core conflict you identified. Acceptance cannot be demanded or forced, yet it is anything but a passive state. It is crucial to establish some measure of acceptance if you hope to ease the conflict in your relationship and facilitate the changes in each other that are really important to you. In these chapters you will learn the important difference between acceptance and resignation and see how even small steps toward mutual acceptance and compassion can improve your relationship.

Part IV, "Deliberate Change through Acceptance," discusses ways in which you can pursue change directly, but in the context of acceptance. As in earlier sections, the core conflict you selected will be the initial focus.

Finally, Part V, "When Acceptance Is Not Enough," looks at those cases when your partner presents special challenges because of his or her own disorder, such as depression, or when your partner mistreats you, such as by having an affair. This section also discusses professional help for individual and relationship problems.

Each chapter in the book relies heavily on examples from couples. To preserve confidentiality, these case examples are an amalgam of the hundreds of couples we have seen in therapy, of couples we have known socially, and even of our own relationships. These examples provide "living evidence" of how our ideas play out in real life. Each chapter ends with a short summary of the main ideas and an exercise that will bring the ideas of this chapter home to your own unique relationship.

Ideally, both you and your partner would read this book and do the individual exercises. It can be helpful to discuss the ideas and relate them to yourselves. But a word of caution is in order: it will be easier to find your partner in these chapters than it will be to find yourself. To prevent the discussions from leading to blame ("You do exactly what they talk about in Chapter . . . "), it is always helpful to focus on applications to yourself rather than applications to your partner.

Whether your partner reads the book or not, it can still be helpful for you to read it. Most of the exercises are designed to be completed alone. Some of the later exercises will prepare you to share your understanding with your partner, whether he or she has read the book or not. These later exercises also prepare you to engage in specific actions that can lead you and your partner to resolve the conflict. While the book will focus you initially on a core struggle that you select, the same strategies can be used for other conflicts.

RECAP

This chapter took a single conflict from a married couple and presented three sides to that conflict: the wife's view, the husband's view, and a more objective view that incorporated both spouses' positions. This three-sided view of conflict gives a taste of what is to come in the next chapter, where we explain conflict from the perspective of the participants.

This chapter also gave an overview of the focus of the book, with its emphasis on acceptance as a path toward resolving conflict, and an overview of the format of the book.

Exercise: Your Current Satisfaction as a Couple

The first step is to evaluate how your relationship is functioning right now. Please complete the 16-item questionnaire below, which was developed by Janette Funk and Ronald Rogge at the University of Rochester in 2007 based on a thorough analysis of items from a variety of questionnaires designed to assess relationship quality. Collecting data from thousands of couples, they were able to show that the items below discriminate best between different levels of relationship satisfaction. Because low relationship satisfaction can result from the absence of positive qualities, the presence of negative qualities, or by some combination of the two, we next ask you to complete the brief Positive Relationship Quality and Negative Relationship Quality questionnaires, developed by Frank Fincham of Florida State University and Ronald Rogge in 2010. After you complete these three short questionnaires, we will show you how to score and interpret them so you know where your relationship currently stands. For this exercise and each of the remaining exercises in the book, your partner can answer the questions separately if he or she is reading the book also, and you two can come back to these questionnaires after working through the book to see how your relationship has changed.

Couple Satisfaction Index

1. Please indicate the degree of happiness, all things considered, of your relationship.

Extremely unhappy	Fairly unhappy	A little unhappy	Happy	Very happy	Extremely happy	Perfect
0	1	2	3	4	5	6

	All the time	Most of the time	More often than not	Occasionally	Rarely	Never
2. In general, how often do you think that things between you and your partner are going well?	5	4	3	2	1	0

	Not at all true	A little true	Somewhat true	Mostly true	Almost completely true	Completely true
3. Our relationship is strong	0	1	2	3	4	5
4. My relationship with my partner makes me happy	0	1	2	3	4	5
5. I have a warm and comfortable relationship with my partner	0	1	2	3	4	5
6. I really feel like **part of a team** with my partner	0	1	2	3	4	5

	Not at all	A little	Some-what	Mostly	Almost com-pletely	Com-pletely
7. How rewarding is your relationship with your partner?	0	1	2	3	4	5
8. How well does your partner meet your needs?	0	1	2	3	4	5
9. To what extent has your relationship met your original expecta-tions?	0	1	2	3	4	5
10. In general, how satis-fied are you with your relationship?	0	1	2	3	4	5

For each of the following items, select the answer that best describes *how you feel about your relationship*. Base your responses on your first impressions and immediate feelings about the item.

11. Interesting	5	4	3	2	1	0	Boring
12. Bad	0	1	2	3	4	5	Good
13. Full	5	4	3	2	1	0	Empty
14. Sturdy	5	4	3	2	1	0	Fragile
15. Discouraging	0	1	2	3	4	5	Hopeful
16. Enjoyable	5	4	3	2	1	0	Miserable

Positive Relationship Quality Rating

Considering only the positive qualities of your relationship and IGNORING the negative ones, evaluate your relationship on the following qualities:

	Not at all	A tiny bit	A little	Some-what	Mostly	Very	Extremely
1. Enjoyable	0	1	2	3	4	5	6
2. Pleasant	0	1	2	3	4	5	6
3. Strong	0	1	2	3	4	5	6
4. Alive	0	1	2	3	4	5	6

Negative Relationship Quality Rating

Considering only the negative qualities of your relationship and IGNORING the positive ones, evaluate your relationship on the following qualities:

	Not at all	A tiny bit	A little	Some-what	Mostly	Very	Extremely
1. Bad	0	1	2	3	4	5	6
2. Miserable	0	1	2	3	4	5	6
3. Empty	0	1	2	3	4	5	6
4. Lifeless	0	1	2	3	4	5	6

SCORING AND INTERPRETATION OF THE COUPLE SATISFACTION INDEX

Scoring the Couple Satisfaction Index is simple; you just add up the points indicated for each answer for each question. Scores range from 0 to 81. The higher the score, the more satisfied your relationship. Based on research conducted with this measure, we offer the following interpretations of three broad ranges of scores, indicating a positive "green zone," a mixed "yellow zone," and a problematic "red zone." See which zone your relationship falls in.

Green Zone (Scores Greater Than 68)

Your score indicates that overall you are happy with your relationship. Your score is similar to or better than that of the average spouse in the United States. Being very happy with your relationship overall is great news for your relationship! Although you may still have a few focused issues you want to work on in this book, you seem to have many strengths that you will be able to build on when resolving those issues. It's great that you're taking the time to strengthen an already-strong relationship and tackling issues before they get too big.

Yellow Zone (Scores Between 52 and 68)

Your score indicates that you are somewhat happy with your relationship but more distressed than the average spouse in the United States. The fact that you're not really distressed (i.e., in the "red" range) is really good news because you and your partner will be able to build on the parts of your relationship that are satisfying as you start working on the issues that bother you. It's much easier to deal with relationship problems before they become too serious. However, your scores on overall relationship satisfaction also suggest that, although there are some things you enjoy about your relationship, you still would like to see things improve. People can score in the "yellow" range for lots of different reasons—for example, feeling like you've lost some of that spark or excitement in your relationship or feeling like some problems are detracting from your happiness in the relationship. Your scores on the positive and negative dimensions will provide you some guidance on which might be true for you.

Red Zone (Scores Below 52)

Your score indicates that you are somewhat to very unhappy with your relationship. Your ratings of your global relationship satisfaction place you in the same range as partners who often seek outside help for their relationship, such as couple therapy. Like many of those couples, you may even be feeling frustrated or hopeless about the relationship. However, it's really great that you are looking for ways to work on your relationship, like doing this book. You also likely have some strengths as an individual and as a couple that will help you improve your relationship—we'll return to those throughout the book. We expect that reading this book and completing the exercises can be helpful in improving your relationship. Additionally, we'll recommend additional resources for your relationship at the end of the book if you decide you'd like to seek additional help.

SCORING AND INTERPRETATION OF THE POSITIVE AND NEGATIVE RELATIONSHIP QUALITY MEASURES

Scoring of the two relationship quality measures is also simple. You just add up the points indicated separately for the two questionnaires. Scores can range from 0 to 24 for each measure. The higher the score for Positive Relationship Quality, the higher the positive qualities in your relationship; the higher the score for Negative Relationship Quality, the higher the negative qualities in your relationship. Based on research with these measures, we indicate some green, yellow, and red zones based on your scores on each of these measures and interpret some combinations of the different zones. Based on these scores, we also offer some suggestions for selecting your core relationship conflict, which you will do in the next chapter.

Positive Quality Green Zone (Greater Than 19); Negative Quality Green Zone (Less Than 4)

Congratulations! Your scores indicate that you experience negatives in your relationship (such as criticism or conflicts) less often than the average spouse in the United States. Additionally, you reported that you also experience frequent positives in your relationship. While there might be isolated or occasional problems that you experience in your relationship, they don't seem to be affecting how you feel about your relationship more generally. Given these strengths, the "core issue" you select to work on in this book will likely center on narrow problems or problems that are just starting. That's great because these types of problems are typically much easier to solve!

Positive Quality Green Zone (Greater Than 19); Negative Quality Yellow Zone (4–6)

Your scores suggest you experience moderate amounts of negatives in your relationship—somewhat more than the typical spouse in the United States. Fortunately, you experience positives in your relationship as much as—or more than—the typical married couple. These positives can help offset some of the relationship negatives. For example, couples who frequently argue can still be extremely happy if they also feel emotionally or sexually connected to their partners. Given your "green" score for positives, it might make sense to select a "core issue" to work on in this book that focuses on reducing a negative (e.g., conflict) rather than strengthening a positive.

Positive Quality Green Zone (Greater Than 19); Negative Quality Red Zone (Greater Than 6)

Your scores suggest you experience a lot of negatives in your relationship—more than the typical spouse in the United States. Fortunately, you also seem to experience frequent positives in your relationship as much as—or more than—the typical spouse. These positives can help offset some of the relationship negatives. For example, couples who argue a lot can still be happy in their relationship if they also feel emotionally or sexually connected to their partners. Given your high score for positives, it might make sense to select a "core issue" to work on in this book that focuses on reducing a negative (e.g., conflict) rather than strengthening a positive.

*Positive Quality Yellow Zone (17–19); Negative Quality Green Zone
(Less Than 4)*

Congratulations! Your scores indicate that you experience negatives in
your relationship less often than the average spouse in the United States.
While there might be isolated or occasional problems that you experience
in your relationship, they don't seem to be affecting how you feel about
your relationship more generally. This is a great strength to have because
it will allow you to focus on strengthening the positive aspects of your
relationship, rather than on remedying the negatives. You also indicated
that you experience relationship positives somewhat less than the typical spouse in the United States but more than people who report being
unhappy overall in their relationship. Given that you don't experience many
negatives in your relationship, focusing on improving the positives in this
book might be the most helpful.

*Positive Quality Yellow Zone (17–19); Negative Quality Yellow
Zone (4–6)*

Your scores suggest you experience moderate amounts of negatives in
your relationship—somewhat more than the typical spouse in the United
States. You also indicated that you experience relationship positives somewhat less than the typical spouse in the United States but higher than
people who report being unhappy overall in their relationship. The combination of these two results suggests that you're dealing with moderate—but not severe—problems with both lack of positives and presence
of negatives.

*Positive Quality Yellow Zone (17–19); Negative Quality Red Zone
(Greater Than 6)*

Your scores suggest you experience a lot of negatives in your relationship—more than the typical spouse in the United States. You also indicated that you experience relationship positives somewhat less than the
typical spouse in the United States but more than people who report being
unhappy overall in their relationship. The positives in your relationship can
help offset some of your relationship negatives. For example, couples
who argue a lot can still be happy in their relationship if they also feel
emotionally or sexually connected to their partners. While there are likely
some relationship positives that could be improved, it might make sense

to select a "core issue" to work on in this book that focuses on reducing a negative (e.g., conflict).

Positive Quality Red Zone (Less Than 17); Negative Quality Green Zone (Less Than 4)

Congratulations! Your scores indicate that you experience negatives in your relationship less often than the average spouse in the United States. However, you also indicated that you were unhappy with the level of relationship positives; your ratings indicate more dissatisfaction with this area than the typical spouse and similar to couples reporting general relationship unhappiness. The good news is that, given your low score on negatives, it's likely that you'll be able to fully engage in this book, avoid fights, and regain some of the connection you've lost. Because a lack of positives seems to be the primary problem in your relationship, it will likely make sense to select a "core issue" to work on in this book that focuses on strengthening relationship positives.

Positive Quality Red Zone (Less Than 17); Negative Quality Yellow Zone (4–6)

Your scores suggest you experience moderate amounts of negatives in your relationship—somewhat more than the typical spouse in the United States. Regarding relationship positives, your ratings indicate more dissatisfaction with this area than the typical spouse, similar to couples reporting general relationship unhappiness. However, the good news is that the moderate amount of negative aspects of your relationship suggests that you'll be able to fully engage in this book, avoid fights, and regain some of the connection you've lost. Because a lack of positives seems to be the primary problem in your relationship, it will likely make sense to select a "core issue" to work on in this book that focuses on strengthening relationship positives.

Positive Quality Red Zone (Less Than 17); Negative Quality Red Zone (Greater Than 6)

Your scores suggest you experience a lot of negatives in your relationship—more than the typical spouse in the United States. Regarding relationship positives, your ratings also indicate more dissatisfaction with this area than the typical spouse, similar to couples reporting general relationship unhappiness. Given that you're unhappy with both the positive and negative aspects of your relationship, you'll want to carefully select the "core issue" that you work on in this book. On the one hand, you'll want to pick an issue that, if changed, will substantially improve your relationship. On the other hand, you want to be careful not to pick something that will be too hard to fix—you're probably feeling pretty emotionally drained from your relationship and might not have the energy right now to tackle a huge change. And don't worry—many couples who were unhappy with both positive and negative aspects of their relationship have found this book helpful!

CHAPTER 2

"You're Wrong!"

RELATIONSHIP PROBLEMS AS FAULTS

> How wonderful to have someone to blame! How
> wonderful to live with one's nemesis! You may be
> miserable, but you feel forever in the right. You
> may be fragmented, but you feel absolved of all the
> blame for it.
>
> —ERICA JONG, *How to Save Your Own Life* (1977)

What starts arguments? What are they about?

Four Triggers for Conflict

Don Peterson, a psychologist at Rutgers University, tried to answer those questions by asking a group of volunteer couples to record important daily marital events. He found that there were four typical events that started arguments.

CRITICISM: THE VERBAL ATTACK

Not surprisingly, the most common trigger for argument was *criticism*. We all know that certain kinds of remarks, those intended to put our partners down, are likely to ignite a conflict. Carol, for example, who was sensitive about her forgetfulness, became only mildly defensive when her husband, Ron, pointed out that he'd found the door unlocked upon arriving home. When he referred to her as a "space cadet," however, she became enraged.

Ron's comment is an example of an obvious and intended criticism. But sometimes criticisms are unintentional. A wife may make what she views as a constructive suggestion or a passing observation, but her husband reacts with hurt feelings and feels either falsely maligned or blamed for something that isn't his fault. When Vivian said to Steve, "You sometimes have trouble dealing with the kids," she may have intended it merely as a statement of fact, given that a temper tantrum by their 4-year-old had recently shattered the evening's domestic tranquility. But to Steve her remark felt like an unjustified attack on him as a father. He believes that at times every parent, including his wife, has trouble handling the temper tantrums of young children. Why does she have to comment on it? What for her was simply an observation was for him a hurtful criticism.

DEMANDS: ILLEGITIMATE REQUESTS

A second common trigger for argument was a *demand* that struck the recipient as unfair or illegitimate. Alicia asked Victor to stay home from his weekly card game with his friends because she was sick with the flu. She thought she would feel better if he stayed with her and took care of her. Victor, however, viewed her request as unreasonable: "I'm not a doctor; I can't help you. Plus, you're not that sick. Why should I give up something that's important to me just because you feel bad?" Similarly, Carol's request that Ron help her revise a report she was writing seemed reasonable to her since she was already stressed out from trying to finish the report for tomorrow's deadline and still had to prepare some evaluations that were also due. But Ron did not see it her way: "You want me to be your assistant because you procrastinated as usual and created the mess that you're in. Why is it my job to bail you out?"

"FOR THE HUNDREDTH TIME . . .": CUMULATIVE ANNOYANCE

Conflicts were also triggered by what Peterson called "cumulative annoyance." If Steve repeatedly forgets to put the dishes in the dishwasher, Vivian gets irritated, and they argue. If Carol is late now and then, Ron can tolerate it, but when she is constantly late, he gets angry. He wonders how she can be so inconsiderate, always keeping him waiting. Carol realizes that she is often late, but she also figures that she has never missed an important event or incurred the wrath of anyone other than Ron. Her coworkers treat her habitual tardiness as an endearing foible. Why can't he?

REJECTION: DISMISSING THE OTHER'S GESTURE

A final common trigger for conflict was a rebuff or a *rejection*. For example, Steve put his arms around Vivian as a gesture of affection, but when Vivian responded with "Not now," Steve got angry: "You say you want me to be affectionate with you, but then you brush me off!" "Yes, in general, I want you to be more affectionate," Vivian retorted, "but can't you accept that I am not always in the same mood as you?"

Ron felt rebuffed when he made a special effort to cook pasta prima-vera, Carol's favorite dish, and Carol said, "Thanks, but I have a bad stom-ach-ache. I think I'll just have some tea and get into bed." Ron wondered out loud, "How can you be so insensitive?" Carol responded defensively, "I just don't feel well, and I'm not hungry!" She couldn't understand why he had to make such a big deal out of her refusal to eat his meal.

History Repeating Itself

In each of these cases an argument begins with the actions or inactions of one partner. In the case of a criticism, an unfair demand, and cumulative annoyance, one partner's actions offend the other. In the case of rejection, it is a partner's failure to respond appropriately that leads to conflict. When such events occur repeatedly, however, each person gets more sensitive to the triggers, such that over time it takes less and less provocation to ignite an argument. Mary does not need to make a full-fledged critical comment about Sandy's dealings with the kids to provoke a reaction from Sandy. After years of enduring critical comments, Sandy may interpret Mary's innocent request "Would you help Max with his homework?" as criticism because it suggests that Sandy *should* have helped Max with his homework or that she *should* have noticed that Max needed help. If Sandy reacts defensively to even these relatively benign comments, Mary may do her best to avoid any-thing that sounds blaming or accusatory. However, even Mary's carefully chosen words at a family outing at the beach, "Remember that Max can't swim well," may contain a hint of judgment (i.e., Sandy won't be careful about watching Max in the water) that comes across to Sandy as criticism.

Similarly, Anna does not need to attempt a passionate kiss with Greg to experience his rejection. After many rejections she rarely makes such obvious gestures to excite his passion. Now even his distracted look when he greets her or his apparent lack of interest when she talks about her day feels like rejection. By now, Greg may be aware of her sensitivity to rejection, so he may try to "psych himself up" to make an enthusiastic response. But she may see through these forced and insincere efforts and feel rejected anyway.

If we were watching these encounters, we might wonder why each per-son had such a strong reaction to such apparently unimportant actions. Why did Ron feel so rejected when Carol's illness made it impossible for her to eat the dinner he had cooked? Why was Sandy so stung by Mary's minor criticism of how she handled the kids? Our confusion would be understandable because we are not privy to the inner experience of these couples, let alone privy to all the past incidents that led to that experience. We would be seeing only a small slice of a long, complicated, and painful history that explains these heightened sensitivities to seemingly innocent remarks.

"Why Is This Happening to Us?": The Search for an Explanation

When any important event occurs in our lives, we seek an explanation. If the event is painful and occurs repeatedly, such as an argument, our search takes on a sense of urgency. We need to understand the event to gain some control over it. If we can accurately determine the cause of the event, we may be able to alter its cause and thus avoid future pain. With some sense of crisis, then, we put on our trenchcoats and, like detectives, search for the culprit. Who perpetrated this crime?

There are two obvious suspects in any relationship conflict: you and your partner. Assuming the conflict did not include other people, you two were the agents in the argument. The culprit has to be one of you. But which one?

Psychologists have conducted extensive research on the kinds of explanations that people develop to make sense of the events in their lives. Perhaps not surprisingly, our analyses tend to differ depending on whether we are looking at ourselves or at others. When we explain our own less-than-desirable actions in a conflict, we tend to look outside ourselves. The pressure of a deadline or the nasty comments of others made us do what we did. Our eyes and ears are directed at the outside world, so we are acutely aware of the external pressures that impinge on us and influence our behavior. But when we explain the actions of others, we generally look to factors within them, such as their personality traits. Because our eyes and ears are focused on them, we may be less aware of the factors in their own world that have influenced them. We see them—and them alone—as the cause of their own behavior. You are late because you are inconsiderate; I am late because of the heavy traffic. It's like the differences noted between biography and autobiography: in telling another's story, we tend to assign more responsibility for sins and errors to the other than we assign to ourselves when we tell our own story.

These human tendencies are constantly at work in close relationships. If a husband and wife both agree that she should ask her boss for a raise but she insists that now is not the time, her husband may explain her reluctance as cowardice while she may blame her boss's mood—she knows when her boss is open to these requests. Similarly, if both husband and wife have agreed to limit their visits to his parents but he immediately accepts another invitation for dinner with them, she may explain his response as personal weakness while he may explain it as guided by his parents' feelings.

In the case of arguments, we are acutely aware of the hurtful actions or inactions of our partners but regard our own hurtful behavior as merely a reaction to our partners' misdeeds.

If we ask ourselves why a painful argument occurred, we are likely to point an accusing finger at our partner. It's our partner who is culpable, and his or her own qualities caused the event. And as for us? No matter how out of line our actions were, we were merely provoked.

Your Partner's Role in Conflict

"IT'S ALL YOUR FAULT": INDICTMENT AND CONVICTION

More trials and guilty verdicts take place in the
heads of married couples than in courts of law.

As we think over our partners' actions, we often conduct a kind of legal inquiry in our heads. We hold a mental trial to evaluate their emotional crimes against us. While limited in its jurisdiction, this court deals with the largest and most profound of claims: high crimes of love and character.

Like everyone else, you undoubtedly have mentally reviewed evidence of your partner's misdeeds and analyzed what these misdeeds mean. Each wrongful action suggests your partner has some bad trait. He didn't listen to your point of view—maybe he is inconsiderate. She did what she wanted to do without taking you into account—maybe she is selfish. He criticized you for things he does too—maybe he is unfair. She angrily interrupted you and called you names—maybe she is hostile.

Your partner's wrongful acts may suggest the absence of positive traits rather than the presence of negative ones. If your partner ignores your feelings, maybe he doesn't care about you. If your partner forgets what you've told her, maybe she doesn't value your input. If your partner doesn't show affection to you, maybe he no longer loves you. If your partner seems uninterested in sex, maybe she has lost her attraction to you. If your partner doesn't spend much time with you, maybe he hasn't made you a priority in his life.

As you think over your partner's recent behavior toward you, you remember similar acts in the past. A recent bit of selfishness brings to mind a string of selfish actions. Recent clues that your partner doesn't really love you remind you of other such evidence. In your mind you review these pieces of evidence, both current and past. They are the exhibits you present in your mental court. They are the incriminating testimony about which your cerebral jury deliberates. A verdict of guilty seems certain.

But a verdict is only the first step toward achieving justice. Next we want our partners to confess their guilt. They need to admit that they are selfish or inconsiderate or lacking in respect and love. At the very least, they should apologize to us. More important, they need to change. They should work on their problem. They should make consistent efforts to be more giving, more considerate, and more loving.

"YOU'RE SICK": THE DIAGNOSIS

Those of us who are more psychologically inclined may search for explanations of our partners' behavior in their personality makeup. Rather than look for moral deficiency, we look for emotional impairment. Rather than holding a court hearing, we conduct a psychiatric examination. Rather than demanding indictment and conviction, we seek an accurate diagnosis.

Often such a diagnosis points to emotional problems. If your partner shows a need for reassurance, appreciation, and love that seems excessive, perhaps he doesn't really like himself and is therefore insecure about whether others love him. If your wife doesn't confide in you or doesn't shower you with affection, maybe she has a deep fear of intimacy with others. If your husband doesn't wish to socialize much with your family and friends, maybe he has a troubling lack of confidence in himself. If your partner is too critical of you, maybe it is because she doesn't accept herself and thus can't accept others.

Your diagnosis of your partner may suggest something even more serious than emotional problems: a specific mental disorder. If your partner is moody and irritable, you may conclude he is depressed. If her accusations concerning you seem wild and unfounded, you may diagnose her as paranoid. If his behavior during arguments seems irrational, you may call him crazy. It is their madness, not their badness, that causes our partners' hurtful behavior toward us.

In our effort to understand our partners' emotional difficulties or mental illness, we may search their past. We often discover clues in the behavior of our in-laws. His family always papers over their differences and never faces their conflicts directly, so no wonder he avoids conflict. Her father always babies her, so now she wants me to spoil her. His parents never forced him to be responsible, so he is irresponsible. Her mother is humorless and often depressed, so maybe that explains her bad moods.

After we have diagnosed our partners' maladies, we naturally want them to listen to our careful analysis of their problems and admit that we are right. Despite our lack of professional training, we genuinely believe that we understand what makes our partners tick. They should face up to their emotional limitations or their mental disorders by accepting our diagnoses.

Once they have openly and nondefensively acknowledged their problem, they will presumably want to improve themselves. We may suggest some self-help books that will buttress our keen insight into what is wrong with them. We may recommend some real therapy for them and perhaps even for their parents and siblings. If needed, we could choose the appropriate therapist for them, and even provide necessary background to the therapist and a tentative diagnosis. Long-term, intensive psychotherapy would undoubtedly be the treatment of choice. However, the cost and length of that treatment may be prohibitive. Perhaps an antidepressant or anti-anxiety medication could restore sanity!

"YOU'RE NOT GOOD ENOUGH": THE PERFORMANCE EVALUATION

We may spare our partners the profound knowledge we have of their personalities and instead evaluate their performance as spouses, partners, parents, providers, or simply people. Rather than search for a diagnosis, we now look for potential inadequacy. Rather than assess for moral weakness, we scrutinize for incompetence. We judge our partners not on their morality or their mental health, but rather on their ability to be a good lover, spouse, or parent.

Our standards for satisfactory performance are gleaned from watching others. If your wife is not physically affectionate but you have seen other wives who shower their husbands with hugs and kisses, you may conclude that she does not know how to express her love properly. If your husband is upset when you go out with friends but you know husbands who encourage their wives to go out with their friends, then maybe your husband is too possessive. If your partner is too clingy and needy, maybe she hasn't developed the ability to be alone or to cultivate friends as others have. Conversely, if your partner doesn't spend enough time with you, maybe he hasn't truly realized that he is now married; his single life is over.

You may conclude that your partner is not mature enough for marriage. She is ill-prepared for intimacy. He never learned to listen attentively or provide support or love properly. Somehow she didn't get the training to be intimate or to tolerate separation, to be sexually open or to be patient sexually, to be ambitious on the job or to prioritize home life, to be open and honest in a close relationship, or to show judgment in what to say and when to say it, or to be spontaneous and free, or to be responsible and committed.

As in addressing judgments of moral inadequacy or diagnoses of mental problems, our partners' first step in correcting their failings is to admit that we are right. They are inadequate spouses. They should acknowledge their deficiencies. Once they do that, they can address their inadequacies in several ways. They can look to other couples for models of proper behavior. If we know other husbands, for example, who are not concerned when their wives go out weekly with their friends, then why should our husbands be concerned? If we have read how often most couples in America have sex, why can't our wives at least meet that standard? Even more important than looking to other couples, our partners can look to us. We, after all, are models of what a good spouse should be: we know how to prioritize our time; we aren't needy; we know how to be physically affectionate. We can lead them back to the Promised Land of a happy marriage—if only they would listen to us.

Your Own Role in Conflict

"POOR ME": VICTIMS

Because we believe we are only reacting to our partners' provocations, we tend to cast ourselves in the role of victim and our partners in the role of villain. If gregarious Rodney spends lots of time visiting with other people at a party, leaving his shy partner, Seth, to fend for himself, Seth will likely be angry and feel like a victim of Rodney's actions. Seth may wonder whether Rodney really cares about him or if he is just incredibly inconsiderate. If Seth voices his distress to Rodney on the way home from the party, Rodney in turn may feel attacked. He may wonder about his partner's insecurity or neediness. Will he always have to look out for Seth? All he did was have a good time at the party. He didn't get drunk or flirt with other men or act inappropriately. Why is he being attacked? He too may feel victimized.

"MAYBE IT DOES TAKE TWO": COCONSPIRATORS

Rodney and Seth illustrate one difficulty with villain–victim casting. If both of you insist you're the victim, you can't hope to take the first step toward resolving conflict. But there is another reason it's hard to maintain the view that you are both innocent victims. A verdict about your partner highlights his or her misdeeds, but it casts a troubling shadow on you as well. If your partner is selfish, inconsiderate, or unfair, why did you two get together? Did you exercise bad judgment? Were you fooled by the classic bait-and-switch trick, seeing your partner's true colors only after you were invested in the relationship? Were you fooled by superficial attractions? Did you encourage or fail to discourage your partner's flaws? Are you a coconspirator in your partner's crimes against you?

Your diagnoses and performance evaluations of your partner can also cast a suspicious light on you. Why did you choose such a damaged or incompetent person as a partner? Did you want or need such a flawed person? If your partner didn't have emotional problems or inadequacies when you two met, did you play some role in fostering these problems? If your partner did have these problems to begin with, why didn't you discern them? Did you contribute to his or her difficulties? Do you share some complicity in your partner's problems? Are you an "enabler," someone who does not have a particular problem but contributes to it in the other by "enabling" it to take place?

"WHAT DOES THIS PROBLEM SAY ABOUT ME?": SECRET VILLAINS

Many of us occasionally stop blaming our partners long enough to wonder whether the way they treat us implies that there really is something wrong with us. If your partner is critical of you, does that mean you are inadequate? If your partner is depressed, does that mean you have not been kind and loving? If she seems an emotional wreck, does that mean you have not been patient and supportive? If he is not attracted to you, does that mean you are unattractive? If she shows little interest in you, does that mean you are uninteresting? If he has so little love to give, does that mean you are unlovable? While you may ultimately discount these possibilities, it is difficult not to wonder about them. You may harbor a nagging fear that you, not your partner, are the real villain.

"Let Me Explain Why We Have So Many Problems": The Battle of Accusations

It's only natural to want to share your conclusions once you have so carefully assessed your partner's misbehavior. If you don't tell your partner about the moral weaknesses or mental problems or inadequacies that you have discovered in him or her, how will your partner learn? Your partner will never be able to change unless someone who knows him or her well is honest enough to reveal these flaws. How your partner reacts to your frankness, however, depends on how and when you broach the subject. If you are bristling from a recent argument, you may tell your partner angrily, even vindictively. Your own distress propels your revelations. Your explanations, although voicing what you believe is true, sound like blame and accusation. Not surprisingly, your partner does not react well to these accusations, however truthful you think they are.

When you are not reacting to an immediate argument, you may try to tell your partner about your conclusions in a calmer, gentler, more respectful way. You may couch your verdict in compassion. You may use your best bedside manner. You may mix positive comments with negative ones in your evaluation.

Even with these extra efforts, you have probably found that your partner seldom reacts positively to your conclusions about his or her faults. Your judgments are not afforded the respect that your care in formulating them should warrant. Your partner may interrupt you. He or she may deny, wholesale, all of your conclusions. Your partner may vigorously defend himself or herself.

As distressing as these reactions may be, even more distressing are the accusations delivered in return. Your partner has gone through his own moral evaluation, diagnostic assessment, and performance evaluation *of you*. She has concluded that it is your faults, your emotional immaturity, and your inadequacy, much more than any of her own, that cause the unhappiness between you. Your partner matches your conclusions with conclusions of his or her own.

What can erupt next is a battle of explanations that quickly turns into a war of accusations. Many of us start out wanting to share our concerns sympathetically or kindly or respectfully, but our partners' reactions put us on the defensive. In the accusations and counteraccusations that follow, neither party would dare voice any fear of having played a role in the problem. To admit that we too may have been villains, or at least coconspirators, would make us too vulnerable.

To protect ourselves, then, any admissions we make are delivered in the service of an accusation. We may, for example, admit to having been blind to our partners' faults early on. We may admit to a lover's foolish optimism that the one we love would eventually change his or her personality. Admissions like these just emphasize the faults in our partners.

During the battle of accusations, we certainly don't feel much closeness and love for our partners. We may even feel active dislike for them. If the argument is particularly heated, we may admit to feelings and attitudes that were once there but are now, regrettably, absent. We may acknowledge "The old feelings just aren't there" or "I don't care that much anymore." The clear references to time ("old feelings" and "anymore") suggest that the feelings and attitudes were once there and that in *those* days appropriate behavior followed quite naturally. But to act in a loving manner given the present feelings would be a lie. And we will not lie. Statements of our integrity often accompany confessions of our lack of feelings: "I have to tell you the truth—I simply don't care anymore" or "I won't lie to you. The feelings just aren't there." The statements often suggest a pressure to engage in dishonesty, presumably to protect the partner in the short run, but a commendable resistance to that pressure for the sake of truth.

Thus, what starts out as an attempt to explain our views of our partner can easily degenerate into a battle of accusations, then into admissions that highlight the accusations, and finally into statements about not caring or not loving the other. These latter comments can be particularly injurious and threatening.

What gets lost in these discussions are the actions or inactions that initially triggered pain in us and led to our attempts at understanding. The fact that we feel so often rebuffed in our attempts to reach out to our partners may never get voiced. Instead, our accusations about their fear of intimacy and their counteraccusations about our insecurity may preclude any discussion of what it is that hurts us. If the conversation deteriorates to "admissions" that we no longer feel the way we used to or that they no longer love us, these discussions may create more pain and hurt than the pain and hurt that led to the discussion in the first place.

Raul and Adreanna often have conflicts over the care of their toddler, Joey. Adreanna is a dedicated, concerned mother who has read a lot about child health and development. She knows that her first responsibility as a mother is Joey's safety and health. Raul takes parenthood in general, and safety in particular, much more casually. He likes to say "Kids learn from their bruises." Given these different stances toward child care, it is not surprising that they have different opinions about how closely to watch Joey and about what kind of activities he should be allowed. In his frustration over Adreanna's views, Raul sometimes diagnoses her as irrational: "You are so neurotically worried about everything. You would raise him in a bubble if you had your way." In her frustration with Raul, Adreanna judges him to be inadequate as a father and lacking in the moral values a parent should have: "You are so preoccupied with your own stuff, you hardly bother to pay attention to Joey. You don't care about his welfare. I'm just grateful he hasn't seriously hurt himself under your watch." With these exchanges of accusations, both will defend themselves and make countercharges. What won't get discussed or at least acknowledged is that Adreanna really does worry when Raul is in charge of Joey and that Raul resents being constantly under surveillance by Adreanna and wants her to trust him. What also doesn't get discussed in these battles of accusation is the specific issue of concern that brought up the conflict to begin with: Should Joey be allowed to play in the backyard by himself, with a parent checking in occasionally, or should a parent be with him at all times? Can Joey climb the stairs by himself, or should someone be right behind him to help him? If the discussion deteriorates into "admissions" of lack of love or caring for the other, these comments may be more painful than the anxiety and distrust that started the discussion in the first place.

"You Always . . .": Burying the Kernel of Truth

What makes one partner in a couple insist on his explanation of the problem and the other insist on hers? First of all, both of you know that there is some truth in your respective explanations. Each of you has witnessed your partner's behavior many times over and seen direct evidence of the characteristic you accuse the other of having. Second, your partner's stubborn resistance to acknowledging any validity in your assertion only makes you press on. How can your partner so willfully refuse to recognize an obvious truth!

Unless one of you is crazy—that is, clearly out of touch with reality—the accusations made by both of you have kernels of truth in them. But those kernels are exaggerated truths, distorted by the heat of the argument and the pressure of your partner's resistance. When you expand on a genuine characteristic, making it more dramatic and excessive than it really is, your partner naturally feels justified in denying the caricature you have drawn. For example, the wife who accuses her husband of overreacting may, in the heat of the argument, claim that he is *always* "out of control." He can vigorously defend such an extreme characterization of him and perhaps even turn the tables on her: "Just who's out of control? You're the one who's overreacting!"

Research in the social sciences provides some support for the truth in our accusations. Studies have shown that partners in bad marriages are more likely to be impulsive, while partners in happy marriages are more likely to be agreeable and conscientious. Even more compelling evidence shows that emotional difficulties are associated with relationship dissatisfaction. For example, neurotic tendencies, alcoholism, and depression are linked to relationship dissatisfaction. Finally, there is even evidence implicating inadequacy as a predictor of relationship problems. Spouses who are less skilled at communication and conflict resolution are more likely to be in dissatisfied relationships. Thus, the spouse who accuses the partner of being bad or mad or inadequate and implicates these qualities as contributing to the relationship problems may have a point.

But these accusations are off the mark in several ways. First, the research shows that traits such as impulsivity and depression only make a good marriage more difficult, not impossible. Being agreeable and conscientious makes a good marriage more likely, but by no means guarantees it. Many couples are able to sustain a fulfilling relationship despite all sorts of personal challenges. Second, the accusation focuses only on the partner's negative characteristics and not on one's own. And as we have said, the accusation is likely to exaggerate the characteristic in the partner. Third, and most important, the accusation, defense, and counteraccusation—the battle of explanation between the partners—does nothing to improve or alter those characteristics under consideration, except perhaps to make them worse.

When all we do is accuse the one we love of misdeeds and character flaws, when we lay blame at every turn, we thwart the very goal we aspire to: change in our partners. Finding fault and exaggerating the human frailties we've identified in this person most dear to us only discourages cooperation and exhausts goodwill toward us. We rarely elicit change from someone else this way. We cannot force change through repeated, futile attacks. There must be a better way.

RECAP

Seen from our own perspective, arguments begin with actions or inactions by our partners that cause us pain. Criticism, unfair demands, cumulative annoyance, and rejection are the kinds of behaviors and responses that may trigger conflict. If these events happen only rarely, we can ignore them. When they happen repeatedly, we try to understand why they happen. We almost always begin our quest by focusing on the other person. What is it about our partners that leads to these painful actions? In our heads we may conduct a kind of legal inquiry into their transgressions and conclude that our partners have certain moral and character deficiencies: they are selfish, unfair, or inconsiderate. If we are more psychologically minded, we may conduct a diagnostic evaluation rather than a legal inquiry, concluding that the one we love has emotional problems such as immaturity, neurotic insecurity, or clinical depression. Or we may instead evaluate our partners' adequacy, determining that lack of training as a parent, lack of skill at communication, or inadequacy at expressing love is at the root of their hurtful behavior.

While we are engaging in this analysis of our partners, we may also wonder about our own contribution to the problems. We may feel like victims but wonder if we are possibly coconspirators. At the very least, we selected a partner with these faults. Might we have also permitted these faults or even fostered them? Could it be that inadequacies in us are also to blame? Although these possibilities may trouble us intermittently, typically we refocus on our partners' culpability rather than our own.

When we finish our analyses, we naturally want to share them, because we believe that informing our partners of their flaws is the best way to get them to work on changing them. But even when we believe we are acting out of constructive honesty and we present our conclusions tactfully, our partners are rarely receptive. Feeling blamed, they are likely to defend themselves and, even more upsetting, share their own conclusions about us. It is our faults, not theirs, that cause the problems. In the battle of explanations that follows, the only admissions that are made are ones that serve to highlight the accusations. Lost are discussions of the concrete events that initially triggered pain. If the battle of explanations is particularly heated, one or both partners may say things that are more painful than the original actions that led to the discussion in the first place. Even if there is some truth in our accusations, albeit exaggerated, that truth often gets lost in the din of battle. Conflict becomes entrenched, if not heightened, and we both dig in our heels and refuse to admit any need for self-change. Thus, actions made in an attempt to stimulate change end up preventing it.

Exercise: Identifying a Core Area of Conflict

The next step in using this book to improve your own relationship is to select a difficult and enduring area of conflict, such as money, in-laws, sex, child rearing, or trust. Throughout the book, you will focus on this area of difficulty as you systematically apply the principles, so it is important that you select it carefully. Please make this selection by choosing the most important, core conflict area in your relationship from the list below. Note that the list does not include one common concern of couples, namely communication. Communication is of course important, perhaps the most important aspect of a couple's relationship, and we will discuss it later at length. However, communication is always about something, about a content area. And here we want you to choose the content area in which you have the most difficulty communicating successfully.

You probably have difficulty communicating about a number of topics, but choose the most common topic below. Write down your core conflict area in the space provided. Then write down a short explanation of that problem area, the explanation that you might have given prior to looking at this book. Your explanation may include some of the fault finding discussed in this chapter—and that is okay. We will later get to a more complete and complex understanding of that problem and how you can make important changes in it. Going through the entire book focused on one core problem will enable you to deal more successfully with that area but should prepare you for dealing more successfully with other relationship problems, either other ones that you have now or ones that may develop in the future.

Common Conflict Areas for Couples

1. Parenting, children
2. Finances
3. Affection
4. Sex
5. In-laws, relatives
6. Household tasks
7. Trust, jealousy
8. Jobs, career
9. Alcohol, drugs
10. Religion
11. Temper, mood
12. Leisure time
13. Goals, aims, major decisions
14. Appropriate behavior or appearance
15. Other _____

Write down your common conflict area, but briefly specify the position of each person. For example, you might write "household tasks" and indicate that you want Bill to do dishes more often, cook occasionally, and help with the cleaning so household tasks are distributed fairly while Bill thinks that his work in the yard and on the car makes up for your extra time in the kitchen. Then write your current explanation of this problem. For example, you might write that Bill does not understand how much you do in the house and how difficult it is while his work outside is not nearly so time-consuming and is a lot more fun for him.

My core conflict area:

_____

_____

My explanation of this conflict:

_____

_____

_____

_____

_____

_____

_____

_____

PART II

A DEEP Understanding of Conflict

THE THIRD SIDE OF THE STORY

CHAPTER 3

"How Can You Be That Way?"

RELATIONSHIP PROBLEMS
AS DIFFERENCES

> Marriage is the process of choosing the right
> woman with whom to be incompatible.
> —EVAN ESAR, *20,000 Quips and Quotes* (1968)

Soon after he reached his 81st birthday, my* father discovered he had colon cancer. The cancer was removed, but the surgeon reported that it had spread and would be terminal. His oncologist predicted that his remaining life would be measured in months. Fortunately, the surgery left him free from pain. During a visit to our home by my parents, I set up a video camera and interviewed first my father alone about his life and then my mother and father together about their almost 45 years as a married couple. They talked openly about their life together and its many ups and downs. Toward the end of the interview, my father spontaneously observed: "I have often been amazed at how different we really are."

My mom and dad were at least as similar as most married couples. They both were Danish immigrants and shared their Danish-American heritage as well as values, such as education and hard work. Yet their individual personalities often pushed them in different directions. Mom was a doer; Dad was a dreamer. Mom was ambitious; Dad was laid back. Mom was a realist; Dad was an idealist. These differences fired their attraction as well as ignited their controversies with each other.

---

*All personal and case examples are from Andrew Christensen.

Differences That Make a Difference

Differences—eternal differences, planted by God in
a single family, so that there may always be color;
sorrow perhaps, but color in the daily grey.
—E. M. FORSTER, *Howard's End* (1910)

The French expression "vive la différence" celebrates the happy way in which the physical differences between men and women mesh, serving as a major source of attraction. But it is not just physical differences that are a source of attraction and pleasure. Different ideas and opinions can enliven conversation between people. A couple may get together because of their spirited discussions about their differing political, religious, or philosophical views. Different roles facilitate the accomplishment of necessary life tasks. Although traditional sex roles had many drawbacks, those roles did allow for a clear division of labor: he worked out in the world; she worked at home. He handled business issues; she handled child care. He managed the upkeep of things outside the house, such as the yard and car; she took care of things inside the house, such as cooking and laundry.

Personality differences may also attract and interest us. Psychological research over many years has suggested five basic dimensions of personality: extroversion (seeking social stimulation), emotional reactivity (strong emotional response to stressful circumstances), interest in new experiences, agreeableness, and organization. Each could easily be a source of attraction. An introvert may find an extrovert appealing since there is less pressure to keep the conversation going, while the extrovert may enjoy the introvert's attentions. An emotionally reactive person may look for calm confidence in another, while the confident one may enjoy the emotional drama of the other. A conventional person may be intrigued by the creativity of an adventurist partner, who in turn may enjoy introducing the conventional one to new experiences. An assertive partner and an agreeable one may find each other a natural fit. A goal-oriented planner and a live-in-the-moment partner may be drawn to each other for the separate strengths they each offer.

Differences that are appealing, however, may also show a darker side. The introvert may resist the extrovert's desires to go out frequently as a couple with others. An emotionally even partner may sometimes find the ups and downs of the other draining (just as the emotional partner finds the evenness boring). The conventional partner may find the adventurist over the top. An agreeable partner may feel run over at times by the assertive other. The organized planner may get frustrated with the spontaneous partner's frequent change in plans. In fact, it is hard to imagine these personality

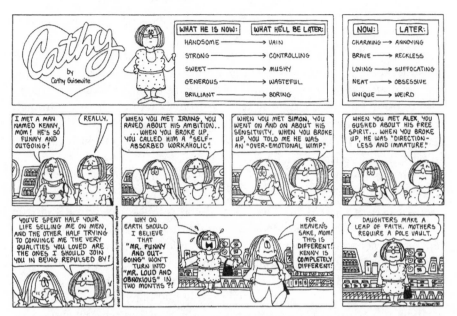

differences not creating difficulty at some point for a couple. They certainly seemed to do so for Debra and Frank, whose stories were told in Chapter 1.

Apart from personality differences, there are other important differences that can attract and repel. Consider desire for closeness and intimacy. Jill may want to spend most of her available time with Bill and share almost everything. Bill may find that appealing at first, a sign of Jill's interest. But over time Bill may need more space, to Jill's dismay. Or consider sexual desire. One may have a strong sexual drive and find the other sexually appealing, an interest that is certainly flattering to the other. However, the partner with the lower drive may eventually find the other's sexual needs demanding and intrusive. Finally, consider a difference in emotional expressiveness. A feeler may find a doer's ability to get things done appealing, while a doer may find the feeler's ability to articulate emotions exciting, helping the doer articulate some of his or her own. But it is easy to imagine the doer's frustrations at the feeler's inactions or the feeler's consternation at the doer's lack of emotional reflection. Just as in personality areas, these initially attractive differences can become a difficulty.

Many differences, of course, were neither original sources of attraction nor bones of contention. They were just part of the package of qualities that made up each person. But now they are a source of conflict. Blake did not feel strongly at first about being more sociable than Sondra, but this difference has since caused them many struggles. Initially Carrie was not particularly concerned that Parker was close to his controlling mother, but his attachment has since led to many arguments.

No matter how widely we survey the range of possible mates through dating, no matter how carefully we select our potential partners through online dating sites or "blind dates" set up via friends and family, the partners we select will be different from us, and often enough these differences will eventually cause us grief.

Ted Huston and Renate Houts, psychologists at the University of Texas, tried to mathematically determine the likelihood of similarities and differences between partners. They studied 168 couples and found that the likelihood that a man and a woman would match each other on the two separate dimensions of leisure interests and role preferences was only 33%. The estimated likelihood of matching on a hypothetical third dimension was about 17%. Matching on more than three dimensions was even less likely. On average, the couples in their study had dated only five different partners more than casually before marriage. This limited exposure, plus the low likelihood of finding a match on three or more dimensions, meant that spouses were incompatible in a variety of characteristics. Incompatibility was a mathematical certainty.

A cynic once remarked that "love is the delusion that one woman [or man] differs from the other." Perhaps the more common delusion of love is that our partners are more similar to us than they really are.

How Our Differences Evolve

I will always cherish the initial misconceptions I
had about you.
—AUTHOR UNKNOWN

Early in our relationships, we may be shielded from differences that make us incompatible. Our initial contacts maximize the opportunities for pleasure and minimize the chances for conflict. We dress up so that we look our best. We choose activities we will both find enjoyable. We are primed to try to impress and please the other. It is only as we begin to spend more time together, to meet each other's friends and families, and move in together that we are exposed to possible incompatibilities. Our moods are brought to light; our habits are revealed; our idiosyncrasies are bared. It is virtually certain that in some of these ways we will not fit well. When we find that the attractions are not strong enough or the incompatibilities are too great with a particular person, we end the relationship.

Fortunately, greater contact not only reveals more incompatibilities but also fosters greater closeness and attraction. We become more comfortable together and feel closer as we share more and more of our lives. Unanticipated areas of pleasure may turn up. We begin to find that life with a partner is a complex balance of positives and negatives. Eventually we make a commitment to someone when the attractions seem strong and the incompatibilities manageable.

Of course, we hope for a happy life together, but in love as in life the only certainty is change. Attraction may fade or love may grow; manageable differences may mushroom into troublesome incompatibilities or big issues may shrink to minutiae. You may expect to spend a lot of time as a couple with your parents, while your husband thinks the occasional Sunday dinner with his in-laws is plenty. Over time your husband may become fonder of your parents and enjoy spending extra time with them, or you may find you need less contact, in which case the difference between you dissipates. But it's just as likely that you could both harden in your positions so that what was a minor problem at first becomes a major problem later.

Incompatibilities may change through individual experiences as well as through shared experiences. Kyle and Joseph were in perfect agreement on how much time they should spend together until Joseph got a job promotion. The challenge, excitement, and pressure of Joseph's new job made him spend more and more of his time working, and Kyle began to feel left out of his life.

Whether incompatibilities are present to begin with or develop over time, they cause difficulty for couples because they mean deprivation or pain for one or both. When Joseph spends less time with Kyle, Kyle feels neglected and unloved. He worries about being a low priority in Joseph's life. However, if Joseph neglects his job responsibilities, he will feel anxious and worried.

If your husband wants less contact with your parents and you comply with his wishes, you may miss this contact and feel guilty about neglecting them. If your husband goes along with you, he may feel bored with your parents or, worse, resentful toward you because you pushed him into going. Incompatibilities have consequences for each partner.

The Light and Dark Sides of Similarities

Similarities are probably more important than differences in determining whom we choose as mates. Research indicates that people choose partners who are similar to themselves in age, background, and values. This is not surprising since our similarities give us common ground for conversation, for laughter, for the people we choose as friends, for activities, and for decision making. As a bonus, similarities beget similarities. Our common interests promote joint activities, which then further our common interests. If we both love politics, our discussion of politics and our attendance at political rallies are shared experiences that may increase our interest in politics. Likewise, if we play cards together, we may become more skilled at these games and find more enjoyment and success in playing cards.

Similarities may also cause conflict, however, although probably less so than differences. Let's consider partners who are similar on the five dimensions of personality discussed above: extroversion, emotional reactivity, interest in new experiences, agreeableness, and organization. Two partners who are both extroverts may agree that they want lots of contact with friends and family but may compete for "airtime" in talking to each other or with family and friends. They might also differ on the friends and family with whom they wish to spend time. In contrast, two introverts may never compete for "airtime" but experience isolation as they have difficulty sharing with each other or making social connections. Two partners who are both emotionally reactive may benefit from the empathy and understanding the other can provide when one is stressed. However, when both are stressed, perhaps neither can serve as the confident, strong one or even have the ability to attend to the other in those stressful moments. In contrast, two people low in emotional reactivity may be level-headed and able to handle stress well, keeping their relationship free of emotional drama. However, this lack of drama may seem as much a curse as a blessing, as their relationship lacks spark or emotional empathy when inevitably one of them gets upset.

Two conventional partners may appreciate the stability and predictability that the relationship provides but experience tedium or boredom in that little new and exciting enters their relationship. In contrast, two artists or adventurers may have a creative, exciting life together, constantly exploring the new and different, only to be distressed later that neither has taken care of the boring but necessary maintenance of their life, such as saving for the future or investing in a home or planning for children. Two agreeable, considerate partners may create a largely conflict-free environment as they are each responsive to the other's concerns. However, they may often have difficulty voicing their true feelings, given their concern about how the other would react, or they may wonder what the other is really thinking or feeling. Their peaceful home comes at a price of some spontaneity and openness. In contrast, two assertive people will never create ambiguity in the other about what each is feeling or thinking. They can create an open, spontaneous household but at a cost of peace and tranquillity. Finally, partners who are both organized, goal-oriented planners may run a tight ship, with all the bills filed and taken care of promptly and possessions all in their proper place, but it may not seem like much of a pleasure cruise, as the plans for tomorrow often trump any joys today. In contrast, spontaneous partners may revel in the pleasures of today, only to be shocked that neither has done appropriate planning for tomorrow.

Similarities in other areas crucial to the relationship can also create their share of problems, not so much by what they incite as by what they block. Two partners who both pursue a close, intertwined relationship may find themselves isolated from others or wondering if their "me" got lost in their "us." Partners who are both apprehensive of conflict and avoid discussion of difficult topics may limit their ability to solve their problems. If both partners are inhibited about physical affection or sex, they may deny themselves sensual pleasures from each other. If partners are both doers or both feelers, they may experience the imbalance and poor decisions that can result from an overreliance on feeling without action or activity unguided by consideration of its emotional consequences. In each of these cases a counterbalancing difference in one partner would be a welcome addition to the relationship.

We Come By It Rightly

When faced with differences or similarities that cause problems, your first impulse may be to find fault with your partner. "Why must you be so different from me?" or "Why can't you be different from me?" As we explained in the last chapter, you may view those problematic differences (or similarities) in terms of morality ("It's wrong for you to be this way") or emotional well-being ("It's a sign of mental illness or emotional immaturity that you're this way") or adequacy ("If you were a better person, you wouldn't be this way"). You may try to change your partner, and your partner may try to get you to change instead.

However, your genetic endowments and your learning histories have combined to make you and your partner who you each are, and change is not easy.

IT'S IN HIS BLOOD (OR HER GENES)

Science is finding more and more evidence for genetic influences on human behavior. Much of what we believed was learned entirely through experience now appears to be influenced in part by our genetic endowment.

One way to study the effects of genes is to look at newborns, who have not lived long enough for the environment to influence them. We now know that newborns start out with different temperaments. Some infants are difficult babies: they are reactive to new stimulation, they are hard to soothe, and they don't sleep regularly. Others are easy babies: they are not easily disrupted by new stimulation, they are easy to soothe, and they sleep regularly. By following infants with different temperaments, scientists have shown that these early tendencies are predictive of later behaviors.

Another way that social scientists investigate the effect of genes on behavior is to compare identical twins, who have 100% of their genes in common, with same-sex fraternal twins, who have only about 50% of their genes in common. They have found that identical twins show greater similarity in personality traits than do fraternal twins. Even when scientists are able to find twin-pairs who were separated at birth and adopted, they are able to show greater similarity between identical twins than fraternal twins.

One group of investigators from the University of Minnesota examined more than 1,500 twin-pairs and found that divorce rates were significantly higher for one twin if the other was divorced. The probability of divorce increased nearly twofold if one had a fraternal twin who was divorced but increased sixfold if one had an identical twin who was divorced. Does this mean there is a "divorce" gene? Hardly. In a later study, the group showed that personality attributes, such as negative emotionality, may be shared by twins, but more so by identical twins, and thus may account for the different divorce rates.

What this research means for you is that your and your partner's personality may not be changed that easily.

WE ARE OUR HISTORY

The past is never dead. It isn't even past.
—WILLIAM FAULKNER, *Requiem for a Nun* (1951)

The past affects both the present and the future. The kind of marriage our parents had determines to some extent the kind of marriage we will have. The way our parents treated us as children determines to some extent the way we will treat our spouses and our children. The kind of culture in which we were raised determines in part the kind of culture we will try to re-create.

A dramatic example is what has been called the "cross-generational transmission of marital instability." What this means is that children are more likely to divorce if their parents divorced. In one study based on five large surveys, Hallowell Pope and Charles Mueller found that people who had divorced parents were 10% more likely to get divorced themselves than people whose parents had never divorced. While this is not a large difference, it is a real difference and one that has been supported by subsequent studies. Presumably this tendency comes from both genetic factors—children inherit the genes of their parents—and environmental factors: the parents' difficult marriage affects the child's own marriage.

Violence in relationships provides another dramatic example of this carryover from the past. Children who witness physical violence between their own parents are more likely to experience violence in their own marriages than children who never witnessed violence in their parents. Children who were abused by their parents are more likely to abuse their own children than are children who were never abused.

But the past doesn't affect us in any simple way. Present experiences constantly modify the effects of past experiences, so that predictability from the past is usually weak. Many children who experience child abuse don't grow up to abuse their own children. Many children who witness violence between their parents don't end up in violent marriages. And many children who witness their parents' own divorce stay with their spouses.

Freudian psychology has popularized the notion that we look for mates who resemble our own parents. We often hear comments like "He married his mom" and "She married her dad." Some of us may notice uncanny resemblances between our own partners and our parents. Connections between our parents and our partners, however, are always complicated. Although there may be some striking similarities between a parent and a partner, there are usually many important differences. Even when one characteristic of our parent influences our choice in seeking a mate, that influence may occur indirectly as well as directly. Consider, for example, a boy who grows up with a demanding mother. He may "learn" emotionally that to get things done you need to have someone around to push you. He may seek a demanding wife and interact with her in ways reminiscent of his relationship with his mother. However, another boy with a demanding mother may experience such negativity from his interactions with her that he seeks a wife who never makes overt demands on him, and he interacts with her in ways that communicate his deep-seated feeling that she better not make overt demands on him. In both cases, the boy's childhood experiences affect his later marriage relationship, but in the first case he re-creates a childhood relationship in his marriage, while in the second case he avoids at all costs the repetition of any semblance of his childhood relationship.

Your experience in your family of origin affects more than just your choice of a mate. The emotional climate in your family of origin or in the larger culture in which you were raised influences what you are comfortable with and thus what you try to create in your own family. If, for example, you grew up in a home where physical affection was expressed freely and openly, while your husband grew up in a family that rarely expressed their love for each other in open physical affection, the two of you will likely have different expectations and comfort levels for physical affection. You may feel neglected and hurt that your husband doesn't put his arm around you more often or hold your hand more frequently. You may often feel disconnected from your husband. For his part, he may feel embarrassed by public displays of affection and uncomfortable with extensive private displays of affection. He likes to watch television with you but doesn't want to hold your hand the whole time.

The level of open conflict is another aspect of emotional climate that we tend to carry over from our families of origin to our adult families. In Melanie's family, open conflict was suppressed. Her father's motto was "If you can't say anything nice about a person, don't say anything at all." Her mother's view was "most problems solve themselves over time." Both parents avoided confrontation. Harsh words were forbidden. The typical result of parental disagreement was tension rather than open argument. The family achieved respect and consideration for each other, but at some cost in spontaneity and openness.

In sharp contrast to Melanie, Nolan's family of origin had a "let-it-all-hang-out" approach to conflict. Members confronted their conflicts directly, voiced their opinions freely, and rarely suppressed any of their feelings. Both of Nolan's parents were strong-willed and opinionated. The family achieved an open, spontaneous emotional exchange but at the cost of peace.

Naturally, Nolan's opinionated, volatile openness often injures Melanie emotionally and makes her feel disrespected and mistreated. He, in turn, often feels guilty for hurting her feelings. Nonetheless, he often gets angry because she won't speak her mind, and he is frustrated when she simply withdraws at the first sign of conflict. Although their differences are striking and problematic, they could enrich each other's lives. Melanie could learn emotional expressiveness from Nolan, while he could learn respect and restraint from her.

Broader forces from the past than our family history influence us today. The culture in which we were raised may exert powerful pressures on us. If the husband comes from a culture that values close contact with one's family of origin, he may view it as a mandatory responsibility to have his widowed mother live with him. To do otherwise would be disgraceful. If his wife comes from a cultural background that emphasizes separation between generations, she may insist that retirement homes be considered as an option. Why should her mother-in-law invade the privacy of their home? Their challenge will be to meet the wife's needs for privacy and separation in their nuclear family while allowing the husband to fulfill his familial responsibilities.

"I Do but I Don't": Confusing Differences

Go away and stop leaving me alone.
—ANONYMOUS

Up to now we have been discussing clear differences between partners: one wants one thing; the other wants something else. The wife endorses one set of values, the husband another. No matter how diametrically opposed the positions, such differences present definite, unambiguous goals for the two. They may fight dirty to reach these goals, but the stakes are clear.

Not all conflicts of interest present such clear-cut choices. Sometimes we think we want something and we articulate our desires clearly, but our behavior suggests something else. We send mixed messages, on one occasion pressing in one direction and on another in the opposite direction. Even a partner who is open to changing for us won't know which changes to make.

Sarah says she wants Hallie to participate equally in child rearing. Hallie reluctantly agrees and genuinely tries to become more involved with their children. However, Sarah's criticisms of her efforts and her unwillingness to relinquish control over the children undermine Hallie's attempts. Part of Sarah wants Hallie to participate equally, since she finds it difficult to take the primary role in child care and still succeed at her job. But another part of her wants to stay in charge of bringing up their children—because she feels she can do it better.

In these situations we see both a conflict *within one person* and a conflict *between two people*. Not only do Sarah and Hallie disagree, but Sarah herself is not sure what she wants. The situation becomes even more confounded and confusing when Hallie also feels ambivalent. Part of Hallie feels she should be an equal partner in raising their children—after all, they are both mothers—especially since Sarah spends as much time at work and contributes as much financially to the family as Hallie does. But part of Hallie feels unprepared for the task: she hasn't had as much experience with children as Sarah has. And, to tell the truth, she takes less pleasure in attending to them than Sarah does.

Consider another example of how conflicts within each partner complicate conflicts *between* them. Harold wants Julie to take better care of him. When he feels down or stressed—which is often—he wants to be pampered, drawn out, catered to. Julie often resists his pressure, feeling she shouldn't have to "baby" him. After all, he doesn't treat her that way when *she* feels bad. But there is something about his open anguish, his inability to cover his hurt, his vulnerability that Julie finds appealing. She feels needed, generous, and strong when she takes care of him. But when she's preoccupied with her own concerns, she finds his demands annoying. Thus she alternates between an angry "Oh, grow up" attitude and a comforting "Ah, sweetie, it'll be all right" attitude.

For his part, Harold feels uncomfortable about the level of support he wants and needs from Julie. It doesn't gibe with his ideas about manhood and often makes him feel "one down" in the relationship. Sometimes, when he just wants to withdraw into his own thoughts, he finds her pampering insulting and intrusive. Thus he alternates between a petulant "Aren't you going to help me?" stance and a defiant "I don't need you!" stance.

Given these mixed feelings within each partner, it's not surprising that the conflict between them is confusing. It's no wonder that they can't elicit or implement any change that either of them wants.

Mixed Blessings

There are no unmixed blessings.
—ANCIENT PROVERB

The personal qualities of our partners are often mixed blessings for us. The presence of any good characteristic is often associated with the presence of a less desirable one.

For example, it's great to have a responsible husband who takes care of business, who is punctual, neat, and orderly. You never have to wait for him, pick up after him, do his chores, check his bookkeeping, or worry whether he'll pick up the kids on time. If he says he'll do it, you know it will get done. But often such husbands demand similarly high levels of responsibility from their wives and children. They may be rigid about following rules and inflexible about adapting to changing circumstances. Their insistence on work before play may create a joyless atmosphere in the household. The "tight ship" they run is rarely a pleasure cruise.

It's also wonderful to have an accepting wife, one who loves you for what you are. She won't criticize you for your inadequacies or pressure you to change. Your foibles create few problems for her. But she may be passive about other aspects of life too. She may not join as vigorously as you'd like in pursuit of the goals you've set for yourself and your family, she may let things slide rather than take corrective action, and her laid-back quality may sometimes feel to you like indifference.

Some positive characteristics are less notable for their other-side-of-the-coin association with a negative characteristic than for their failure to include some other positive quality. For example, it's good to have a husband who is devoted to his family, who enjoys spending hours with the children after school and on weekends, playing sports and taking them places. He readily assumes his share of the kids' doctor and dental visits and delights in helping them, playing with them, talking with them. But such a man is unlikely to be a cutthroat power player at work. He may have neither time nor inclination to drive himself to greater heights (and higher salaries) at his job.

By the same token, it may be great to marry a career woman whose prestigious job adds substantially to the family income. Her career provides interesting material for conversation, is a source of pride, and allows upward mobility. However, she may not have the time or the interest to do certain "wifely" things that her husband also desires, such as preparing great meals, taking a personal interest in the laundering of his shirts, and assuming the major role in child care.

Obviously, it's possible to be responsible without being rigid, to be accepting without being passive, and to combine career, marriage, and parenting successfully. However, the development of one characteristic often precludes or at least limits the development of another. Certainly, limitations of time and energy prevent us from being good at everything. Therefore the characteristics of our partners, though often blessings, may be mixed ones.

Because of this, we may complain that our partners don't help out enough at home, even while we continue to push them to earn promotions at work. We may complain about their being controlling, yet gladly turn over more and more responsibilities to them. We certainly want them to find us sexually desirable but may find their frequent overtures annoying.

Yes and No

Even if desirable qualities in our partners came unaccompanied by undesirable ones, our incompatibilities might cause confusion. Often your feelings about a single characteristic are mixed. You may be attracted to your partner because of a particular attribute but at times find the same attribute distasteful. Your ambivalence may arise from your own internal conflicts about a particular characteristic. You may experience certain desires in yourself while finding these feelings emotionally or morally repugnant.

Lucy, for example, has always felt shy and uncomfortable about her sexuality. Discussions of sex embarrassed her, and sexual situations inhibited her. Surprisingly, she found herself attracted to Terry, who seemed just the opposite. He loved to tell ribald jokes, often made suggestive remarks, and vigorously pursued Lucy sexually. Her reactions to his sexual frankness were mixed. At times she found his behavior provocative and arousing, but at other times she found it disgusting.

Jorge has mixed feelings about wealth. Raised in the 1960s when materialism was scorned, he had since tried to lead a simple life. As values changed in the 1970s and 1980s, he held on to his philosophy, often lamenting society's "conspicuous consumption," "technological fixes," and "insatiable materialism." Yet he also yearned for certain possessions: the latest smartphone, a superb audio system, and a fast car. When he met Wanda, he found himself enjoying her posh condominium and stylish sports car. Even though he teased and criticized her for her materialism, he took full advantage of it himself.

Our desires may create conflicts not because these desires, in themselves, repel us, but because they don't fit our image of ourselves. Consciously accepting these longings would damage our self-esteem. Chim, who wants to be protected and taken care of in a relationship, chose Ben partly because he seemed strong and dependable. Throughout their relationship Ben has come to her rescue financially, taken charge of practical details such as car repairs, and pressured her to do long-range planning (by making investments, buying insurance, and making a will). Such a relationship doesn't fit Chim's view of herself as a liberated, independent woman, so she criticizes Ben for treating her "like a child."

Cecil hates paperwork of any kind. He'll gladly work on the car or in the yard for hours rather than spend 10 minutes with bills, budgets, or bank statements. Jessica has taken charge of the paperwork in their relationship, partly because she enjoys it and partly because Cecil avoids it. However, being uninformed about finances doesn't fit Cecil's view of manhood. Jessica's greater knowledge and control over their budget makes him feel weak in the relationship. When she informs him of their financial situation and recommends that they save more or spend less, he often resists, making vague accusations about her inability to control their budget. Sometimes he makes impulsive purchases, partly to demonstrate his financial independence.

Our ambivalence may arise less from internal conflict about a characteristic than from envy and competitiveness. We may seek in our partners those characteristics we lack yet feel angry that they possess those qualities while we do not. For example, James has always had difficulty asserting himself. He went along with the wishes of others, rarely voicing his own desires but often feeling resentful about being "taken advantage of." He found himself attracted to Darlene in part because of her frankness. She spoke her mind and "took shit from no one." James envied this quality in her yet criticized her for being insensitive to others and taking advantage of them.

Ray loved social gatherings of any type: parties, business lunches, dinners with friends. An entertaining conversationalist, he was sought out by others as much as he sought them out. Ray's husband, Boyce, was more reserved and uncomfortable socially. It took Boyce a while to "loosen up" with friends. Boyce envied the social attention Ray commanded but put down his skill as "superficial charm."

Ambivalence may develop over time as you become more familiar with your partner's qualities. As is illustrated with the "Cathy" cartoon earlier in this chapter, over time, once-appealing characteristics can show a darker side. What you once saw as unkempt charm now seems more like sloppiness; what you once viewed as a relaxed, easygoing attitude toward life now looks like laziness; what you once regarded as loving caretaking now seems like controlling behavior. You're finding fault and demanding change, and your partner quite naturally cries "Foul!"

Whatever its source, ambivalence adds confusion to any conflict with your partner. You generate mixed messages, sometimes supporting a characteristic of your partner, sometimes complaining about it. These changing responses cause confusion not only because they are contradictory but also because you present them *indirectly*. If you directly told your partner, "I don't like this" and then said, just as directly, "I do like this," he or she could comment on the contradiction and attempt to clear up the confusion. But you may not be fully aware of the ambivalence and present at least one side of the contradiction indirectly.

Lucy may criticize Terry's sexual vulgarity as bad taste yet actually reward his suggestive comments and jokes by making ineffectual protests that draw attention to his antics. Cecil may complain about Jessica's financial management and control but continue to force her to take charge by refusing to get involved with their finances himself. Boyce may minimize Ray's social skill by labeling it "superficial charm" yet depend on him to "break the ice" and bring him into the social swim. As these examples illustrate, we directly communicate the negative side of our ambivalence: don't do that or don't be that way. Yet at the same time we often indirectly communicate the positive side of the ambivalence—by acting in such a way as to reinforce the characteristics in question.

Ambivalence in *both* partners about the *same* issue creates even greater confusion. Each one has mixed feelings about an issue, has limited awareness of the confusion, and sends contradictory messages. No wonder they fail to resolve their conflict.

Consider, for example, Chim's ambivalence about being taken care of by Ben. She wants to be an independent woman, and so she criticizes Ben for treating her like a child. Yet she makes impulsive financial decisions that get her into situations from which she needs Ben to rescue her, and she avoids practical planning for her life, depending on him to do it for her. For his part, Ben wants her to need him, enjoys taking care of her, and seeks opportunities to exercise his considerable abilities in attending to the practical side of life. Yet he wants her to express appreciation for his efforts, insists on control of these practical areas if he has to take responsibility for them, and expects her to carry out the tasks he allocates to her without giving him any static. When she does give him static—which she often does when she sees him assigning her errands to take care of *her* life—he complains about her lack of responsibility. Or, when he is overwhelmed by his own responsibilities and finds the addition of hers a burden, he may tell her to "grow up." Thus Chim accuses Ben of treating her like a child and Ben accuses Chim of acting like a child; both are genuinely angry at each other's behavior, but both support and maintain these characteristics in each other. Their conflict is confused by the ambivalence of both about the issue of caretaking.

RECAP

In this chapter we have considered relationship problems as differences. Although we seek out partners who are similar to us in many ways, we also seek out partners who are different from us. And things that are initial similarities may grow to be differences, and vice-versa, over time. We all have unique genes and unique social histories that shape who we are. Thus we can never find a clone for a partner and, even if we did, we'd probably be unhappy with that clone. Inevitably we will find a partner whose differences from us or similarities with us cause problems.

These differences are the stuff of arguments. They are the content on which we engage, the relationship problems we face. And because the differences and similarities that lead to apparent incompatibilities often are the result of powerful genetic and historical influences, they are not easy to change.

Although some differences from your partner are defined and clear-cut, others may be more nebulous and slippery, adding confusion to your conflicts. The good qualities you like in your partner may be part of a natural constellation that includes some qualities that you don't like. Your partner's personality is inevitably a "package deal," and you have no "line-item veto" whereby you can cancel some qualities but keep others. Even a single quality in your partner may evoke complex and ambivalent reactions in which you are drawn to the quality at times but bothered by it at others.

Exercise: Personality Differences in Your Relationship That Might Make a Difference

In the following exercise, you will look at your personality and interests and consider which one of these traits is different for you and your partner and is related to your core conflict. The personality traits below are hardly the only areas in which partners are different, but they are common areas. This process will get you started on the D phase (the Difference or similarity related to your core issue) of a DEEP understanding of this issue.

Please complete the three brief questionnaires on the next three pages and score them as indicated.

Five Dimensions of Personality Measure*

Instructions:

Here are a number of personality traits that may or may not apply to you. Please rate each statement to indicate the extent to which you agree or disagree with that statement. You should rate the extent to which the pair of traits applies to you, even if one characteristic applies more strongly than the other.

I see myself as:	Disagree strongly 1	Disagree moderately 2	Disagree a little 3	Neither agree nor disagree 4	Agree a little 5	Agree moderately 6	Agree strongly 7
1. Extroverted, enthusiastic	Disagree strongly 1	Disagree moderately 2	Disagree a little 3	Neither agree nor disagree 4	Agree a little 5	Agree moderately 6	Agree strongly 7
2. Reserved, quiet	Disagree strongly 1	Disagree moderately 2	Disagree a little 3	Neither agree nor disagree 4	Agree a little 5	Agree moderately 6	Agree strongly 7

Extroversion Score (1–2) = _____ (Higher scores mean greater extroversion)

	Disagree strongly 1	Disagree moderately 2	Disagree a little 3	Neither agree nor disagree 4	Agree a little 5	Agree moderately 6	Agree strongly 7
3. Sympathetic, warm	Disagree strongly 1	Disagree moderately 2	Disagree a little 3	Neither agree nor disagree 4	Agree a little 5	Agree moderately 6	Agree strongly 7
4. Critical, quarrelsome	Disagree strongly 1	Disagree moderately 2	Disagree a little 3	Neither agree nor disagree 4	Agree a little 5	Agree moderately 6	Agree strongly 7

Agreeableness Score (3–4) = _____ (Higher scores mean greater agreeableness)

(cont.)

*Adapted from Gosling, Rentfrow, and Swann (2003). Copyright 2003 by Elsevier. Adapted by permission.

Five Dimensions of Personality Measure (cont.)

5. Dependable, self-disciplined

Disagree strongly	Disagree moderately	Disagree a little	Neither agree nor disagree	Agree a little	Agree moderately	Agree strongly
1	2	3	4	5	6	7

6. Disorganized, careless

Disagree strongly	Disagree moderately	Disagree a little	Neither agree nor disagree	Agree a little	Agree moderately	Agree strongly
1	2	3	4	5	6	7

Organization Score (5–6) = _____ (Higher scores mean greater organization)

7. Calm, emotionally stable

Disagree strongly	Disagree moderately	Disagree a little	Neither agree nor disagree	Agree a little	Agree moderately	Agree strongly
1	2	3	4	5	6	7

8. Anxious, easily upset

Disagree strongly	Disagree moderately	Disagree a little	Neither agree nor disagree	Agree a little	Agree moderately	Agree strongly
1	2	3	4	5	6	7

Emotional Reactivity Score (7–8) = _____ (Higher score means greater calmness, less emotional reactivity)

9. Open to new experiences, complex

Disagree strongly	Disagree moderately	Disagree a little	Neither agree nor disagree	Agree a little	Agree moderately	Agree strongly
1	2	3	4	5	6	7

10. Conventional, uncreative

Disagree strongly	Disagree moderately	Disagree a little	Neither agree nor disagree	Agree a little	Agree moderately	Agree strongly
1	2	3	4	5	6	7

Interest in New Experiences Score (9–10) = _____ (Higher scores mean greater interest in new experiences)

Emotional Expressiveness Measure*

Instructions: Using the scale provided as a guide, indicate how much you agree or disagree with each of the following statements by selecting the appropriate choice.

	Disagree strongly 1	Disagree 2	Neither agree nor disagree 3	Agree 4	Agree strongly 5
1. I am able to describe my feelings easily					
2. It is difficult for me to reveal my innermost feelings, even to close friends	Disagree strongly 1	Disagree 2	Neither agree nor disagree 3	Agree 4	Agree strongly 5

Emotional Expressiveness Score (1–2) = _____ (Higher scores indicate greater ease and interest in discussing feelings)

Desire for Closeness Measure**

Instructions: Please answer the following questions regarding your relationship.

1. On the whole, would you like more independence or more closeness in your relationship?

More independence 1	2	3	No change 4	5	6	More closeness 7

2. Given the limited amount of free time you have, would you prefer to spend more time with your partner or more time alone or with friends?

More time with partner 1	2	3	No change 4	5	6	More time alone or with friend 7

Desire for Closeness Score (1–2) = _____ (Higher scores mean greater desire for closeness)

*Adapted from Bagby, Parker, and Taylor (1993). Copyright 1993 by Elsevier. Adapted by permission.
**Adapted from Christensen et al. (2006). Adapted with permission from the author.

You have rated yourself on two sample aspects of each of the following personality traits: extroversion, agreeableness, organization, emotional reactivity, interest in new experiences, emotional expressiveness, and desire for closeness. The full measure of each of these traits would require you to rate yourself on more items and to do more detailed scoring, but this abbreviated version should give you an idea of what is meant by these variables. Your score on these variables is important for our purposes to the extent that (1) it differs from how your partner might have answered these questions and (2) it is related to the core issue you identified earlier. Do you believe that you and your partner are substantially different on one of the personality variables above and that that difference is centrally related to the core issue you identified? If not, consider other variables on which partners often differ, such as closeness with family of origin, libido (sexual interest), and leisure interests. If none of these seem central to your core conflict, think about what fundamental difference between you and your partner is related to the core conflict. Write down that difference below. If you think a similarity, rather than a difference, is key to your conflict, you may write that down instead.

Fundamental difference (or similarity) between my partner and me that is related to our core conflict:

_____

This is the first step in your DEEP analysis of your core conflict. We will come back to this difference later as we explore your conflict.

CHAPTER 4

"You Know How to Hurt Me"

RELATIONSHIP PROBLEMS
AS EMOTIONAL SENSITIVITIES

You always hurt the one you love.
—DORIS FISHER AND ALLAN ROBERTS,
SONG TITLE (1944)

A Roman divorced from his wife, being highly
blamed by his friends, who demanded, "Was
she not chaste? Was she not fair? Was she not
fruitful?" holding out his shoe, asked them
whether it was not new and well made. "Yet,"
added he, "none of you can tell where it pinches
me."
—PLUTARCH, *Parallel Lives: Aemilius Paulus*
(CIRCA 100 A.D.)

It is not hard to see how fundamental differences (or similarities) between people, such as in their personality traits, can create relationship problems. A couple where one partner is a saver and the other a spender needs to develop a reasonable way of spending money together. A couple where one partner wants more closeness and the other more independence needs to decide when to spend time together and when to spend time apart. A couple in which one partner is outspoken while the other is reserved needs to develop ways of communicating comfortably. A couple in which both like to be in control needs to work out areas where each is in charge. What may not be nearly as obvious is what is happening emotionally with the partners when they deal with these conflicts. Often their emotional reactions are strong and at times confusing. What else is going on besides the simple fact of their differences or their conflicting similarities? What happens to couples who get upset by their differences?

More Than Meets the Eye: Surface and Hidden Emotions

What is obvious is the emotions that appear when partners struggle with these differences—we call these "surface emotions." The saver gets irritated at what the spender has spent. The independence seeker gets angry when the partner complains about the lack of time together. The reserved partner shuts down when the other gets opinionated. The partners who both want to be in control get furious with each other for pushing for the very thing they want. Often these surface emotions mask deeper emotions that the partners don't express—what we call "hidden emotions." The saver may feel anxious and worried that they will have too little money and could be thrown into bankruptcy by some unforeseen expenses. The spender may feel that his or her freedom is being curtailed or at least challenged. The independence seeker may feel suffocated by the closeness seeker, who feels disappointed or abandoned. The reserved partner may feel walked on by the opinionated partner, who feels he or she can never get a straight answer. The couple who both would like control may each feel anxious that they have little or none.

We may conceal some emotions, our hidden emotions, because we may be only dimly aware of them. People seeking control may have only a hint of the anxiety they feel when they have to cede it to others. Or we may find the hidden emotions embarrassing. People wanting greater closeness may be embarrassed by their loneliness or fear of abandonment. Or we may fear hurting our partners if we reveal our true emotions. People who feel suffocated by their partners may want to protect the partners from that knowledge. Or we may not feel entitled to some feelings. A reserved man may not feel it is manly to experience the intimidation he feels with his opinionated partner. For any or all of these reasons, we may camouflage some hidden emotions with our surface emotions. If we feel initially threatened by abandonment, we may reveal anger rather than fear. If we feel slighted or unrecognized, we may withdraw in irritable silence rather than express any open hurt. If we feel not in control, we may aggressively attempt to seize control rather than express any anxiety about loss of control. If we feel invaded or intruded upon, we may distance ourselves and shut down emotionally rather than express our growing claustrophobia.

Surface emotions are often harsher than hidden emotions. We may express anger rather than hurt; resentment rather than disappointment; irritation rather than shame or guilt. The surface emotions often serve a protective function, portraying the self as strong and invulnerable rather than open and vulnerable and thus subject to further injury. Sometimes hidden emotions are masked not with an alternative emotion but with no apparent emotion at all. Rather than express the rejection we feel, we shut down; instead of voicing our envy or jealousy, we act as if we don't care. Rather than describe the aching loneliness we feel, we retreat in disinterest. And finally, sometimes hidden emotions trigger neither an alternative emotion nor a withdrawal but rather animated action. Instead of expressing any anxiety to our partners, we take charge of the situation and tell them what to do or how to do it. Instead of voicing our distrust, we interrogate our partners about their whereabouts. Instead of revealing the neglect we feel, we demand more time with our partners.

Unfortunately our visible, surface emotions often mislead our partners. They don't know what is going on with us. These emotions may also mislead us. If we feel embarrassed by the genuine hidden emotion, we may feel relief at expressing an alternate one. If we are concerned that expressing our genuine hidden emotion, such as feeling overwhelmed or intruded upon, may injure our partners, then expressing a different emotion may also lead to relief. So we express visible emotions that seem safer for all but hide our initial genuine reactions, which seem more threatening to us or our partners. The safety we gain comes at the steep price of confusion for us and our partners.

Let's consider a case of surface and hidden emotions in detail. Jack and Avery go to a cocktail party with friends of hers from work. Always more outgoing than Jack, Avery immediately gets engaged in the party and has a great time laughing and joking with her colleagues. Meanwhile Jack awkwardly tries to make conversation with some people he doesn't know well and with whom he doesn't feel like he has much in common. He feels abandoned by Avery and envious of her social skill and charm. Avery notices Jack and senses his discomfort but is not sure what to do and gets caught up in the fun of the party. On the way home from the party, Avery is anxious that Jack did not enjoy the party and is fearful that he may blame her, but she doesn't want to open the proverbial can of worms and so simply says hopefully "I thought the party was really fun." Jack feels too vulnerable to share his experience of social awkwardness and abandonment, so he expresses disapproval of the party and remarks, "I thought it was boring, with everyone just focused on work." Then Avery and Jack get into an argument about whether the party was a good one or not and how much people should focus on work at a social event. Their genuine emotions remain hidden, and thus they have the wrong discussion, triggered by their surface emotions. Unfortunately, they end up just arguing and miss an opportunity to understand each other better, which could help them handle the next party better.

A Soft, Sensitive Spot

Strong emotional reactions to differences or similarities, whether those strong emotions are surface ones or hidden ones, suggest sensitivities or vulnerabilities in each of us. Unless the triggering event is one to which virtually all people would have a strong emotional reaction, our emotional reactions point to our personal soft spots. This is especially the case when the triggering event is relatively small, one that others might easily ignore. Yet in reaction to this small event, we, seemingly out of context, explode emotionally, as if some combustible material inside us, some personality plutonium, reached its critical mass and blew up. These sensitive spots provide the emotional energy or fuel behind the conflict over our differences and similarities.

Although *explosion* is an appropriate analogy for the force of many emotional reactions, the connection between the provocation and our response suggests something more akin to an allergic reaction. What is to most a mildly negative experience, such as a bee sting, or a curative one, such as penicillin, or even a pleasurable one, such as the smells of spring or the taste of a particular food, can cause strong negative, allergic reactions in others. Their bodies react with fits of coughing and sneezing or with rashes and itching or much worse. An anaphylactic reaction can lead to death without quick medical intervention. One person's meat is truly another's poison.

Viewing some of our emotional reactions as "psychological allergies" is appropriate for at least two reasons. The provoking event is an innocent one, or at most a mildly annoying one, for many people, whereas we have a special sensitivity to that kind of event. Similarly, just as the body's exaggerated, protective response to an allergy can create difficulty and in some cases threaten life itself, so our efforts to defend and protect ourselves from psychological allergies can create difficulty and in some cases threaten our relationships.

In the midst of an argument Hector mentions that he and Clarice ought to divorce. For him, this statement merely indicates his anger at the time; he has no intention of divorcing Clarice. For many couples such comments would be unpleasant and might be responded to in kind ("Yeah, well why don't you just move out?"). However, for Clarice, such a comment is deeply troubling. Her sensitivity to abandonment and rejection makes it impossible for her to dismiss Hector's remark. She is hurt and scared, but mostly furious. Her reaction is to pack up and leave that very night. She will protect herself by rejecting him. She will implement his plan before he can. It takes Hector several difficult days of coaxing her back before she returns. But her strong reaction to his comment makes Hector genuinely question their marriage much more than the argument that led him to suggest divorce.

Our reaction in these situations is so intense because we take the provoking event so personally. Like a heat-seeking missile that finds the engine of an aircraft, the seemingly innocent event finds our soft spot. It exploits our vulnerability. It finds the weak spot in our defenses, where we lie openly exposed. Ironically we expect our partners to be careful to avoid this sensitivity, even though we may be taken by surprise by it ourselves. We are offended; they are remiss.

Why do we have these emotional sensitivities? Where do they come from? Although psychological research indicates that we may be born with certain tendencies, such as a tendency toward anxiety or emotional reactivity, it normally requires particular life experiences to activate this tendency and these life experiences shape the particular sensitivity that we will have. The bumps, bruises, and wounds we experience throughout life leave their marks. Having been injured before, we are more vigilant about being injured again and may feel more pain if we are. We have been shaped by our experience to be sensitive.

Naturally some of the emotional sensitivities that lead to our strong surface and hidden emotions in our relationship come from our past experience with our partners. Our contact with them has created injuries that alert us to possible future ones.

Relationship Events That Create Sensitivities

We can certainly understand the reactions that people have to egregious actions by their partners. If a wife betrays her husband by having an affair, we can understand the husband's sensitivity to issues around fidelity—his anxiety when she goes out, his suspicions when she gets a call from someone unknown to him. Or if a husband physically abuses his wife, we can understand her anxiety if she brings up a topic of disagreement or her intimidation when he gets angry. We will discuss these special cases in Chapter 16.

However, most of our sensitivities develop from less dramatic actions by our partners. The crimes of the heart are usually misdemeanors. Although partners will sometimes do horrible things, most of the events that create conflict in relationships are relatively small infractions. Yet these events can create sensitivities to future such events. Let's consider three kinds of relationship events.

"YOU WEREN'T THERE TO CELEBRATE WITH ME"

In the early years of their marriage, Susan spent most of her time raising three children. Tom was heavily involved in his work as an architect. When their youngest child was 8, Susan started law school in the evenings; 5 years later she got her degree. She was offered a job with a fine law firm and wanted to take the position, but Tom asked her to postpone it for a while. He had taken on extra responsibilities as head partner and needed help from her at home to entertain colleagues and clients. She agreed. Here is how she describes her reaction to that decision and subsequent events:

> "I was relatively satisfied with my decision. I was able to help Tom and at the same time do interesting law work. My volunteer work was well recognized in the legal community. A year and a half later, I was to receive a special award for my contribution to Legal Aid. I was really happy and looked forward to the award dinner, which many lawyers I respected would attend. But that evening, I was very embarrassed when Tom never showed up at the banquet; the chair reserved for him next to me near the center of the table stayed empty all evening. I was even angrier when I returned home that night to discover him watching television and to hear him tell me that he had been just too tired to attend the dinner.
>
> "That incident brought matters into focus. It forced me to realize how much the two of us had been drifting apart. I realized how much effort it now took me to ask Tom about his work and how rarely he inquired about mine or even listened when I did tell him about an experience. I also realized there wasn't much of a spark in our sex life. I started actually reveling in my extra 'space' when Tom was away on a trip. I began to feel resentful about the imbalance in our lives: Tom, at the peak of his career, expecting me to continue making sacrifices while giving me little in return. I became resentful about doing the bulk of the housework; resentful about Tom's taking me for granted; resentful that, after all the years I'd listened to his stories and supported his career, Tom now didn't give a damn about my career." (in Levinger, 1983, pp. 317–318)

This incident—Tom's failure to attend the banquet—set off a train of events that ultimately led to the failure of their marriage.

"Finally, I figured I'd had enough. I received another good job offer and decided to take it without consulting Tom. I also told Tom that I'd probably want to separate from him. When I told him that, he seemed stunned. He said I was the most important person in his life and asked what he could do to keep me. I was so shocked at his insensitivity, though, that I blurted out: 'Nothing. There's nothing you can do to keep me, if you can't even figure out how unhappy I've been.'

"After I moved into my own apartment, I began to feel a lot better physically. The headaches and backaches I'd been having went away, and I felt good to be on my own. At the same time, I felt bad about the breakup and felt bad for our kids. Sometimes I worry about my future alone. But I think I made the right decision." (in Levinger, 1983, p. 318)

When probed after the separation, Tom revealed that on the day of the banquet he had lost an important competition for a major design contract, yet he insisted at the time that the only reason he had skipped the banquet was that he was tired. He did not seem to understand that his absence had hurt Susan or that he may have been threatened by an award for her on a day of failure for him. Susan, too, was incredulous at the suggestion that Tom might be threatened by her success. She saw Tom as being so far ahead of her professionally as to be invulnerable.

This true story dramatically illustrates how relationship problems— and in this case relationship dissolution—are created when one partner fails to come through for the other. This failure to be there when it counts most causes the other embarrassment and humiliation and makes him or her feel unimportant. Our story also illustrates how partners can have limited understanding of their own sensitivities and hidden emotions or their partner's, a lack of knowledge that allows them to attribute the other's behavior to the worst instincts. Tom had no sense of how important this recognition dinner was to Susan; she had no sense that he could feel threatened by her success.

"YOU WEREN'T THERE TO SUPPORT ME WHEN I NEEDED YOU MOST"

We are more likely to need our partners during moments of despair than during moments of glory. When threatened with illness, coping with the death of a loved one, or dealing with a failure, we feel most vulnerable and in need of our partners' help and support. At these crisis points we may need heroic actions from them. Their failure to come through for us may leave us deeply wounded and angered inconsolably. The experience may etch a memory that won't be erased easily.

Wendy had chest pains late one night when Delia was on a business trip. When Wendy called Delia at 3:00 A.M. and told her of her pains, Delia encouraged her to go to the emergency room but assured her that the pain was probably due to stress or possibly just in her head. Reminding her that she often had various aches and pains, Delia said, "Don't let your hypochondria get the best of you." Wendy took Delia's reassurances as veiled attacks and asserted that she had never awakened in the middle of the night with chest pains and had never before called Delia about them. When she got off the phone, Wendy wasn't sure whether she was more upset with Delia or with the threat to her health. Impulsively she called for an ambulance— *someone* had to take seriously the pains that scared her so much. After all, her father had died of a heart attack at 59. In the ambulance and at the emergency room, Wendy was struck by the irony of her feelings: hoping on the one hand that her pains were nothing and on the other that something was wrong with her so she could justify her call to 911 and vindicate herself with Delia. She got a little of both: the doctors found some irregularities in her heartbeat that required follow-up but no evidence of a heart attack. Now Wendy felt justified in being furious at Delia: she hadn't been there for her when she really needed her, when something really was wrong.

When Mara's mother died, Walter decided not to go to the funeral. He had an important business meeting that day, one that could lead to a new and large account for him. He explained to Mara that he had never gotten along with his mother-in-law, so to attend the funeral would be sort of a sham. Furthermore, he hated funerals. Mara was surprised and hurt by his decision but could not argue with his logic. Walter's decision not to go to the funeral was just another upset that got muddled in with all the rest, and it was only at the funeral that she realized clearly that she needed him there for her. Whatever his feelings toward her mother had been, it was her feelings that mattered now. She was terribly hurt by his absence at this difficult moment for her.

"NOT ONE BIG THING, BUT A THOUSAND LITTLE THINGS"

We can understand and perhaps excuse powerful and dramatic reactions to stunning events, such as a failure to show up at an honorary dinner or a funeral. Fortunately, such events in marriage are rare. More common are daily slights, ordinary injustices, and routine disrespects that hurt and anger us. He doesn't respond when she reaches for his hand. She shows little interest when he talks about his day. His kisses seem perfunctory. She seems bored by his stories.

At times we voice no overt reaction. Surprised by the intensity of our response, we try to convince ourselves we are overreacting and end up suffering these hurts in silence. At other times, however, we react strongly. We make sarcastic comments: "I didn't realize I was so boring to you." We accuse: "You don't care about me. You can't even bring yourself to touch me." We make attacking suggestions: "Maybe you should find someone who will capture your interest better than me." We storm out of the room: "I don't want to be in the presence of someone who has no interest in or love for me."

When we do react strongly, our partners are likely to respond in kind, either defensively or offensively: "Is it a crime to yawn?" "Look, I'm tired tonight." "We are not adolescent love birds." "Here you go again!" "You are so demanding." "You can't take not being the center of attention."

Why such seemingly small actions can provoke such big reactions may be explained by our history. A chronic pattern of daily neglect, in which each single incident might be explained easily, can eventually create powerful reactions of hurt and anger. In John Updike's novel S., Sarah Worth leaves her physician husband of more than two decades not because of any egregious actions on his part but because of his "genteel atrocities of coldness and blindness toward me." In a letter to him, she describes the "nearly twenty-two years of mental and emotional cruelty you with your antiseptic chill have inflicted on me." In a letter to her adult daughter, she tries to justify her leaving: "Well, I recently tried an experiment. I didn't tell your father a thing about my day. And *he never asked.* Not once, day after day of biting my tongue—he utterly didn't notice. That settled it. So absent from his perceptions, I might as well be absent in fact." A long history of neglect—of inattentive acts, each one small and easily dismissed if considered in isolation but powerful in their totality—led Sarah to leave her husband and the material luxury they had.

Sensitivities That Originate in Prior Relationships

Although we may become sensitive to certain triggers as a result of the way our partners have treated us, more often we enter these relationships with sensitivities that were generated in earlier relationships that we had with our parents, our peers, or our earlier romantic relationships. Our partners do something relatively trivial, but it has a significant impact on us because of the raw nerves that were exposed in earlier encounters with other people. Although partners will sometimes take egregious actions, most of the events that create conflict in relationships are relatively small infractions. As we noted earlier, the crimes of the heart are usually misdemeanors. Yet the reaction can be intense, because the infraction touched on a sensitivity.

Below we describe a number of common sensitivities in people that can help explain their strong reactions, their psychological allergies, to their partners' seemingly insignificant behavior. These sensitivities occur around universal themes of security, freedom, admiration, approval, and control. We describe these sensitivities and possible reasons for their development in earlier relationships.

"DON'T EVER LEAVE ME"

Compared with animals, we humans have an exceptionally long period of dependency on our parents. We are born totally dependent, unable even to roll over or raise our heads. Even after a year, we can barely walk or feed ourselves. It takes almost two decades before we are recognized by society at large as adults capable of handling our own affairs.

Developmental psychologists have studied the attachment of infants to their primary caretaker—usually the mother. Because infants' physical survival, as well as their emotional well-being, depends on their caretaker, they have an automatic reaction to separation from her. They don't take it lightly if she leaves them alone, particularly in an unfamiliar place. They use her as a secure base from which to explore the world; if anything scary happens to them, they rush back into her arms. Psychologists speculate that if the caretaker is responsive to distress, if she handles separation sensitively so that the infant is familiar with his or her new surroundings and new caretakers before she leaves, then the infant develops "secure attachments." The infant learns that others can be trusted, that others will be there when needed, that abandonment is not a possibility.

On the other hand, if the caretaker is not responsive to distress, if she does not handle separation sensitively, and especially if she is rejecting, the infant will not develop a secure attachment. He or she will *not* learn that others can be trusted, that others will be there for him or her—because they weren't. Some genetic predisposition may amplify these distressing experiences for the infant.

Psychologists tend to weight early experiences more heavily than later ones, because these early experiences are the foundation of learning on which the infant builds its model of what the world is like. However, later experiences certainly modify earlier ones. Infants exposed to inconsistent caretakers early on may later be exposed to more reliable ones and learn

greater trust and confidence. Unfortunately, early experiences tend to predict later ones. Children don't have the luxury of "trading up" their caretakers. Usually the one who was inconsistent and rejecting when they were
infants is still around to be rejecting and inconsistent when they are older.

If you emerged from a history of caretaking that didn't inspire trust or
confidence and had perhaps a genetic predisposition that magnified these
unfortunate experiences, you may be an adult with a vulnerability to signs
of abandonment or rejection. Separations from your partner may be difficult for you. The simple business trip that takes your partner to another
state for a week may be threatening to you. Reunions may be tinged with
anger: "Why did you leave me in the first place?" You may be especially
sensitive to signs of love or commitment. Your partner's temporary preoccupation with other matters may feel like a message of rejection. Your partner's desire for time alone or time with friends may feel like abandonment.
You may have exquisite radar that detects your partner's slightest interest
in potential rivals. Your partner's mild flirtation or sidelong glance at an
attractive other may feel like betrayal. Your partner, unfortunately, did not
grow up like you and is mystified by your attitude.

"HELP, I'M TRAPPED"

The trouble with wedlock is that there's not enough
wed and too much lock.
            —CHRISTOPHER MORLEY

A vulnerability to feelings of entrapment, like a vulnerability to feelings of
abandonment, makes love a fearsome activity, but for very different reasons.
Those with a sensitivity to entrapment are on guard for signs that their
partners may smother, overwhelm, or intrude on them.

This pattern of vulnerability may also begin early in life. Perhaps you
had a parent who showered you with love, but the hugs and kisses and
expressions of love were triggered by your parent's needs rather than your
own. So you often got hugs and kisses whether you wanted them or not.
And if you resisted, maybe you got messages that made you feel guilty, as
if you didn't love your parent or weren't a good, grateful child. Maybe reci-
procity of love was demanded. Thus your early experiences showed you that
love has claws. Closeness with another is a needed but troubling experience.

Apart from your own childhood experiences, you may have developed
or aggravated your sensitivity to entrapment through your adult romantic
relationships. Through some combination of chance and design, you had
a partner who intruded on your space, demanded your love, overwhelmed
you with his or her feelings, and made guilt-inducing comments about your

failure to reciprocate. Closeness with another raised danger signals even as it provided love and support. Closeness seemed to offer a luxuriously furnished prison, golden chains, a velvet coffin.

Love consistently raises the question "How much of me do I have to give up to be with you?"

"I AM SOMEBODY"

I feel like a nobody to everybody. I want to be
somebody to somebody.

As children we seek recognition from our parents. We look expectantly for the "Good girl!" and the "That-a-boy!" for our accomplishments. We want attention for the pictures we draw, applause for the balls we hit, laughter for the jokes we tell, and compliments for the grades we get. Although most parents naturally provide this kind of recognition to their children, some may be so preoccupied with their own lives that their child gets little notice. These parents may experience their children's bids for attention as irritating annoyances. As a result, the children get little concrete evidence that their achievements really matter to anyone. It is not clear that they are special in anyone's eyes.

The presence of more than one child in the family complicates the recognition of children. Parents' attention, compliments, and applause must be shared. Children inevitably compete for this parental recognition. But often the playing field is not level. One child may be more verbal or more athletic or more humorous or more social or more physically attractive than the other and therefore may have a built-in advantage for recognition. Parents may favor a particular child because he or she looks or acts like them or otherwise has some attractive feature they value. As a result, parents will never mete out exactly equal doses of recognition to their children. In some families the inequities may be obvious and dramatic.

Little overall parental recognition in childhood, or little recognition relative to a sibling, may sensitize you to issues of recognition in adult relationships. If your experience throughout childhood was that others in the family were getting an unfair surplus of attention, you might be on guard to see that the same doesn't happen in your marriage. The opposite is true too: an overdose of attention and recognition in childhood may lead you to expect a heavy diet of attention and recognition in adulthood.

Sensitivity to recognition may spring from adult relationships as well as childhood ones. If you have been with unresponsive partners, who have been stingy with their praise, you might well be on the lookout for personal slights. If your partner seemed to hog the attention, you might have felt hurt and envious. If your partner seemed to value his or her own accomplishments and to slight yours, you may have felt competitive.

Whatever its origins, some of us will be sensitive to recognition in our relationships. We may feel hurt if our partners are not enthusiastic about our successes or make too much of our failures. We may need our partners to serve as cheerleaders for whatever we attain. We may want to be looked up to and honored for our accomplishments. We may want our partners to listen to our stories of what we have done and the clever way we did it. We seek admiration as much as love from our partners, because admiration seems the most tangible evidence of love. When we don't get it, we seek change in our partners, a request that may feel like a significant imposition to them.

"TELL ME I'M OKAY"

Carl Rogers, one of the early giants of psychotherapy, told a story about a preschool girl with whom he had worked. To start a conversation with her, he asked her what her name was. She replied: "Alice Don't." Rogers surmised that she had been told "Alice, don't!" so often that she had incorporated that parental warning not only into her self-concept but into her very name.

One of the main tenets of Rogers's theory of personality development was that children need validation and approval from their parents. They need messages that they are okay children. According to Rogers, if they get many messages that they are not okay, or if they have to do everything right to get approval, then their development will be harmed.

Whatever the merits of Rogers's theory, experiences of approval and disapproval with our parents early in life and in other close relationships later in life will likely affect our concerns about approval in our adult romantic relationships. Those of us sensitive about approval may seek reassuring messages from our partners that we did or said the right thing. We may have difficulty taking action without approval from our partners. We may feel upset if they do not support our actions or are irritated by the pressure we put on them to express approval. We may also confuse legitimate disagreement with disapproval. If our partners disagree with our views or our actions, we may experience such disagreement as disapproval of our very selves.

If you are vulnerable about receiving approval from others, you may be especially sensitive to criticism. For you, criticism represents obvious disapproval. You may have thin skin. You can sense the implied criticism even in an innocuous remark. If your partner sighs and says, "Well, I better do the dishes now," you may hear the overtone "You should have already done them." If your partner voices frustration that he or she has too much to do, you may hear an implication that you should have done more. Your antenna is tuned to the criticism frequency, and you can pick up even the weakest signal. However, if you respond to a verbal criticism with a question of "Why did you have to say that?" you may elicit yet another criticism of "Why are you so sensitive?"

"I'M IN CHARGE"

An older couple I once worked with described the following incident. The husband had recently retired from his job of some 30 years and was having difficulty finding daily activities to keep himself occupied and interested. One day, late in the morning, he wandered into the kitchen and began fixing himself a peanut butter sandwich. His wife noticed what he was doing, rushed into the kitchen, and ordered him out. It was not yet time for lunch, which she had already planned. Furthermore, if he was hungry now, she would fix him something. But above all, he should get out of *her* kitchen!

The husband was a bit dumbfounded by the strength of her response. After all, he was just trying to fix himself a simple sandwich. He certainly wasn't trying to take over food preparation in general or her kitchen in particular. However, she saw his action as an incursion into the territory she had controlled all of their marital life. She was also anxious about his difficulty in finding meaningful retirement activity and hoped he would find something soon, but not the activities that were hers. He may have lost his territory through retirement, but he was not to take over hers.

Issues around control come up from time to time for all of us, particularly when an area of control that we cherish seems threatened. However, some of us may be especially sensitive about power and control. We may feel threatened even when the challenge to our control seems less obvious. We don't want to appear weak or under someone else's thumb, particularly our spouse's thumb. Our anxieties about life are soothed whenever we are in control but ignited whenever others are. We want to be in the driver's seat, literally and figuratively. If our partners express a strong opinion, we may feel they are trying to take over. If they assert their rights, we may view the assertion as an attempt to abridge ours. Delegating work to others may be difficult because we fear that they won't do it as we would—indeed, they often don't.

In the process of raising children, parents must constantly make decisions about how much control to maintain and how much to relinquish. It is the job of parents to protect their children, both physically and psychologically. Therefore, they must limit their children's independence until their children can manage particular situations on their own. When and in what situations can toddlers play by themselves or bathe by themselves? When can you let children walk to the store by themselves? When can teenagers be allowed to take the family car out for the evening?

Even little children want control. They want things their way. They want to do things by themselves. Some appropriate measure of control is certainly important for children's well-being and their appropriate development. It is clearly important to their satisfaction. Once my wife and I allowed our toddler son to maintain control of some M&M candies we bought for the family. We assured him that he could be the "boss of the M&Ms." He beamed with the pride of ownership and power. Carefully and judiciously he passed out the candies to his parents and his sister. After that incident he would occasionally ask, "Can I be the boss of the . . . ?" He wanted to reexperience the power of having control.

Given the struggle between parents, who must protect their children by exerting control over their behavior, and children, who want independence and control for themselves, it is not surprising that some people might emerge from this struggle with sensitivities about control. Perhaps an overprotective parent exerted excessive control that created anger and rebellion. Perhaps a permissive parent failed to exert sufficient control so the child became used to little accountability and maximum independence. Experiences such as these might lead one to exert control over a partner or to fear and rebel against such control by a partner.

As noted earlier, this list of psychological vulnerabilities is intended simply to illustrate the kinds of sensitivities people may bring to or develop in their relationships. The list is certainly not meant to be exhaustive. Nor are the categories mutually exclusive. It is possible for someone to have sensitivities in more than one of the areas. Furthermore, there are many other specific sensitivities that may trouble partners in relationships. For example, one member may be embarrassed about how little formal education she has had, another may be sensitive about his hair loss, another about his weight, and another about how poorly her children have done in school.

It is impossible to get through life without becoming sensitive to certain issues. People who never overreacted or underreacted to any event, who took all the vicissitudes of life in stride, who had only the reactions that make logical sense and seem conventionally appropriate would be strangers to all of us who must struggle daily with the "slings and arrows of outrageous fortune." And these automatons would probably not be very sympathetic to our struggles.

Handle with Care

The finest qualities of our nature, like the bloom on fruits, can be preserved only by the most delicate handling.
—HENRY DAVID THOREAU, *Walden* (1854)

In our areas of vulnerability we will be especially alert to how we are treated. Our feelings are close to the surface and easily disturbed. So we are vigilant, lest those feelings be ignited.

A fascinating study by Dartmouth College researchers Robert Kleck and Angelo Strenta illustrates how we can be hypersensitive to others' behavior when we feel vulnerable. They told a group of women that they were interested in studying how other women would react to them if they were disfigured by a facial scar. With the women's permission, they used theatrical makeup to create an authentic-looking scar. Then they had the women examine the scar with a hand mirror so they could see how authentic the scar appeared. After the women had finished examining the scar, the experimenter applied a "moisturizer" to "keep the makeup from cracking." In fact the so-called moisturizer actually removed the scar, but without the women's knowledge. Then each of these women, thinking she was showing a disfiguring scar, talked with another woman who saw no disfigurement and had no idea of what had gone on before. The conversations were poignant. Thinking they looked horrible, these "scarred women" were very self-conscious. Compared to a control group of women, who were led to believe that their conversational partners merely thought they had an allergy, the "scarred women" rated their partners as more tense, distant, and patronizing. Neutral observers who watched the videotapes of these interactions could see no difference between how the "scarred women" and the "allergy women" were treated. Clearly a sensitivity about the scar made these women interpret the behavior of their conversational partners differently.

Something analogous to what happened in this experiment may occur with psychological vulnerabilities. A heightened sensitivity may lead us to misinterpret our partners' response or lack of response to us. If, for example, a husband is sensitive about the interest and attention his wife gives to his accomplishments, he may react angrily if his wife does not ask him about his job interview as soon as he gets home from work. She may reply honestly, albeit defensively, that she has been both aware of and concerned about his interview, but given her own frustrating drive home from work, she was not at that exact moment thinking of his job interview. An argument might easily ensue in which he claims she doesn't really care about his efforts to find a better job and she claims he is overly sensitive.

When we are sensitive about some issue, we want to be handled with care. Our fragile feelings need to be cushioned from the bumps and jolts of normal handling. We expect those who love us to treat us with special consideration.

Our partners may feel we are asking too much. They may invoke a fairness argument: "I don't ask you to treat me that way." They may list instances in which we were not so sensitive to them and they didn't get upset. The wife who forgot to ask about her husband's job interview may charge, correctly, that he often forgets to ask her about important events at her job and certainly doesn't do so immediately upon his entry into the house. Such reactions, although understandable, fail to acknowledge that one is sensitive in a particular area while the other is not. It is a bit like someone with a normal ankle saying to someone with a sprained ankle: "I don't have to limp. Why should you?"

When Vulnerabilities Collide

Dealing with sensitive areas can be challenging under the best of circumstances. We may feel burdened by the demands of handling our partners' feelings with such care. We may feel like parents dealing with an immature child. We may fear that accommodating them will increase their demands so that we, like they, become slaves to their sensitivities. For example, the wife who was scolded by her husband for failing to ask about his interview may fear that if she makes an effort to show him extra attention, his needs for special consideration will increase, his demands for immediate response will become insatiable. However, often the special care that we can give our partners may soothe their vulnerabilities and make them more responsive. They may become more giving to us because they feel cared for and want to reciprocate. Their sensitivities may, paradoxically, be less of an issue for them than for us.

As challenging as it is to handle a partner's area of vulnerability when we are doing well, it becomes even more formidable when our own sensitivities come into play. If a particular incident or issue taps both of our sensitivities, then conflict is liable to result. Consider, for example, a wife, Ruth, who is sensitive about abandonment ("Don't ever leave me") and her husband, Gaylord, who is sensitive about entrapment ("Help, I'm trapped"). If each of their sensitivities gets aroused by the same incident, conflict will likely follow. Let's say that the stressful circumstances of his life at work and with Ruth have made Gaylord feel a strong desire for space, for separateness from Ruth so he can calm down, while similar stressful circumstances have aroused fear in Ruth that their relationship is falling apart. She needs the reassurance of closeness with Gaylord. When Gaylord informs Ruth that he is making plans to spend the weekend hiking with his best friend, she may explode: "How can you leave when things are so bad between us?" He replies, "That is exactly why I want to leave." And a battle ensues.

Consider a second example, but one in which partners share the same sensitivity. Clayton and Carmen are faced with a cross-country move that must be completed by the end of the month so they can start their new jobs. Both are anxious about whether they can accomplish all that they need to do in that time frame. Clayton in particular fears that the furniture he inherited from his parents may get damaged during the move. Carmen is especially worried that the files from her home office will get lost or disorganized in the process. Both cope by taking charge, by exerting control. But theirs is a divided command. They argue about which mover to choose, about who should do what, and about why the other is being so resistant. The stress of their communication is just as bad as the stress of their move.

Provocation or Vulnerability?

Between the obvious cases of provocative action that would upset most of us and the obvious cases of psychological allergies in which only those with a particular sensitivity would get upset, there is a vast, unmarked land of mildly provocative actions and well-tuned vulnerabilities. Which is the most important cause of the hurt and anger: the mildly provocative action or the reactive vulnerability?

Couples often battle over this issue in the "action–reaction conflict." You blame your partner for a particular action that triggered upset, but your partner suggests that it was your reaction, not his or her action, that was the problem. For example, you charge your partner with being "too critical," and he replies that you are "hypersensitive." Or your partner accuses you of not being affectionate, and you reply that she is "too insecure." When one of you charges the other with being impolite, the accused replies that the accuser is "too uptight."

Who is right?

Both are. For an interpersonal problem to occur, one partner must do something or not do something that has the potential to sting. But the other must have some exposed skin tender enough to respond. Without a provocative action (or inaction), there would be no problem. However, even if there were a dastardly act, if there were no tender, exposed skin, it could be sloughed off and no problem would occur.

For June to be critical of Ward, she must make a statement that could be interpreted as critical. She might say something obviously critical, in an angry tone, such as "You don't do your share of work at home." Or she might say something more innocent, such as "I've got to clean up the mess the boys made," which carries the implication that Ward should have cleaned up after them. But her statement by itself, even the obviously critical statement, is not sufficient for Ward to feel criticized. He could respond to her statement about not helping out at home as if June were upset and simply "blowing off steam." Ward might experience her comment as "She is not primarily attacking me but simply expressing her frustration." Or Ward might agree that he does in fact not help out enough at home and that she is merely stating, albeit harshly, what they both know to be true. "She is simply pointing out a characteristic of mine," Ward says to himself, "that I don't spend enough time doing household chores and leave them to June. And she is really frustrated by it now." He might even openly agree with her and validate her view of him. If Ward responded in any of these ways, we might say that criticism didn't even occur between them. Or, at the very least, the critical comment did not create an interpersonal problem.

If, however, Ward was sensitive about approval from June or was sensitive about how much he helps out at home, he would respond very differently. He might defend himself by listing all the things that he does at home or by describing all of his other responsibilities. He might counterattack her for what she doesn't do at home. Even if June made the more innocent comment that "I've got to clean up the mess the boys made," Ward could respond with defensiveness and counterattack. If Ward responded in these ways, we would know that criticism had occurred. And that an interpersonal problem had been created.

Who is responsible for this conflict between Ward and June? Clearly, both are. Ward's sensitivity to criticism combined with June's critical comment create their struggle. And so it is with most conflicts: they start from a volatile combination of a provocative behavior and an exposed vulnerability.

But just because partners share responsibility for an interpersonal conflict does not necessarily mean that they share this responsibility equally. Mutual responsibility does not necessarily imply equal responsibility. A problem may result more from the husband's criticism than from the wife's hypersensitivity. If the husband's friends, family, and coworkers all experience him as critical, but none of the wife's friends, family, and coworkers experience her as hypersensitive, we could confidently place more of the responsibility on the husband.

Spouses cannot easily obtain information about how most other people respond to their mates. Even if they could obtain this information, it would never be as clear-cut as in the preceding example. Even people who are critical in many of their relationships show considerable variability. With some people, they criticize a lot; with others, they criticize very little. Some people handle their criticism well, and it does not create problems; other people handle it poorly, and it creates serious problems. Therefore, to accept that both are responsible for a problem, but to argue over who is more responsible, is to quibble over a fruitless question that is virtually impossible to answer.

RECAP

Our sensitivities are often the powder keg for conflict. Dramatic incidents of neglect, when our partners are not there when we need them, or stunning examples of provocation, where our partners do something that embarrasses, humiliates, or betrays us, will certainly create conflict. But the more common, everyday instances of neglect and provocation, many of which are suppressed or ignored, can eventually cause conflict as well. The power of these events lies not just in the actions or inactions of our partners but in our own sensitivities to these events. We may have vulnerabilities developed through our past experience that, like psychological allergies, make us especially reactive to possible threats of abandonment or entrapment, lack of recognition or approval, or loss of control. We argue over incompatibilities that get their power from the vulnerabilities in each of us. If our sensitivities collide with those of our partner, the pain and consequent struggle may be even greater. We want to be handled with care in our special areas of vulnerabilities. However, because we are only dimly aware of them or feel embarrassed by them, we are not open about our sensitivities. When they are activated, the visible emotion we express may camouflage a hidden emotion that we don't express, so as to protect ourselves or our partners.

Exercise: Surface and Hidden Emotions

The first step out of the trap that surface and hidden emotions can create is to identify our own emotions, our own sensitivities, and the history that may have shaped them. It can also be helpful to think about your partner's emotions. In the exercise below, you will be asked to identify the surface and hidden emotions that you experience when your core conflict occurs as well as those your partner may experience. Then you will be asked to write about why this core conflict is a sensitive issue for you by referring to past experiences that have shaped you. This process will get you started on the first E phase (the Emotional Sensitivity related to your core issue) of a DEEP understanding of this issue.

Think about the core conflict you identified. What are the surface emotions that you usually reveal? What are the surface emotions that your partner usually reveals? Below is a list of common emotions to help in your selection. Although any emotion can be revealed or hidden, the emotions on the left are the most common surface emotions, while the ones on the right are the most common hidden emotions.

Angry
Angry
Offended
Frustrated
Pissed off
Irritated
Mad
Resentful

Disrespected
Disrespected
Insulted
Mocked
Brushed off
Inferior
Insignificant
Mistrusted

Defensive
Defensive
Untrusting
Guarded
Possessive
Closed off

Controlled
Controlled
Bossed
Lectured to
Powerless
Restricted
Claustrophobic

Jealous/Envious
Jealous
Envious
Misled

Lonely
Lonely
Isolated
Estranged
Empty

Afraid
Afraid
Cautious
Intimidated
Anxious
Overwhelmed
Worried

Guilty
Guilty
Embarrassed
Regretful
Sorry
Shameful

Sad
Sad
Disappointed
Hurt
Dejected
Humiliated
Depressed

Neglected
Neglected
Rejected
Uncared for
Unloved
Cast aside
Passed over

When we are struggling with the core issue that I have identified, the surface emotion I tend to show is _____; the surface emotion my partner tends to show is _____. (If you or your partner usually doesn't show any emotion, just write "little or no emotion").

Now consider the hidden emotions that you experience. Use the lists above to help with your selection. When we are struggling with the core issue that I have identified, what I'm typically feeling underneath is _____.

Although you cannot know for sure what your partner is feeling underneath, why don't you take a guess? When we are struggling with the core issue that I have identified, my guess is that the emotion my partner is typically feeling underneath is _____.

Now consider the core conflict you have identified and the surface and hidden emotions you experience. What past experiences have made this issue a big deal for you? Try to remember one or more experiences in your family of origin, your adolescence, or other romantic relationships as well as any important experiences in your current relationship. Here is an example: I am sensitive about being consulted about decisions because my parents tended to make all the decisions for me, even as an adult. I often felt that I didn't have much input into important decisions about me, like where I was going to go to college. In my current relationship, my partner sometimes tries to surprise me with gifts or trips, but then I feel that I don't have much input into them.

Some past experiences that have made the core conflict I identified an important and sensitive issue for me are:

_____

_____

_____

_____

_____

Putting It Together

We have now identified two pieces of the puzzle of your core conflict: Differences and Emotional sensitivities. It is important to note that although these are separate pieces of the puzzle, they influence each other. If there were no relevant emotional sensitivities, then the difference would be more manageable. If there were no relevant differences, then the emotional sensitivities would not be so problematic. The fact that the two coexist makes your core issue so difficult.

Up to now, we have focused on factors *within* you and your partner. Your separate genetic endowments and your unique social histories have created the two of you, complete with the differences and emotional sensitivities that are now part of you. Next we turn to the environment in which the two of you function to see how it can influence your core issue in ways both good and bad.

CHAPTER 5

"Can't You See I'm Stressed Out?"

RELATIONSHIP PROBLEMS
AS EXTERNAL CIRCUMSTANCES

> Man is a creature of circumstance.
> —GILBERT SELDES, CITED IN B. F. SKINNER,
> *Beyond Freedom and Dignity* (1971)

> The circumstances of others seem good to us, while
> ours seem good to others.
> —PUBLILIUS SYRUS

I (A. C.) once heard a social psychologist give a broad and succinct summary of two major findings in the field by saying that (1) situations influence people's behavior and (2) people are not aware of this fact. Study after study has shown that circumstances dramatically affect people's behavior, yet people often explain others' behavior with reference to their personalities alone.

Psychologist Stanley Milgram provided perhaps the most dramatic example of how situations can influence behavior. In the context of a study purportedly designed to explore the effects of punishment on learning, participants were asked to monitor the performance of another participant in a different room and to press a switch to give the participant an electric shock whenever he or she made a mistake. In reality the other "participant" was a confederate of the experimenter and was never actually shocked; his or her reactions were staged. The actual participants found themselves in a situation in which a scientific experimenter was encouraging them to apply increasingly high and apparently dangerous levels of electric shock to, they

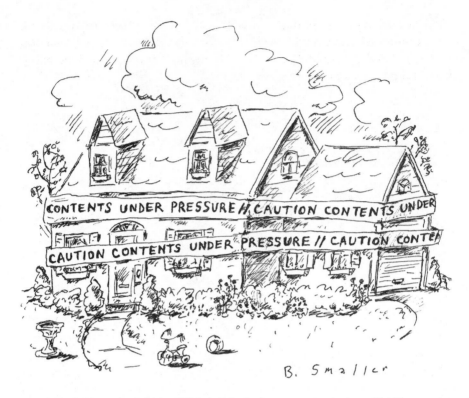

believed, a fellow human being. Despite hearing screams of pain from the next room, which they thought were cries from the participant in reaction to the shocks, the great majority of these generally upstanding Americans showed considerable emotional distress but nonetheless complied with the experimenter's directives. Even though they were not people who normally hurt others, they neither refused to give the shocks nor asked that the study be terminated. They engaged in seemingly dangerous and aggressive behavior in response to the situation in which they found themselves.

Fortunately, most of us will not find ourselves in a situation where we are encouraged to engage in hurtful treatment of others. In fact, even a study such as the one just described could probably not be done today because of the emotional stress to participants. But even though we may be spared such a situation, we will be influenced by our circumstances more profoundly than we may believe. Whatever our genetic endowment or historical background, our present circumstances will also powerfully affect our behavior. These present circumstances may minimize or exacerbate personal differences with our partners and sensitivities to our partners, differences and sensitivities that initially resulted from our genetic backgrounds and personal histories.

External Circumstances and Differences

Sometimes our current circumstances work in our favor, minimizing the differences we have with our partners. Consider Dawn and Felicia, for example. Dawn is more of a loner than Felicia. She came from a small family, feels uncomfortable in crowds, and prefers either solitary activities such as reading and playing computer games or doing things just with Felicia. On the other hand, Felicia comes from a large family, feels comfortable in a group, and enjoys loud parties and team sports. When they finished graduate school and both found a job in Felicia's hometown, these differences became less of a problem because Felicia could meet some of her social needs through the large network of family and friends in her hometown without either pressuring or threatening Dawn.

Unfortunately, present circumstances may create or exacerbate rather than alleviate personal differences. Consider the stereotypical situation of the traditional breadwinner husband and the mother/housewife at the end of a working day. He often comes home overstimulated from a day of dealing with people and their problems and wants nothing more than to collapse in front of the television. She is exhausted from a day of housework and handling their children but has had little adult social contact. She wants to talk with her husband and go over the problems of the day that she has been unable to share with anyone. Whatever their general personal inclinations to talk over issues at the end of the day, their separate circumstances create different needs for adult conversation.

Daily circumstances can affect not only how *much* we want to talk to our partners but also *how* we talk to our partners. If the breadwinner husband doesn't spend much time with his children, he may not be sympathetic to his wife's difficulties with the children. No one can give advice on child rearing like those who don't have children, and he may almost fall into that category. He may dismiss her problems with them with facile advice about being firm and consistent with them. But let him spend a day with the kids and see how he does! Similarly, because she is not employed outside the home, the mother/housewife may be unsympathetic to her husband's work difficulties. She may express frustration that he won't put some reasonable limits on his boss's demands. Why does he always complain about his boss? Why can't he stand up to him? If only she could spend a day with his boss! Our different daily circumstances may deprive us of our ability to understand and empathize with our partners' worlds, and consequently we don't take their difficulties seriously.

By "present circumstances" we mean much more than simply the daily events in each person's life away from the other. We mean their current position, abilities, and status as well. Roland believes that signing a prenuptial agreement would be a statement of lack of trust between him and Marianne. He urges that they "believe in their love for each other" and go into the marriage without financial preconditions and stipulations. Marianne believes that a prenuptial agreement is a realistic precaution to take in the face of today's high separation and divorce rates. She argues that "love is not incompatible with realism." While there may be personal differences in the level of Marianne's and Roland's romanticism and realism, their different financial situations also led them to their different positions. Marianne comes to the relationship with significantly more assets than Roland and would thus stand to lose more if they eventually divorced. Roland can literally "afford" to be more romantic than Marianne.

Status and ability may affect not only a spouse's reactions to entering a relationship but also his or her behavior in that relationship. Juan and Angela have very different reactions to thoughts and discussion of possible separation and divorce. Juan finds those thoughts and discussions a realistic exercise, given the conflicts the two of them are having. He loves Angela and doesn't really want a divorce, but finds the idea of staying in a loveless and conflictual relationship for the rest of his life unbearable. Angela, on the other hand, finds the discussion of possible separation and divorce threatening. For her, bringing up the topic implies a lack of love and commitment. She asks, "Why are we even discussing this just 2 years into our marriage?" Although there may be many factors that account for these different reactions, their current ability to attract others is one of them. Juan is a gregarious guy who loved the world of dating and found it very easy to meet others. If he and Angela did divorce, he would find alternative relationships quickly. In contrast, Angela is painfully shy and found the whole world of dating quite unpleasant. She could not easily replace Juan. There is nothing comforting to her about the idea of divorce.

Because we are two different people, we come from different situations and place ourselves in different situations than our partners. These situations can minimize our differences and increase our compatibility or further accentuate our differences or even create new differences. What is certain, though, is that neither we nor our partners will remain static.

External Circumstances and Emotional Sensitivities

External circumstances affect not only differences between partners but each of their sensitivities as well. Consider, for example, a sensitivity about trust and fidelity. Having a partner who works from home might minimize the fear that he or she will find a more attractive other or stray from the relationship. In contrast, having a partner who travels extensively in work or who has contact with many attractive singles could exacerbate that distrust. External circumstances can sometimes allay sensitivities so they don't impinge on the relationship. Partners who have a strong need for recognition but find great success in their career may be less demanding of recognition from their mates. However, if they experience failure or lack of recognition in their careers, they may be particularly needy of that from their partners.

External circumstances can not only exacerbate emotional sensitivities but at times create them. Having a partner who is not committed to the relationship or one whose love is inconsistent may, over time, create a fear of separation or doubt about your ability to hold on to a partner even if you were not scarred by your history. Having a partner who is unfaithful naturally leads to distrust, a distrust that might grow exponentially as incidences of unfaithfulness occur.

Now here is the complication—sometimes it works the other way. Existing vulnerabilities can sometimes *create* circumstances that trigger that very vulnerability. Consider, for example, a sensitivity about rejection. Having such a sensitivity would lead you to react strongly to slight signs of rejection, such as a partner who at times is not affectionate or who is preoccupied. You get upset or angry when your partner is not responsive to you. Yet those strong reactions will likely create or intensify doubt in your partner as to whether he or she wants to continue being with you. As a result of this doubt, your partner may then show less commitment or clear rejection, which in turn retriggers your vulnerability. So the process works like a feedback loop: minor rejection by one may stimulate a vulnerability and strong reaction in the other, which in turn may cause greater rejection and lack of commitment, which in turn triggers greater vulnerability and stronger reactions.

Consider an example. After the early stages of their relationship, when Dylan pursued Shawna intensely, Shawna was usually the more involved and committed one in the relationship. She was the one to press for marriage with a reluctant Dylan. Now, 2 years into their marriage, Dylan is voicing greater doubts about their relationship. He misses the freedom of the single life. He is attracted to many other women. He is frustrated by the daily grind of their relationship. His vocal doubts and his wandering eye create anxiety in Shawna, even panic at times. She loves Dylan and has come to depend on him, but she has always felt some insecurity with him. In her anxiety, she pushes Dylan for reassurance; she becomes clingy at times, and at other times she attacks him for his immature desire for the single life at 35. Unfortunately, Shawna's behavior only strengthens Dylan's feeling of being trapped in the relationship. Dylan loves Shawna and reluctantly gives her reassurances, but they feel phony to him—and to her. He tolerates her clinginess at times, but it feels uncomfortable to him. He hates her criticism, although he fears it may in part be accurate. All of her reactions combine to make him even more doubtful about the relationship, and his growing doubts, in turn, create greater anxiety in her.

The Worst Kind of External Circumstances: Stressful Circumstances

> Pressure and stress is the common cold of the psyche.
> —ANDREW DENTON

> Stress is the trash of modern life—we all generate it, but if you don't dispose of it properly, it will pile up and overtake your life.
> —DANZAE PACE

> The time to relax is when you don't have time for it.
> —AUTHOR UNKNOWN

We often talk about our lives being "full of stress" or of being "stressed out." It is important to distinguish between stressful circumstances (or stressors) and stressful reactions. Stressful circumstances are events outside of us such as job or school demands, legal problems, debt, conflict with family or friends, even traffic and noise. We normally think of stressful circumstances as being negative events, but they can also be positive events. A promotion may lead to more money and prestige in the company but entail much more responsibility and thus more stress. Stressful reactions are the way we respond to those circumstances, both physically and psychologically. We respond physically to stressful circumstances with greater arousal, such as higher heart rate, blood pressure, and perspiration. This arousal provides us with the necessary energy for the well-known "flight-or-fight" reaction. We respond psychologically to stressful circumstances with quicker reactions, snap judgments, and heightened emotions. For example, if our partners ask us for help when we are in circumstances that are low stress, such as on vacation, we may show no rise in heart rate or blood pressure and respond graciously and generously. However, if our partners ask for the same help when we are in stressful circumstances, like finishing a report that has a looming deadline, we may experience an increase in heart rate and blood pressure, may make the snap judgment that our partners are being inconsiderate, may respond irritably or angrily, and may summarily reject the request.

Psychologists typically divide stress into two major categories: major life stressors and daily stressors. *Major life stressors* include important transitions that happen to most of us: for example, having a child, moving, getting a new job, retiring, or suffering the death of a parent. Major life stressors also arise from unexpected negative events, such as an illness, accident, disability, business failure, and financial loss. *Daily stressors* are chronic conditions we have to deal with, such as a difficult child, a contentious boss, noisy neighbors, limited financial resources, or a long commute.

Both kinds of stress typically train our attention on the stressor and how to cope with it. If we are faced with an imminent business failure, we go over and over in our minds what went wrong, what we are going to do next, and how we will make ends meet financially. If we have a difficult child, we may struggle with our mixed feelings of love and anger toward the child, we may think about how to handle him or her, and we may wonder about what the future will bring. This narrowness of attention means that we neglect other aspects of our world. We may ignore our partners or be unresponsive to another child's needs. The stressor has commanded most of our psychological resources, so we have less to give to anything else, even our partners.

Stressful events may activate well-learned patterns of coping. If we have learned to cope with stressors socially, we may want to share our problem with others, to elicit reassurance and support from them, and to feel that we are not alone in this. If we have learned to cope independently, we may pull back from others and become totally preoccupied with our own thoughts as we try to work it through. In this case, social contact is a burden, not a relief. If we have learned to cope with anxiety by exerting greater efforts to order and control our life, we may map out plans, make lists of things to do, and organize the papers on our desk.

The extent of our stressful reaction depends on how we perceive the stressful situation. If we see the situation as one in which we have little control and that is likely to have negative consequences for us, then we are likely to feel stressed. However, if we perceive the same situation as one in which we have considerable control over the possible consequences, then we are likely to experience limited stress. For example, students facing a final exam in a course required for their major but in which they have not done well and do not understand the material are likely to experience strong stressful reactions. They have little control over an outcome that has consequence for them. In contrast, students facing the same exam who have done well on previous exams and who understand the materials well are likely to feel limited stress.

The extent to which we experience a stressful reaction has an interesting, surprising, and nonobvious impact on our behavior in relationships. Of course, when we experience low levels of stress, there is little impact on our relationships. At moderate levels of stress, such as a frustrating day at work, we may feel irritable and impatient with our partners but may not be clear why and may not be able to adjust our relationship behavior well. We may be irritable with our partners without any explanation of the source of that irritation, leading them to wonder what they did wrong or what is wrong with us. In contrast, at high levels of stressful circumstances, such as a minor automobile accident or losing an important document, we may be clear about the source of distress and communicate that clearly to our partners. This knowledge about the source of distress and clear message to the partner—I am upset about the car accident—can often protect the relationship from that stress. Partners know they are not the stressor and can often be a source of comfort or assistance in ameliorating that stressor. Finally, at severe levels of stress, like losing a job, we may know what the stressor is and know it is not our partner but be so upset by the stressor that we cannot compartmentalize our reactions or protect our relationship from its effects.

Stress and Differences

When stress is low and we are comfortable, confident, and relaxed, we can more easily tolerate the differences that exist between us and our partners and, as needed, accommodate those differences. Relaxed and comfortable introverts are more understanding of their extroverted partners' need to socialize and might be more willing to accompany them than were these introverts experiencing stress themselves. Similarly, savers are more tolerant of their spender partners when they are relaxed and comfortable. When stressed, we are more attentive to our own concerns and less attentive to our partners' concerns. This narrowing of attention, plus the impatience and irritability that often come with it, may complicate any attempt to work out the differences or reach acceptable compromises.

Stress not only makes differences more difficult to manage but can also intensify differences through deprivation. Money problems will make savers even less accommodating and understanding of their spender partners than they usually are. A decline in the stock market or an expensive repair that depletes the bank account deprives them of the financial buffer they need to feel comfortable. Similarly, stressful workdays that involve overwhelming social contact usually make introverts need more time alone than they ordinarily require. The overdose of difficult social contact is remedied for them only by an extra dose of time alone.

Perhaps the biggest impact of stress on the differences we have with our partners is on how we deal with stress. Those who deal with stress by talking it out with a trusted other will need that outlet even more as their stress increases. In contrast, those who respond to stress by withdrawing from social contact to lick their wounds and consider their options may withdraw even more with greater stress. One can easily imagine a talker and a withdrawer in a relationship facing a joint stress and dealing with that stress in very different ways that intensify their differences. Talkers want to share their concerns with their intimate partners, intensifying the withdrawer's need for time alone. Withdrawers want to withdraw to get their needed recovery and perspective, leaving their talkative partners with an even more intense need to share their thoughts and feelings with someone.

Sometimes stress leads us to seek solace in activities that themselves are part of important differences we have with our partners. The saver might find solace in examining the stock funds and bank accounts even when experiencing stress unrelated to finances. A highly organized person may find it soothing to organize the household when some stress, such as job stress, makes her feel out of control. If the saver and the organized one are in relationships with a spender and a messy one, respectively, then their efforts while under stress could intensify differences unrelated to the stress.

Stress and Emotional Sensitivities

Stress can not only exacerbate differences but also expose emotional sensitivities. When things are under control and we feel comfortable, our sensitivities often lie dormant. Even though we may be vulnerable to feelings of abandonment, in good times we can encourage our partners in their separate pursuits. Even though we may be vulnerable to feelings of entrapment, we can enjoy intimacy and commitment. Even though we may often want to be in charge, we can be loose and casual.

Stressors may affect our emotional sensitivities in two ways. First, a stressor may directly hit our vulnerability, like an arrow into Achilles' heel. If Donna is sensitive to feelings of abandonment and rejection, an incident at work in which a coworker snubs her may be especially difficult for her. It raises her general fear that she is not likable. If Michael is sensitive to issues of control and has a boss who breathes down his neck and gives him little independence, he may react strongly because he feels like he has no power of his own. These events for Donna and Michael, although occurring in their work places, may carry over into their respective relationships. Donna may be especially needy of support from her partner or reactive if he shows any sign of rejecting her. Similarly, Michael may attempt to exert a power over his home life that he doesn't feel in his work life. Of course, a stressor will create greater relationship distress when it occurs within that relationship. If Donna's partner voices doubts about their relationship or Michael's partner takes control of something that he wants to be in charge of, the reactions by both will create greater disruption in their relationships than similar stressors at work.

Second, a stressor may affect our sensitivity indirectly. It doesn't hit us in our soft spot, but by hitting us at all it weakens us and makes us cope in ways associated with our vulnerability. For example, even when Donna has a stressor that has nothing to do with interpersonal rejection, such as the stress of an oncoming deadline, her needs for interpersonal support may increase. She may need increased love from her husband not because her own sensitivity to rejection has been challenged but because she can cope better with any challenge if she gets support from those close to her. Similarly, any anxiety that Michael faces, whether it involves control or not, may increase his own efforts to exert control. An upcoming deadline may make him organize and schedule because he then reduces his own anxiety about the deadline.

Thus, stressful events, particularly those that hit us in a soft spot, increase our needs even as they make us less able to accommodate the needs of those around us. This double-barreled effect may be manageable if only one of us is under stress. When we both are under stress, conflict may be inevitable. Rather than living up to Hemingway's ideal of "grace under pressure," we may grate under pressure. And the grating may be with our partners, who love us most and who could support us most—if they weren't also so stressed.

RECAP

Although what we and our partners bring to a conflict is highly influential, the external circumstances in which we find ourselves also influence this conflict, for good and for bad. Sometimes external circumstances may serve to reduce the differences between the two of us or to cushion the emotional sensitivities of one or the other. However, sometimes circumstances do just the opposite, accentuating our differences or exposing our emotional sensitivities. The worst kind of external circumstances are stressful circumstances, which can narrow our attention on our own concerns, eclipsing our attention to our partner's concerns. These stressful circumstances may accentuate our differences and heighten our emotional sensitivities, especially when our normal response to stress is different.

Exercise: What Role Does Stress Play?

This exercise will help you achieve a better understanding of the role stress is playing in your life. Below you will be asked to complete a measure of your stress, adapted from a longer questionnaire developed by Sheldon Cohen, Tom Kamarck, and Robin Mermelstein, which you can then score and interpret based on the information we provide. Then you will be asked to think carefully about the specific stresses you and your partner are under and how those stresses impact your differences and emotions. This process will enable you to complete the second E phase (the External stressors related to your core issue) of a DEEP understanding of this issue.

Perceived Stress Scale

The questions in this scale ask you about your feelings and thoughts during the last month. In each case, indicate by circling how often you felt or thought a certain way.

	Never	Sometimes	Very often
1. In the last month, how often have you felt that you were *unable* to control the important things in your life?	0 1	2 3	4

	Never		Sometimes		Very often
2. In the last month, how often have you felt confident about your ability to handle your personal problems?	4	3	2	1	0
3. In the last month, how often have you felt that things were going your way?	4	3	2	1	0
4. In the last month, how often have you felt difficulties were piling up so high that you could not overcome them?	0	1	2	3	4

SCORING AND INTERPRETING THE PERCEIVED STRESS SCALE

To determine your total score, simply add up your scores on all four items. Then read below for the interpretation of your score.

Scores of 0–3

You told us that, overall, you feel pretty confident and able to handle stress in your life and you feel in control of stressful situations. That's good news because it suggests that you might not have to buffer your relationship from your stress very often. However, that of course doesn't mean that you don't get stressed out in particular circumstances, and in those times you'll need to consider the issues discussed in this chapter.

Scores of 4–8

Your results show that you feel you are able to handle stressful situations and control important things in your life most of the time. However, there seem to be certain times in your life when things start to feel out of control, as if you might not be able to handle them. While it's great that it doesn't happen all or even most of the time, when you are feeling stressed out, it can have a big impact on you and your relationship, as you learned in this chapter.

Scores of 9–16

Your score indicates that you are dealing with a significant amount of stress in your life. Therefore, the material in this chapter is going to be especially important for you. As you work to strengthen your relationship it will be important to keep in mind the role stress might be playing. Later we will talk about how to protect your relationship from the impact of stress.

IDENTIFYING SPECIFIC STRESSORS

You have looked at your overall level of stress. Now let's consider the specific stressors that most often affect the core conflict you have identified. Which of the common stressors below is most likely to heighten difficulties around your core conflict? Which is most likely to heighten difficulties around your core conflict for your partner? Choose up to three from each column. Then pick the most important stressor from each column.

Stressors that affect the core conflict for me

_____ Job/school

_____ Children

_____ Extended family

_____ Health

_____ Friends

_____ Legal problems

_____ Life transition (e.g., move)

_____ Finances

_____ Other

Stressors that affect the core conflict for my partner

_____ Job/school

_____ Children

_____ Extended family

_____ Health

_____ Friends

_____ Legal problems

_____ Life transition (e.g., move)

_____ Finances

_____ Other

IMPACT ON DIFFERENCES AND EMOTIONS

Now that you've identified the top stressors for you and your partner, take a moment to think about how stress affects how you deal with differences and emotions. For example, does stress make your differences more pronounced? Do you have differences in how the two of you respond to stress? Also, do the stressors you identified above impact your emotional sensitivities directly, or does the stress just make it more difficult to deal with those sensitivities?

_____

_____

_____

_____

Putting It Together

You have looked at your overall level of stress as well as at the specific stressors that affect you and that affect your partner and that separately or together may heighten your struggle over your core issue. At this point, you have a pretty good idea of the first three aspects of your DEEP analysis of your core conflict: how D (Differences), E (Emotions), and E (External stressors) affect the problem. It is important to see how each part affects the other two. Stress may exacerbate differences and emotional sensitivities; emotional sensitivities can make differences and stress harder to handle; differences can make emotional sensitivities and stress more difficult to manage. One important remaining piece is the P—the Patterns of communication that you get into when you try to resolve your core struggle.

CHAPTER 6

A Cure Worse Than the Disease

RELATIONSHIP PROBLEMS AS PATTERNS OF COMMUNICATION

> Bad solutions don't merely fail; they create an even bigger problem.

All that Anika had wanted from Ralph was a sympathetic ear. All that Ralph had wanted was to finish installing his new computer software before getting involved in a conversation. But when the two parted that night, they were both so hurt and angry they couldn't even look at each other, much less talk.

The couple started out alone together in their living room. Anika was fidgeting on the couch, worrying about a problem she was having with her boss, while Ralph was hunched over his laptop in a chair across from her. After a couple of attempts to get his attention—deep sighs, queries like "So what's going on with your computer?," and vague comments like "What a day . . . "—met with no response, Anika stopped thinking about work and started fuming about how unresponsive her husband was. Her choice, she figured, was to get mad and walk out right now or try to explain to him why she was so upset. She chose the latter: "Ralph, if you could just look up at me for *one second,* I really need to talk to you."

Ralph looked up with a grimace and heaved a big sigh of his own. From years of experience with this "dance," he knew this was the beginning of a harangue about his lack of sensitivity. Why couldn't she just see that he was preoccupied and frustrated and would be much more open to whatever she wanted to discuss once his mind was free of this computer problem? As Anika tried to explain what upset her about him, he tried to break in and explain to Anika that she gets upset too easily and should relax and learn to "go with the flow." "You always patronize me!" Anika snapped back. "Why are you always so insensitive?" Ralph's protest that he wasn't insensitive opened the floodgates to Anika's list of examples from their history together: the time his mother was upset with him for how he had mishandled his father's terminal illness, the time he left her to deal with euthanizing their dog alone because he was at work, the time he had tried to make a joke out of his having forgotten their 10th anniversary. . . . Ralph countered with evidence of her "gross overreactions," such as the incident just yesterday when she had yelled at the kids over nothing. In response, she claimed that living with Ralph was like living in an emotional desert. He countered that maybe she should find someone else and then stormed out of the room.

Clearly, both partners had a hand in this conflict. Just as clearly, their efforts at dealing with the initial problem of Ralph's inattention to Anika created an even bigger problem. In fact, in the turmoil that was generated during this argument, they temporarily forgot the initial problem.

A slogan of the 1960s, popularized by a speech by Eldridge Cleaver, charged "If you are not part of the solution, you are part of the problem." In relationships, it is somewhat different. In an attempt to be part of the solution, you can sometimes end up not only being part of the problem but making that problem worse.

Throughout Parts I and II of this book we have seen couples encounter problems, make efforts to cope with these problems, and then face reactive problems—difficulties created in the process of trying to solve the initial problem. In the preceding example, the initial problem was a difference in desire for conversation or connection, triggered in part by Ralph's focus on his new software and Anika's desire to talk about a work problem, all of which led to hurt and angry feelings. Perhaps the initial problem was emotionally fueled by Anika's vulnerability about being abandoned or neglected and Ralph's sensitivity to criticism. Anika's stress over problems at work that day created a sense of urgency in her, while Ralph's excitement about his new software contributed to his distraction.

In response to the initial problem, the couple made efforts to solve the difficulty. Anika tried to solve the problem by sharing her feelings with Ralph and later by presenting evidence of his "insensitivity"; Ralph tried to solve the problem by pointing out to Anika that her emotions are too intense and later by presenting examples of her overreactivity. These efforts at coping were not only unsuccessful but created a reactive problem as well, a subsequent problem that was bigger than the initial one. Now they must cope with the hurt and anger that each feels as a consequence of the other's attacks—Anika's sense that Ralph really doesn't care about her feelings and Ralph's sense that Anika will hurl unjustified accusations at him at the slightest provocation. Moreover, there is now a breach in their relationship that this argument created—Ralph's vague suggestions that maybe Anika "should find someone else."

Why does this happen? Often we're so caught up in the heat of the moment that our arguments feel like they happen *to* us rather than being something we actively participate in. To better understand the anatomy of an argument, let's break it into its three main components: the content of the initial problem, the process of how we deal with that initial problem, and the reactive problem created by our failed attempts to solve the initial problem.

The Initial Problem: The Content of Conflict

As we've already discussed, our differences (or similarities) and emotional sensitivities are like flammable material. If kept in a cool, dark place in separate containers, they create no problems. But if those differences and emotional sensitivities meet in a provocative incident, particularly when exposed to the heat or friction of stressful events, they ignite. With Ralph and Anika, the combination of his new software and her problems at work, as well as the fact that they were both tired from a long day at work, triggered the combustion. The immediate consequence when sensitivities and incompatibilities are triggered is negative feelings such as hurt, disappointment, and anger. Anika was first hurt and disappointed that Ralph was inattentive to her—these were her hidden feelings. What she expressed to him, however, was the surface feeling: anger.

The initial problem that a couple faces—a triggering event or circumstance, the activated difference and emotional sensitivity, and the immediate reactions of each—provides the *content* of their interaction. The initial problem is what each thinks about during conflict, what the two discuss during argument. These initial problems set the early agenda for conflict discussions.

Typically, couples focus on the triggering situation rather than the broad differences between them or the emotional sensitivities within each partner. For example, even though Gary favors a relaxed, take-it-easy lifestyle while Jana is ambitious and wants to get ahead financially, they rarely if ever discuss this broad difference between them. Instead, they are much more likely to discuss disturbing incidents that reflect this incompatibility. They may disagree about whether to take an expensive vacation, which Gary prefers, or to do something more economical and save their money, which

Jana prefers. A conflict may get started when Jana gets up early on a Saturday morning to get a head start on what she wants to accomplish rather than spending the morning lazing around in bed with Gary. Gary's comment that his sales record this year is going to be lower than last year's may precipitate an argument about how much effort he is putting into work. In each of these three instances, Gary and Jana are discussing a *triggering event*, which is a manifestation of their somewhat incompatible approaches to life.

We care deeply about the content of our conflicts. We are invested in having sex tonight, in not going to the in-laws' house this weekend, and in getting more attention from our partners. We want the freedom to take the weekend off for a hike with a friend or the power to buy the new sofa for the living room. We care because the content of the conflict represents the problem we face: a partner who differs from us on an important matter, who mishandles our emotional sensitivities, and who is not responsive to our stressful circumstances.

Attempts to Solve or Cope with the Initial Problem: The Process of Conflict

Any particular initial problem can be coped with in a variety of ways. Gary and Jana could debate their choices of vacation, with each presenting the advantages of his or her own point of view. They could bargain and negotiate their choices, such as by proposing that one choose the kind of vacation they take this year and the other choose it next year. In contrast, Jana or Gary could each make plans unilaterally and inform the other of what was done. Jana could criticize Gary for his irresponsibility in proposing to deplete their savings with one vacation. Gary could criticize Jana for her stinginess and inability to enjoy life. Gary could withdraw in anger until Jana supports his point of view. Combinations of these and other approaches are also possible. The point is that the *content of conflict*, provided by the initial problem, is distinct from the *process of conflict*, which is how couples cope with the initial problem.

Gayla and Josh disagree about housekeeping. Gayla feels comfortable only when her home is completely organized and spotless. Also, her self-esteem is tied up with the state of her home: if friends dropped by and her home was less than spotless or disorganized, she would be embarrassed. But Gayla believes in equality, and so she wants Josh to share in the housework. In contrast to Gayla, Josh finds clutter somewhat comforting. If he lived alone, his house would have to be positively unsanitary for him to feel embarrassed about it when others visited. Although he generally endorses the ideology of equality between men and women, he certainly doesn't want to do half of the housework if it means doing the housework to Gayla's high standards. Furthermore, he feels his work on the cars should count in the housework equation. All of these differences define the initial problem that Gayla and Josh have about housework.

Gayla and Josh could cope with this problem through different patterns of communication. They could negotiate detailed schedules of who has to do what when. They could tease each other about her compulsivity and his slovenliness. Or, in a more complicated scenario, Gayla could do most of the housework herself but experience a building resentment that eventually led to an emotional outburst that spurred Josh, already feeling guilty, into action. He would help a lot for a while but then drift back to doing little until Gayla took over completely and the pattern repeated itself. The important thing to note is that the process of Gayla's and Josh's conflict isn't an attempt to purposely punish each other; instead, it's a way to try to cope with the content of their initial problem.

We may recognize but ignore the process of conflict, or we may lack awareness of it. Fixated on our angry and hurt feelings, we don't attend to the way we cope with these problems. Given our problems, we can't imagine other ways of interacting. Carlos knows no other way to deal with his greater sexual appetite than to keep the pressure on Jan. If he doesn't push, he fears, they will have no sex life at all. Lori knows no other way to deal with Manny's lack of involvement with the kids than to criticize his lack of involvement and complain about being a "single mother." If she didn't complain, she fears, he would forget about his role as father entirely. And so the pattern continues.

We have seen how the content of conflict typically comes from the differences (or similarities) between partners and their emotional sensitivities, often as triggered by stressful circumstances. The process of conflict is how the couple attempts to solve this conflict through their interaction. Unfortunately, these "solutions" often make the problem worse. They are toxic cures that aggravate the illness. They are treatments that are worse than the disease. Their intent is to create change for the better; their result is to create change for the worse. Below we detail specific types of toxic cures.

ACCUSATION, BLAME, AND COERCION: MOVING AGAINST THE OTHER

The classic ABCs of heated argument are accusation, blame, and coercion. We hold our partners responsible for the initial problem, and we pressure them to change as a means of fixing the problem. We could also add a D to the ABCs, for defensiveness. If our partners charge us with any complicity in the problem, we defend ourselves (and then likely counterattack when we see an opening).

We may blame our partners for a particular action, perhaps something that triggered the initial problem. Or rather than accusing them of specific behaviors, we may charge them with broad, negative personality characteristics. We engage in the fault finding described in Chapter 2, analyzing our problems and concluding that they are caused by the moral weaknesses, mental problems, or personal inadequacies of our partners. We accuse our partners of being bad, we blame them for emotional instability, or we chastise them for incompetence. Of course, they may defend themselves and countercharge us.

Coercion goes beyond mere attack of our partners. In coercion, we force our partners to do what we want by barraging them with aversive behavior. We make demands, threaten, nag, criticize, complain, and induce guilt until our partners give in. Then we sometimes get what we want, and they get peace. When that happens, our coercive efforts are reinforced because our partners comply with our demands; our partners' compliance is reinforced because we cease our coercive actions. And so the pattern becomes entrenched.

Coercion has a seductive appeal because it produces such immediate responses. But like an addictive drug that requires increasing dosages to achieve the same effect, higher levels of coercion are required to get our partners' response. During the early stages of romance, slight indications of dissatisfaction may have drawn our partners' attention and prompted them to try to fix the situation. But over time our partners may habituate to our coercive attempts, they may deliberately ignore them, and they may even actively resist them. While an edge to the voice was all that was necessary early on in the relationship, now screams and yells may be required to get a reaction.

The immediate rewards of coercion are often dwarfed by the ultimate costs. Although our partners get peace by giving in, they may find our demands more and more onerous. They may become upset with themselves for being weak, for complying with our demands. They may become more and more angry and resistant when we push them.

Coercion breeds countercoercion and punishment. Our partners don't just respond to our coercive attempts; they initiate their own. And they punish our failures to satisfy their own needs. A vicious cycle of mutual coercion and punishment quickly develops. However successful these coercive and punitive efforts are in the short run, they erode the positive feelings and loving atmosphere in the relationship.

AVOIDANCE, DENIAL, AND WITHDRAWAL:
MOVING AWAY FROM THE OTHER

Avoidance is a time-honored method for dealing with problems. Look the other way. Get involved in something else. Problems are unpleasant, so don't face them; they will probably clear up on their own. Discussing them directly might make matters worse.

Avoidance works in the short term. What we choose to do when we avoid problems gives us more pleasure (and is easier) than facing problems. No matter what the program, watching television will provide more relaxation than discussing incompatibilities or trying to soothe emotional sensitivities. However, we often carry with us a nagging sense of discomfort about the problem when we avoid it.

We can achieve the benefits of avoidance and also weaken the nagging discomfort if we minimize, dismiss, or even deny the very existence of the problem. There is nothing really wrong. Everything is fine. Therefore, there is nothing to discuss. We can withdraw.

Avoidance, denial, and withdrawal may work in the long term as well as in the short term. Sometimes problems develop from some unique combination of circumstances; discussion might complicate or prolong a problem that will disappear with changing circumstances. Mary notices Lou's flirtation with another woman at her company picnic. She feels hurt by his actions but avoids discussion. Then she denies to herself that his actions were even inappropriate. He is just a solid all-American man, one who had a couple of drinks in him and a pretty woman in front of him. Since he doesn't repeat his behavior at future parties, Mary's (and Lou's) avoidance and denial are innocent enough. Discussion might have increased the tension between them, although it might also have led to greater understanding and appreciation between them.

Sometimes long-standing problems improve over time. Changing circumstances and individual growth diminish the problems that were once avoided and denied. Dave often resented Leo's attachment to his mother, but except for some occasional sarcasm and innuendo, neither brought up the matter for discussion. However, as they developed their individual careers and their own life together, Leo's attachment to his mother and Dave's resentment about it lessened. The avoided problem did improve on its own.

These examples are, however, the exception rather than the rule. Avoidance and denial are more likely to nourish problems than to stifle them—especially when those problems tap into important differences or emotional sensitivities. Changing circumstances are usually not so fortuitous or individual growth so benign as to erase chronic difficulties. More often, tension and resentment rise in both partners. Even though they may refuse to discuss a problem and deny that it exists, their emotions force a discussion of sorts. Indirectly, through their moods or through unrelated minor arguments, they communicate their dissatisfaction. However, without direct discussion, the partners may easily miscommunicate, get confused, and make the problem even worse.

Barbara feels unhappy about her sexual relationship with Sol. She sees him as a selfish lover, insensitive to her needs but vigorously pursuing his own. She doesn't discuss her dissatisfaction directly with Sol but withdraws from sexual interaction with him. She shows less interest in making love and is not responsive when she does. Sol feels distressed by her withdrawal and disinterest and wonders if she is "frigid," but he too avoids discussion. He reacts with more forceful initiations and more vigorous pursuit, which provides further evidence for Barbara that he is a selfish lover. She withdraws even more, which provides further evidence for Sol that she is frigid. Their avoidance of the problem makes it worse.

WATCHFULNESS, INTRUSION, AND INFRINGEMENT: HANGING ON TO THE OTHER

Rather than moving against our partners with accusation, blame, and coercion or moving away from our partners with avoidance, denial, and withdrawal, we may move toward our partners, but with concern and anxiety. If we fear they may leave us, we may watch them closely, intrude into their privacy, or infringe on their territory. Consider Jane and Nancy. Because of her physical beauty, Jane easily attracts other women's attentions and had many girlfriends prior to Nancy. Throughout their relationship, Nancy was more committed to the relationship and more interested in getting married. Knowing Jane's attractiveness to other women and sensing her lack of equivalent, reciprocal commitment to her, Nancy fears she might lose Jane. When she's out of town, she sometimes asks a friend to drive by their house late at night to make sure Jane is home and no strange cars are in the driveway. When she is not looking, Nancy sometimes checks Jane's cell phone to see who has called her and whom Jane has called. When they go out together, Nancy tries to stay away from bars or other public settings where women might look at Jane and be attracted to her. When Jane wants to spend an evening by herself or with friends, she questions Jane on the specific plan for the evening. Thus Nancy both shields Jane from exposure to other women and keeps her under surveillance in case she is tempted to contact other women.

When there has been a betrayal of trust in a relationship, such as when one partner has had an affair, watchfulness, intrusion, and infringement are often the results. The betrayed partner has understandably lost trust in the other and, to prevent another betrayal, may keep an anxious watch over that other. Because Ricardo had an affair on one of the many trips required by his job, Clara gets worried whenever he leaves again. She calls him often while he is away and questions him about his activities and plans. Ricardo protests that his one-night stand was meaningless and that he revealed it to Clara soon after. He tells her he feels interrogated while he is away but she wants to protect herself from another betrayal and does that through investigation of his actions while he is away.

Moving toward the other anxiously can be driven not just by betrayal or lack of commitment, but by emotional sensitivities. If Dyshona fears abandonment by those close to her, based on her own personal history, then she might engage in fearful watchfulness of Dan or infringe on Dan's privacy, even if he has never betrayed her and is fully committed to her. However, some of his own traits, such as his desire to spend time away from Dyshona with his friends or his desire to spend time alone, could activate her fears and thus her anxious movement toward him.

Keeping others under surveillance, intruding into their lives, and infringing on their territory can get some temporary satisfaction. You get immediate answers, and your fears may be temporarily assuaged. However, its long-term effects are often disappointing. There is an old proverb that says "Never trust a man who never had a chance to steal." If you limit others' freedoms out of your fears of what they might do, you never get to have the trust-building experience of seeing that they do return to you and that they don't betray you. Furthermore, your intrusions may backfire, creating the very thing they were intended to prevent. Anxious interrogation of partners may lead them to share less and less because the experience is so unpleasant and because they fear your reaction if they share even innocuous information. In extreme cases, the intrusiveness may reduce the partner's commitment or desire to stay in the relationship, thus triggering the abandonment that the intrusiveness was designed to prevent.

ALLIANCES AND COALITIONS: MOVING AGAINST THE OTHER WITH OUTSIDE HELP

Russ found it hard to talk to Shanna about any problems between them. Being uncomfortable with such discussions, he came on critically, and she then reacted coolly, showing no interest in pursuing the matter. Her attitude could be summed up in her favorite cliché: Let sleeping dogs lie. Since

Russ had always had a close relationship with his mother, he started telling her about his problems with Shanna. His mother made some discreet but pointed suggestions to Shanna, who initially responded with polite tolerance. Then, as the suggestions kept coming, Shanna became colder and colder toward her, finally telling her mother-in-law to keep her nose out of other people's business. Russ and Shanna began fighting about his mother, with Shanna criticizing her and Russ defending her. Russ and his mother preoccupied themselves with laments about Shanna's problems and inadequacies. Shanna felt ganged up on; Russ's mother felt rebuffed; and Russ felt caught between his wife and his mother. What had been an ordinary problem between Shanna and Russ became an entangled conflict among the three of them.

When we experience difficulties of any kind, but especially interpersonal difficulties, we seek the support and counsel of others. We want an ally to listen to our point of view, to validate our position, to support our efforts, and perhaps to give us advice. This universal tendency to seek personal cover in a storm can restore calm to our emotions, give reassurance to our shaken confidence, and provide direction and motivation for our efforts to deal with the difficulty. But this alliance in the face of adversity may become a coalition against the supposed cause of the adversity. The one experiencing difficulty may initially seek an alliance for individual support, but then he or she enlists the new ally in the struggle against the romantic partner.

Unfortunately, the alliance with the supporter often disturbs the alliance with the romantic partner. So, how do these understandable efforts to seek support from others go awry? First, others may fuel the fires of discord. They may encourage our tendencies to blame and punish our partners for difficulties that are caused mutually. If we voice desires to leave the relationship, they may encourage us in that pursuit. If later we make up with our partners, our allies may be confounded and question our wisdom. We recently cast our partners as villains and contemplated escape from them. Why have we changed so dramatically? Second, others may actively interfere in our relationships with our partners. However well-intentioned, they may take it upon themselves to assist us directly through words or actions delivered to our partners. Usually these efforts backfire: our partners get angry at us and our allies for "butting in." Third, others may provide substitute benefits that weaken our relationship. The husband who seeks reprieve from the troubles with his wife by having intimate conversations about his marital problems with another woman may find temporary solace and comfort. However, the intimate conversations with the other woman may lead to a closeness that excludes his wife. If his wife discovers this other relationship, she may be angered by the betrayal of their confidential marital problems and suspicious that something else is going on. Even if she never discovers his other relationship, the fact that another woman is meeting his needs weakens his relationship with his wife. Fourth, the involvement of others may create problems for these unsuspecting supporters. The most obvious and frequent example occurs when parents use children as allies in their marital difficulties. The alliance may put the children in a position of divided loyalty, which leads to anxiety and stress. The children may feel that they must "choose sides" in the conflict. They may feel that they have to see one parent as good and the other as bad. If parent–child alliances become too intense, the closeness may inhibit the children's development. Children need time with peers and emotional freedom from parents to develop attachments with their peers. If children spend most of their time with a parent or if they worry about a parent or their parents' marriage, they will not experience enough freedom to develop their own independence.

Our understandable and human efforts to reach out for family and friends in times of relationship struggle may relieve our stress and ease our difficulties. We may find temporary solace from our troubles and strength to renew our efforts at solving the problems. We may gain emotional release from the tension, new perspectives on the problems, and new ideas for solving them. However, if our family and friends directly interfere with our relationship, if they promote adversarial views of the problems, and if they offer a continual source of benefits and satisfactions that we should be receiving from our partners, these well-meaning supporters may make our relationship problems worse.

The Reactive Problem: A Worse Problem, an Additional Problem, a Relationship Rift

If at first you don't succeed, try, try, again.

We have been discussing the communication that occurs in a single conflict or argument. One incident by itself rarely constitutes a relationship problem. A single argument may be unpleasant, but it won't propel a couple onto the therapist's couch or send them to the relationship self-help section of their local bookstore. It's repetition that transforms arguments into relationship problems. We use the same toxic cures to try to solve the same problem—again and again. The repetition of toxic cures creates the reactive problem, which is usually much more troubling than the content of the original problem or the process of a single argument.

Repetition does not necessarily mean that we apply the same toxic cures in the same way. As we flounder around in the problem, we will enact many variations on the same "solution." We repeat the same dance but with different steps. Consider Valerie and Brad's jealousy problem. Brad tries to cope with his jealousy of Valerie in several different ways: sometimes he interrogates her closely about her actions ("So what were you and Bill discussing at the party?"), occasionally he barks out a demand ("I want to *meet* these so-called business partners before you have lunch with them"), or sometimes in the presence of others he hovers over her, trying to be a buffer between her and imagined suitors. These are his attempts to solve the problem of jealousy. For her part, Valerie often evades his accusing questions, tries to escape from his hovering presence, and occasionally in anger at Brad flaunts her attractiveness and provocatively seeks the attention of other men. However varied, his behavior reflects a hovering, heavy-handed, suspicious watchfulness, while her behavior varies between avoidance of Brad and his questions on the one hand and taunting, angry flirtatiousness on the other. Their attempted solutions to the problem of jealousy have created a vicious cycle of interaction that, far from solving the problem, sustains it.

If we realize, even dimly, that we are in a vicious cycle of interaction, we may focus on the question "Who started it?" We both got caught up in a negative pattern, but who started the thing in the first place?

Naturally, we disagree. We each see ourselves as reacting to the other's negative behavior. I think it started with your ignoring me; you think it started with my criticism. I think it started with your coldness; you think it started with my preoccupation. But who is right?

We are both right and both wrong. Once we are in a relationship, we can never "start fresh." Our current discussions are affected by our past ones. We may decide that a particular argument has nothing to do with any dispute from the past, but that simply isn't true. What past event we choose as a starting point will be somewhat arbitrary.

Wife: I come home, I greet you happily, and you scowl at me.

Husband: You don't call all day, and then you come home and give me this "innocent" greeting. And you expect me to respond?

In this example, the husband and wife see the argument beginning at different points. The wife thinks the argument started when she got home.

He thinks it began earlier in the day, when he expected a phone call. She didn't think she had to call. She was not attempting to appease him with an especially cheerful greeting. Furthermore, she didn't leave that morning ruminating about any unsolved problem from the past. She had no hangover from any previous interaction. For her, the argument really did start when she got home. But for him the argument started when she failed to call. He expected her to call, and when she didn't he got upset. So, there are two beginnings to this argument: his and hers. The interaction genuinely started at different points for them.

Deciding when an argument begins and ends gets even more complicated when the arguments are repetitious, when they are part of vicious cycles of communication. The preceding example was an isolated instance. But consider Phillip, who often nags Jennifer to pick up her things and keep the house neat and orderly. She often resists his efforts and complains about his "nagging." He says to himself, "I have to nag her because she resists doing what she ought to do. If she wouldn't resist, I wouldn't need to nag her." In his view the problem begins with her resistance and is followed by his nagging. Of course, she says to herself, "I resist him because he nags at me. If he didn't nag, I wouldn't resist." In her view, the problem begins with his nagging and is followed by her resistance.

We can think of our relationship as a long, continuous film. When we discuss it, we show parts of the film. We can't show it all, so we select portions. But this editing of the film—these decisions about where to start and end the episode—are up to the editor. Every editor chooses a different beginning and a different ending. We usually start the film with our partners doing something to us and end it with our justifiable reaction. We are good; they are bad. Not surprisingly, our partners start the episode with our behavior and end with their understandable reaction. They are good; we are bad.

However the interaction gets started, whenever the film starts rolling, we may get into some version of our vicious cycle of interaction. These vicious cycles not only sustain our problems and prevent their resolution, they may exacerbate those problems and create additional problems. This exacerbation of the existing problem and/or creation of a new one is called the reactive problem. While each cycle is unique, we've found that reactive problems tend to fall into three broad negative patterns: escalation, polarization, and alienation. As we repeat the same unsuccessful solution to our problems, persisting in wanting our partners to change, our tensions may escalate, our positions may become polarized, and we may become alienated from each other.

ESCALATION

As we cope ineffectively with the initial problem, created when our differences and emotional sensitivities are triggered, often within a stressful situation, we often generate a worse problem. The argument escalates: our tension increases, our voices become harsher or louder, our emotions are amplified. The volume goes up, literally and figuratively. We started out with a small conflict; now it is a big conflict.

Escalation often occurs through a kind of "short-circuiting" of the interaction. As we experience a vicious cycle of behavior repeatedly, we tend to anticipate its occurrence. Then we sometimes respond to our anticipation as much as we do to our partners and get into the cycle more quickly and intensely than we would have otherwise. For example, consider a pattern of criticism and defensiveness. Erik is often critical of Alicia, particularly concerning her messiness and lack of organization. She tends to respond with defensiveness, trying to convince him that she has been too busy to put things away or trying to show him that she has her own organization system. As this pattern repeats, Alicia will anticipate Erik's criticism and become defensive even before he has been critical. For example, she may try to explain why her papers are on the couch even before he has noticed them there. For his part, Erik may anticipate that things will be out of order and get angry at Alicia even before he has seen anything out of order. When their responses are short-circuited like this, they are primed for emotional reactions. They may have a more intense encounter than otherwise because their anticipations have set them up for it.

Arguments can escalate not only vertically, with an increase in tension, but also horizontally, with an expansion of focus. New issues are raised during the conflict, some legitimately related to the original topic, some brought in just to "get back" at the other. In Anika and Ralph's argument, Anika brought up Ralph's handling of his father's terminal illness; Ralph brought up Anika's handling of the kids. In what is often called "kitchen sinking," everything but the kitchen sink is brought into the discussion.

A common direction in which arguments escalate is toward the process itself. Although couples are often focused on the content of their incompatibilities and hurt feelings rather than the process by which they cope with these problems, at times their interaction becomes so painful for one or both of them that it becomes a focus of discussion. At times when Lori criticizes Manny for not being involved with their children, he may criticize her for her criticism: "All you do is complain and criticize. Can't you think of something better to do with your time?" She may defend her behavior—"I wouldn't have to complain if you would do something around here"—or she may attack him: "You can't take any criticism, can you, even when it is 100% deserved?" At this point they are arguing about the way they argue. They are criticizing each other for being critical. Now the process of their interaction, the way they cope with their problem, has become the content of their discussion. Their solution to the problem has become the problem. The "cure" has become the disease.

POLARIZATION

When we cope with our problems ineffectively, we often become polarized in our positions. We get more rigid, fixed, and extreme in our views. Although we might have been open to listening and trying to understand our partners' position prior to the argument, once the argument gets under way we stop listening. Instead we become more convinced of our own positions. In the heat of an argument, we engage in what psychologist John Gottman has called the "summarizing self syndrome." We restate our own positions or we state them somewhat differently, and then we summarize all that we have said. As we listen to ourselves making repeated arguments in favor of our own views, we become more and more convinced of the correctness of those views.

Not only do we become more convinced of our own views, we may also become more extreme in those views. Although early in the discussion we may feel justifiably that we have an important point to make, as the argument progresses we may feel that our point is the only point worth making. Our point is self-evident. Only a fool would argue against it. Any other ideas are at best irrelevant and at worst a devious attempt to undermine truth.

Sometimes the argument itself provides us with evidence that makes us more convinced about the rightness of our views. As the argument between Anika and Ralph escalated, Anika became more convinced that Ralph cares little about her. He certainly showed no caring during the argument; instead, he completely dismissed her concerns. For his part, Ralph found incontrovertible evidence that Anika overreacts to problems by the fact of her increasing upset during the argument. So both found evidence in the argument that polarized their positions.

Polarization over time may also occur in more subtle ways. Repeated conflict over an issue and pressure about an issue may squelch our inherent interest or spontaneous desire. Consider Enrico and Rosa's differences in desire for sexual contact. Because of these differences, Enrico initiates sex with Rosa far more than she does with him and more than she would like him to. Often Rosa declines, but his hurt response makes her feel guilty. Over time, she gets apprehensive about his requests, at times even dreads them. She begins to question her own sexual interest, particularly her interest in Enrico. All of this dampens whatever inherent, spontaneous sexual interest she had in him. When she forces herself into sexual contact with Enrico even when she doesn't want to, the whole experience takes on a negative emotional tone for her. Thus, as a result of their repeated conflict over sex, Rosa's interest in sex decreases and their incompatibility increases.

Deprivation may also play a role in polarizing a couple. As you are both unable to get your needs met, those needs can become intensified. For example, if sexual contact happens less and less, Enrico may find his desires for sex increasing. Apart from simple deprivation of this special experience, Enrico may find his desires for sex increasing just because it is being denied to him—a pleasure denied is a desire intensified. Meanwhile Rosa finds her sexual desire decreasing because of Enrico's pressure. Their persistent attempts to solve their sexual incompatibility have made the incompatibility greater. Their repetitive solutions have created a bigger problem.

ALIENATION

After conflicts escalate and positions become polarized, partners may eventually end the discussion in despair. They can't get through to each other. The other doesn't "get it." Further conversation about the matter is hopeless. Each retreats to his or her own corner and shuts down. Further conversation, if there is any, is tense and stilted. Partners have become alienated from each other.

Sometimes in the heat of the argument comments are made that trigger alienation. Right before he stormed out of the room, Ralph suggested that both he and Anika should find someone else. This comment catalyzed her concerns about his commitment to the relationship. Consequently, she withdrew from him for days.

Although alienation often occurs after escalation and polarization, it can happen much earlier in the conflict. When partners avoid dealing with an important problem, they often end up feeling distant from each other. They have prevented an open argument from erupting, but they haven't given themselves a chance to air their feelings or to express their views about an important matter. Because the issue is important to them, they think about it. They make conjectures about the other's motives and reactions. They have conversations in their head rather than with each other. Any actual discussion between partners often feels distant and disingenuous.

As our problems escalate and become polarized over time, we may feel trapped by these problems. How can we ever solve them? Even if our "solutions" don't create a bigger problem, their ineffectiveness can create despair.

We may question our relationship. Are our partners really right for us? We may say things in anger—a threat to leave, a harsh accusation—that create a rift in the relationship. Feeling trapped and hopeless about ever solving the problem and angry with our partners for the problem, we become alienated from them. It is not just a problem we have in the relationship. The relationship itself is now a problem.

RECAP

In this chapter we put together the components of conflict discussed in earlier chapters to create a complete DEEP analysis of conflict. Earlier in Part II, we saw how our problems with our partners are often readily understandable if seen in the light of the Differences (D) between us, the Emotional (E) reactions and sensitivities we bring to the relationship, and the External (E) circumstances, particularly the stressful circumstances, in which we encounter. In our effort to cope with these initial problems, we respond reflexively with dubious methods that only cause further problems. These methods tend to get reinforced because they all provide some occasional benefits. Moving against the other with accusation, blame, and coercion may vent angry feelings or force a temporary solution; moving away from the other with avoidance, denial, and withdrawal may provide temporary refuge from the problem; hanging on to the other with watchfulness, intrusion, and infringement may give temporary reassurance; moving against the other with outside help through alliances and coalitions can provide some immediate support for a problem. However, far from solving the initial problem, these strategies are often toxic cures that over time lead to vicious cycles or patterns (P) of interaction. In turn, these patterns or cycles of interaction may escalate the conflict, polarize and alienate us, and eventually cause us to question our relationship. The solutions that were designed to "cure" the initial problem create reactive problems that can finally undermine our very relationship.

Exercise: What's Your Problematic Pattern?

Below you will be asked to select the most common strategy you use to solve the core conflict you identified earlier. Then you will be asked to select the most common strategy your partner uses to solve this core conflict. Finally, you will put these two strategies together to create what you believe is the pattern of interaction between the two of you. This process will enable you to complete the P phase (patterns of interaction) of a DEEP understanding of your issue (the questionnaire is based on Christensen, 2011).

A. During our core conflict my partner is most likely to (circle the number of only one category below and check the behaviors that your partner engages in within that category) . . .

   1. Move against me by . . .
     ____ Criticizing, blaming, fault finding, attacking, finger pointing
     ____ Demanding, nagging, pressuring, reminding, pushing
     ____ Controlling, competing, showing who is right
     ____ Arguing, escalating, exaggerating

   2. Move away from me by . . .
     ____ Withdrawing, escaping, avoiding, distancing, shutting down
     ____ Hiding, evading, being secretive, misleading
     ____ Dismissing, minimizing, denying my concerns, resisting my efforts
     ____ Defending, justifying, explaining self

   3. Hang on to me by . . .
     ____ Pursuing, clinging, hovering, not letting me go
     ____ Intruding, invading, being nosy
     ____ Questioning, investigating, monitoring, keeping watch over me

   4. Move against me with the help of others by . . .
     ____ Telling things about me to family and friends that make me look bad
     ____ Seeking support from others who don't support our relationship
     ____ Allying with others against me, getting others to intervene in our relationship

B. During our core conflict, I am most likely to (circle the number of only one category below and check the behaviors that you engage in within that category) . . .

   1. Move against my partner by . . .
     ____ Criticizing, blaming, fault finding, attacking, finger pointing
     ____ Demanding, nagging, pressuring, reminding, pushing
     ____ Controlling, competing, showing who is right
     ____ Arguing, escalating, exaggerating

2. Move away from my partner by . . .

_____ Withdrawing, escaping, avoiding, distancing, shutting down

_____ Hiding, evading, being secretive, misleading

_____ Dismissing, minimizing, denying partner's concerns, resisting his/her efforts

_____ Defending, justifying, explaining self

3. Hang on to my partner by . . .

_____ Pursuing, clinging, hovering, not letting him/her go

_____ Intruding, invading, being nosy

_____ Questioning, investigating, monitoring, keeping watch over my partner

4. Move against my partner with the help of others by . . .

_____ Telling things about my partner to family and friends that make him/her look bad

_____ Seeking support from others who don't support our relationship

_____ Allying with others against him/her, getting others to intervene in our relationship

C. Now put these two pieces together and write out a short description of the most likely scenario when you and your partner struggle with your core issue. Even though the pattern is cyclical and it is impossible to know who starts it, start with your behavior. Write it as if to your partner, but don't show it to him or her yet (e.g., "I move away from you by withdrawing and defending myself while you move against me by criticizing and blaming me").

_____

_____

_____

D. Now think of a recent example of this pattern and write a short description of it (e.g., "Yesterday I defended myself about being too busy to have cleaned up the dishes when you pointed out that I had left dishes in the sink").

_____

_____

_____

Putting It Together

Now that you have completed the DEEP analysis of a core problem, it would be good to look at each part of it again. Go back to the exercises at the end of Chapters 3, 4, and 5. Does it seem like you have your differences identified correctly, your emotional reactions and sensitivities targeted appropriately, your relevant external stressors determined, and your pattern of interaction selected correctly? Please make any revisions you'd like to your DEEP understanding. Now write out a short description of your DEEP understanding of your core issue in your own words but as if you were going to show it to your partner. We don't want you to show it to him/her yet; that will come later. But try to frame it as constructively as possible, avoiding any kind of unilateral blame. Here is an example of what we have in mind.

EXAMPLE OF A DEEP UNDERSTANDING OF A CORE ISSUE*

The core issue in our relationship that disturbs me the most is our struggle around my mother **(statement of core issue).** I think a key difference between us that contributes to this issue is our different views and experiences with our families of origin. My family fostered greater closeness with family members, whereas I think yours fostered greater independence **(statement of D—the Differences that contribute to the core issue but stated constructively so both sides of the difference are framed in a positive light).** When we struggle about this issue, I think I show the surface emotion of frustration or irritation, but what I am often feeling underneath is disappointment that I may lose my close contact with her as she now is getting older and needier, concern that she will be hurt and rejected, and a little guilt that I am not a good child of hers **(statement of E—the surface and hidden emotion the writer experiences).** I think I am sensitive about being a good child and not abandoning her **(further elaboration of E by describing the writer's emotional sensitivity).** I think the stress of my career and our own family, which limits my available time, make this an even bigger problem for me. I think the stress of your career and our own family, which limits your available time, makes you want to spend as little time as possible with extended family **(statement of the second E—the external stress in both self and other that may contribute to the problem).** Finally, I think our pattern of interaction has often been mutual moving against each other with me trying to convince you of my mother's good qualities and criticizing you for your lack of extended family connection and you criticizing my mother and the way she reared me

*Key features are listed in parentheses in **bold** type.

(statement of P—the pattern of communication that occurs during this issue). But recently, the conflicts have been so frustrating to us both that we have moved away from each other, avoiding this topic as much as possible and not sharing our feelings or concerns **(further elaboration of P—how the pattern of communication has changed over time).**

Now it is your turn. Write your full DEEP analysis in your own words:

_____

_____

_____

_____

_____

_____

_____

_____

_____

_____

_____

_____

_____

Next Steps

You won't necessarily see your relationship transformed just because you have a new understanding of your core conflict. You may, however, see glimmerings of change between you and your partner. Perhaps you view your partner's foibles a little more philosophically than in the past; maybe you have a sharper awareness of your own emotional vulnerabilities as well as your hidden and manifest display of them. Maybe you see more clearly how external stress can affect you and your partner and how you each contribute to patterns of frustrating or painful interaction between you. Maybe you even catch yourself occasionally nipping an argument in the bud, or your soft spots aren't quite as sensitive as they used to be.

How much (if any) improvement you already notice in your relationship may depend on whether you and your partner have been reading this book together. Because all conflict between partners takes two, improvements may be greater when both of you are altering your perspective. If your partner is not reading the book along with you, you may want to encourage him or her to read Part I and II before you move on to Part III. However, if your partner is unwilling to read the book, it is still helpful if you go it alone. Later in the book we will show you ways that you can involve your partner, such as by constructively sharing your DEEP analysis with him or her, even if he or she isn't reading the book.

Wisdom is the first step toward acceptance in relationships. At this point you should have a wiser view of your core conflict from this DEEP analysis of it. In Part III we will show you how to use this DEEP understanding to create greater acceptance in your relationship. In so doing, you may lessen the conflict that plagues your relationship, particularly the reactive conflict. Equally important, you may increase the intimacy between the two of you. And, as an added bonus, your partner may spontaneously make some of the changes you were unsuccessful in producing with your toxic cures. If not, Part IV will help you create specific changes in your relationship.

PART III

From Argument
to Acceptance

CHAPTER 7

The Delicate Balance

ACCEPTANCE AND CHANGE

> God grant me the serenity
> to accept the things I cannot change;
> courage to change the things I can;
> and wisdom to know the difference.
> —REINHOLD NIEBUHR, *The Serenity Prayer* (1943)

In the movie *Blue Sky*, for which she won an Oscar, Jessica Lange portrays the emotionally volatile wife of an army nuclear radiation expert (played by Tommy Lee Jones). In one scene, they and their two daughters enter the dilapidated house that will be their new home on an army base in Alabama. Upset at the move and the condition of the house, Lange has a major emotional outburst. She tears down the curtains, storms outside, jumps into the car, and screeches away. Tommy Lee Jones runs after her, eventually rescues her, and brings her back home. The next morning as she sleeps, the girls are still upset about the incident. Jones tries to comfort his daughters and explain his perspective to them. He assures them of his own and their mother's love for them. He uses the metaphor of water to explain their mother. Just as water can be liquid or steam or ice, so their mother has many shifting properties. He tells them, "I made a decision a long time ago just to love her basic properties." Jones clearly experiences pain from his wife's emotional outbursts, yet he is able to tolerate that pain, recover from that pain, and accept that pain. He is even able to make humor out of the situation with a pun about nuclear fishing (fission) in the water that is his wife. He sees her specific behaviors in the larger context of her whole life—as just one of her shifting properties. And he sees her behaviors in the context of their life together: her emotional dynamism has made her the provocative, charming, and challenging person she is. In his dealing with her emotionality, he never seems weak or submissive, but strong and loving.

This movie dramatically illustrates what we mean by *acceptance*. When we talk about "accepting" your partner, we mean tolerating what you regard as an unpleasant behavior of your partner, probably to understand the deeper meaning of that behavior, certainly to see it in a larger context, and perhaps even to appreciate its value and importance in your relationship.

In sharp contrast to this example of acceptance is an example of submissiveness. In the movie *Mr. and Mrs. Bridge*, Paul Newman's and Joanne Woodward's characters are having dinner together at a country club when a tornado threatens. Everyone seeks shelter in the basement except Newman and Woodward, because Newman wants to finish his dinner. Distressed by the danger, Woodward wants to seek refuge but waits as her husband eats. As the wind wails and crashes outside, Newman comments, "They never give you enough butter." Woodward anxiously searches at other, now abandoned tables for more butter for Newman's bread. Finally, when her fear of the tornado surpasses her fear of offending him, she hesitantly questions, "Don't you think we might be better off downstairs in the basement?"

Newman replies, "Now look here, for 20 years I've been telling you when something will happen and when it will not happen. Now, have I ever, on any significant occasion, been proved wrong?"

The tornado subsides, and Newman is proved right again, but Woodward's weak voice of hesitant protest is muffled further.

Newman's stubbornness in the face of the tornado and his insensitivity to Woodward's anxiety are painful for her and dangerous to them both. However, she submits to his control and suffers with only the weakest of protests. Hers is not acceptance but submission.

Submission comes from a position of weakness, acceptance from a position of strength. Submission means enduring aversive behavior from your partner because you have or believe you have no alternative. Acceptance, in contrast, is tolerating aversive behavior because you choose to—you see that behavior as part of a larger context of who your partner is and who you are. Acceptance does not mean that you lack power to protest or are fearful of protest. Rather, acceptance means that you regard the negative behavior, as Jones did, as part of the many shifting properties of your partner. Your partner's scalding steam and cool comforting waters are just different manifestations of the same property that he or she is.

In its highest form, acceptance can promote more than just tolerance: it allows you to see beyond your partner's negative actions in the moment to the good intentions from which they spring or the positive consequences they sometimes have. This does not mean that you never resist your partner's aversive behavior, never argue about it, or never try to limit it. But it does mean that you can go beyond it.

Sarah wants to be updated on important developments in Jack's job, a desire that Jack would accept, but she also wants to express her opinion about these developments and encourage actions that she deems appropriate, two desires that upset Jack. She is particularly interested in how Jack is being treated by his superiors at work, and she often nags him to stand up for himself and demand his due. Her involvement in his work annoys Jack and causes many arguments. It also makes Jack feel devalued, as if he can never do enough to satisfy her perceptions of what is right. And he recoils from the idea that he should be fighting at his workplace to meet *her* expectations for *his* job.

Yet he also knows that were it not for Sarah, he would have accepted job assignments without insisting on the necessary support to carry them out. He would have gone several years without a pay increase simply because he was hesitant to ask for one. And he might even have lost his job to another. He knows that without Sarah's discriminating judgment, his naive trust in the goodwill of others would have gotten him into trouble. So Jack has mixed feelings about Sarah's critical questions and nagging concerns. Jack often disagrees with Sarah's comments and must take care to maintain a boundary defining what Sarah can and cannot control, but he has learned to listen to her opinionated views because he knows she usually has his best interests at heart, she understands his weaknesses, and she has insight into others' attempts to take advantage of him. In short, he accepts her criticism, nagging, and pressure about his work.

Acceptance versus Change

Acceptance and change are fundamentally different but linked events. A conflict ignites for a couple when one member, the *agent*, does something undesirable to or fails to do something desirable for the other, the *recipient*. Sarah was the agent of the problematic behavior of nagging and pressuring; Jack was the recipient of this behavior. *Change* occurs when the agent performs the unpleasant action or inaction less frequently or less intensely—for example, when Sarah does not nag or question or criticize Jack's work as much as usual. In contrast, *acceptance* occurs when the recipient reacts less negatively to the agent's behavior, is more tolerant of it, and has greater perspective about it. Acceptance occurs if Jack develops more tolerance for Sarah's behavior, perhaps because he sees its importance for their relationship and for him personally. The roles of agent and recipient shift back and forth as couples engage in conflict. Although Sarah is the agent of the problematic behavior of nagging and pressuring, were Jack to accuse Sarah of interfering in his work, Jack would be the agent of this accusation and Sarah the recipient.

Acceptance and change represent two ways to solve relationship problems. Although they are very different strategies, they can achieve the same goal: ending the conflict. For example, Denise is distressed because Frank rarely initiates any affectionate physical contact. If she sits beside him on the sofa, he will instinctively move away, as if to provide them both with more space. Yet the space in between them is precisely what Denise wants to bridge. One way to resolve this problem would be for Frank to become more openly affectionate with Denise, by holding her hand more often, kissing her more frequently, hugging her more intensely, and cuddling with her at night. These changes would all solve the problem, especially for Denise. If Frank felt comfortable with these changes and if the changes endured, then the problem of lack of physical signs of affection would truly be eliminated from their relationship. In a second possible solution Denise could become more accepting of Frank's difficulties with physical affection. She might see that he expresses his love for her in other ways than through physical affection: he works hard for her and the family, he is available to help her in times of need, and he listens attentively to her concerns. She might realize that he was raised in an unexpressive family, that he has never been very affectionate to anyone, and that he feels uncomfortable giving and receiving physical affection. And she may be reassured by the thought that Frank's lack of physical affection doesn't mean that he doesn't love her or isn't attracted to her. This greater acceptance would certainly solve the problem, especially for Frank. If Denise were truly accepting, so that Frank's lack of physical signs of affection was comfortable for her on an ongoing basis, then the problem would be solved for her as well.

If Frank and Denise solve the problem in the first way, then Frank makes a change: he becomes more physically affectionate. If they solve the problem in the second way, Denise makes a change: she becomes more accepting of Frank's lack of physical affection. Her change is not so much a behavioral change—although she may respond differently when Frank is not affectionate—as it is a change in how she receives or reacts to his behavior. It is a change in her attitude about his behavior, in her emotional reaction to his behavior, and in her interpretation of his behavior. We call this significant change she has made *acceptance* and reserve the term *change* for the type of specific behavior change Frank would make if he increased his affection. In an important sense both are changes, but we will use the terms *change* and *acceptance* to distinguish them.

This leads us to principle number 1 for solving problems: *A relationship conflict can be resolved through either change or acceptance.*

But which solution should couples choose? Frank would, of course, choose that Denise accept him as he is, and Denise naturally would choose that Frank become more affectionate. Each would prefer that any movement toward a solution be made by the other.

Most of us would like to hear the message "I love you the way you are" from our partners. They should see our foibles as endearing, or at least, in the shadow of our strengths, easily forgivable. Alongside the fantasy of being accepted exactly as we are, we may also harbor the fantasy of changing our partners. Our ideas for change would improve them and make life easier for us. This fantasy is captured in the old joke that asks what three things the bride thinks of as she walks down the aisle in church on her wedding day. The answer: Aisle, altar, hymn ("I'll alter him"). Therefore, each of us sometimes sends out the message "You should accept me as I am, but you should change to accommodate my needs." We may feel this message is justifiable because "your negative features are deeply disturbing; mine are merely inconveniences."

Let's suppose that Frank and Denise, after open communication about their affection problem, agreed on either change by him or acceptance by her. Would that be the end of the issue? Only if Frank's new affectionate behavior felt comfortable to him or Denise's new acceptance could be reconciled with her need for open signs of affection. Otherwise, given Frank's history, he might have a hard time keeping up his new level of affection, and after a few days or weeks of effort fall back into his old patterns. Similarly, Denise might make a good start of accepting Frank the way he is but end up feeling resentful and returning to her old angry pursuit of greater physical affection.

Theoretically, relationship problems can be solved through unilateral change by one person or unilateral acceptance by the other, but that kind of one-sided solution often does not work. Fortunately, there is a third solution.

The Third Solution

The third way to solve this affection problem and most other human relationship problems is through a combination of acceptance and change. Frank could make some changes regarding his infrequent displays of affectionate behavior *and* Denise could become more accepting of Frank's ways of showing love, which often don't include physical affection. This third possibility offers a number of advantages. The burden for solution falls on both partners: both give, but both also receive. Their actions may create a positive cycle that encourages and motivates each. If Denise sees some change on Frank's part, some effort to be more openly affectionate, she may find it easier to accept his overall limited ability to provide physical affection. A lack of any change in one partner, however, often proves to be a barrier to the other's acceptance of problematic behavior. Likewise, if Frank experiences Denise as being more accepting of his lack of open affection—as less negative and applying less pressure about it—he may find it easier to be somewhat more affectionate. Often another's pressure to change becomes a major barrier to change, whereas another's acceptance facilitates and even encourages change.

Frank and Denise have one other big area of conflict. Frank complains that Denise criticizes him too much, that she constantly monitors and evaluates him, usually negatively. Clearly Denise could cut back on her surveillance and criticism, or Frank could become more accepting of Denise's criticism. But because either unilateral approach could foster resentment in the party making all the changes, the third option might be best: Denise becomes less critical *and* Frank becomes more accepting of Denise's criticism. Denise's change would thus encourage Frank's acceptance, and Frank's acceptance would encourage Denise's change.

The benefits of this double-barreled solution go beyond their problem of criticism. Often relationship problems are linked: one person's problematic behavior is intimately connected to the other person's problematic behavior, such that solving one has mitigating effects on the other. Denise's criticism and Frank's lack of affection are linked in a vicious cycle of communication. Denise is often critical of Frank because of his lack of affection. Likewise, Frank finds it difficult to be openly affectionate with Denise because of her criticism. A solution to one problem would go far in solving the other one.

Frank and Denise started out their life together with differences in their desire and need for physical affection. These differences may have been inflamed by sensitivities in one or both—perhaps a fear in Denise of being neglected or abandoned or a fear in Frank of being suffocated or overwhelmed. At times stress may have exacerbated their differences and their sensitivities, as when Denise's work demands make her more desirous of affection or when Frank's work demands make him seek escape. Denise tried to solve this initial problem by being critical of Frank, and Frank reacted by being even less affectionate. This pattern of communication polarized the two of them so their initial differences in the expression of affection grew into a bigger incompatibility.

Another important difference characterized Frank and Denise. She started out their relationship being more outspoken, more likely to voice her likes and dislikes, than Frank. Because of his own sensitivity to criticism, this difference was a problem for Frank. When Denise was stressed, she was particularly likely to voice her views; when Frank was stressed, he was particularly uninterested in those views. He tried to solve the problem by withdrawing from Denise, and while this often provided some temporary respite, it ultimately made her even more critical of him. Their pattern of communication thus made the problem of criticism even worse.

If Frank and Denise tackled their affection and criticism problems through the bilateral, third alternative solution, they might gain greater improvements in both problems than they could expect for either problem with a unilateral approach. Solving the criticism problem will leave Frank less "on guard" with Denise, and thus he might be more physically responsive to her. Solving the affection problem will neutralize at least one major criticism of Denise's.

This brings us to principle number 2 for solving problems: *The best solutions to most problems involve acceptance by one member and change by the other.* This two-pronged approach not only makes both partners part of the solution and serves to motivate both partners, but may affect the solution of other, linked problems as well.

Acceptance and Change: The Chicken or the Egg?

Even in solutions that involve both acceptance and change, a question that couples often encounter is "Which comes first?" Should I wait for my partner to show some evidence of change before I begin to accept my partner's behavior? Or should I try to accept my partner's behavior, partially in hopes that it will lead my partner to change? While there are definitely certain situations that may require change, let us introduce principle number 3 for solving problems: *For most problems, acceptance is the best starting place.* Acceptance is important in its own right because it makes us feel comfortable and "at home" with our partners. We are loved, flaws and all. We can drop pretense, relax, and just be ourselves. Somewhat paradoxically, however, acceptance is also important as a major route to change. The kinds of experiences that promote acceptance also promote spontaneous change in couples. When we feel accepted, when we don't feel defensive, we are better able to hear our partners' concerns and appreciate their struggles. We may change to accommodate our partners, not out of force or pressure or coercion, but because we see and experience them differently. We change because we care for them and want them to feel better. When they feel accepted by us and hear our concerns, they may do the same for us.

Because it requires less effort and comes naturally, spontaneous change can be more gratifying than deliberate change. You don't feel as if you've given up something by compromising. You avoid the work of negotiation. Spontaneous change feels inner-directed: you change because you feel like it, because you want to. It is given freely, without strings.

Planned, deliberate change can be more complicated. Sometimes easier to achieve than acceptance in the short run because much behavior is under our voluntary control, planned change may be tough to sustain because it often comes with tangled emotional strings. You may, as we've discussed, be able to see the sense in making a change and appreciate the fairness of it, but if it treads too heavily on your core characteristics and ingrained sensitivities, you could resent and regret it in time. Or you could simply return to your old ways.

So we strongly advocate working on acceptance first, not only to promote acceptance, but also because acceptance may generate spontaneous change and thus reduce the need for planned change. But if planned change is needed, and it often is, we will describe in Part IV how to orchestrate deliberate change in ways that are likely to be most effective.

What <u>Should</u> Be Changed Because It <u>Shouldn't</u> Be Accepted?

Is there anything that should *not* be accepted? Are there any behaviors that should and must be changed, no matter what? Physical violence—especially when it results in fear or injury—should not be accepted in any couple. Even violence that was intended to just vent frustration and not harm the partner can escalate or accidentally result in physical injury and sometimes death. Even if it doesn't cause physical injury, the resulting fear it creates can linger, sometimes for years. Therefore, it's not surprising that even low levels of physical aggression are predictive of higher rates of relationship distress years later—even if couples don't consider the physical aggression a problem in and of itself.

Although low levels of physical aggression such as shoving, pushing, and throwing things are often exchanged by both partners, severe violence and aggression meant to control the partner—often called battering—is typically perpetrated by men. To accept this type of physical aggression is clearly not acceptance but submission. Women in these relationships often feel they have no choice; many may have little power to stop the violence they endure. Ending physical violence, either by leaving the relationship or by stopping it from happening in the relationship, is no simple matter.

Chapter 15 will address violence. For now, however, how do you determine what else is unacceptable?

Many would put emotional, psychological, and verbal abuse together with physical abuse as unacceptable behaviors for any couple. This kind of abuse is harder to define than physical abuse. Some language, such as threats and degrading names, is clearly abusive. No one should accept comments such as "You do that again and I will bust your face" or "You worthless bitch." Beyond these obvious examples of verbal abuse, however, it is impossible to establish clear-cut, universal criteria of what is abusive and what is not. A shouting match with name calling may feel abusive to some couples but may be merely a heated argument to others. The "silent treatment" may feel abusive to some but a relief to others. What seems like criticism to one member may feel like abuse to the other. To define emotional, psychological, and verbal abuse, we need to take into consideration both the actions of the agent and the reactions of the recipient. Even though these actions cause no physical harm, they are distressing to most, but for some they are truly damaging. Because of the importance of emotional, psychological, and verbal abuse and its association with physical abuse, we discuss it further in Chapter 15.

Other than physical violence and obvious cases of verbal abuse, it is difficult to list specific acts that no one should accept. Most might argue that no couple should accept infidelity, yet even this is not a universal rule. Some couples accept extramarital sex openly and others accept it implicitly. Many spouses have learned to forgive a partner who was unfaithful. Thus, the list of unacceptable actions must be individualized. Each spouse has the right to identify the actions that are totally unacceptable to him or her.

The danger is that a list of unacceptable actions will grow to the point that it includes every negative or unpleasant behavior. Melinda may insist that disrespect, rudeness, coldness, public humiliation, insensitivity, dishonesty, and selfishness (to name a few) are all unacceptable to her. Such a list mixes what is truly unacceptable to Melinda with what is merely unpleasant for her. This kind of list defeats its own purpose: it makes it less likely that her husband will make changes in either group. The list is so long that it implies that he is a major villain, perhaps the sole villain in their relationship.

A declaration that some action is unacceptable carries with it a moral force. When Joe tells Patrice that he can no longer accept her "public humiliation" of him, he is telling her that her actions are morally wrong, that she is at fault for taking these actions, and that she must change unilaterally. He frames his declaration in such a way that his reaction to her actions is not relevant. Whatever he might have done to provoke her actions is immaterial. Her public humiliation of him is so onerous that it dwarfs any negative actions of his. She must stop it forthwith.

Change by the perpetrator is the only antidote for so-called unacceptable behavior. Yet this antidote is often a cure worse than the disease. Describing behavior as wrong and thus unacceptable often creates barriers to change rather than facilitating change. The perpetrator often does not view the behavior in question as wrong, resists being accused of wrongdoing, and rebels against the notion of making unilateral change. A perpetrator who does change may resent the initial accusation and subsequent pressure that forced the change. Also, the communication sets up an inequality, with the partner "in the right" occupying the high moral ground and the partner "in the wrong" inhabiting the moral swamp. Such a position is not comfortable for the "lesser" partner and not likely to be tolerated well.

A story about Abraham Lincoln and his volatile wife, Mary Todd, illustrates that even behavior that might be defined conventionally as unacceptable does not have to be viewed in that intractable way. As we have explained, an interpersonal problem depends not just on some provocative behavior but also on a vulnerability to that behavior. Lincoln was outside talking to a congressman about the important political matters of the day. Mary Todd stormed out of the house, ruthlessly castigated Lincoln for something he had done, and then stormed back inside. Aghast that a wife would behave so outrageously in public, the congressman looked to see Lincoln's reaction. Lincoln was undisturbed by the incident and explained to the incredulous congressman that such outbursts made his wife feel so much better that he hardly wanted to put a stop to them.

This kind of action by a wife would have certainly been considered "public humiliation" by most of Lincoln's male peers and thus deserving of the most serious sanctions. Most men today might also experience such an act as public humiliation. Lincoln, however, was not humiliated, either publicly or privately. His reaction made Mary Todd's action something therapeutic for both of them rather than something bad and unacceptable.

Not only must "negative actions" be defined in terms of the recipient's vulnerable response as well as the perpetrator's provocative action, but negative actions must be considered in context. People are rarely disrespectful, rude, cold, insensitive, or selfish "out of the blue." Often their behavior is part of a vicious cycle of negative behavior. As we saw in the last chapter, partners may differ on where they define a starting point for a conflict. The victim may feel that the partner "attacked out of the blue," while the partner may view his or her attack as simply a reaction to some previous behavior by the other.

When viewed in this way, much of what partners call "unacceptable behavior" in each other can be described more accurately as components of the negative patterns of communication between them. Certainly, spouses have the right to declare specific actions of their partners "unacceptable." In a later chapter we will describe ways to create change in unacceptable behavior. However, "unacceptable behavior" is harder to change than merely problematic behavior that is part of a vicious cycle between members of a couple. Problems are more manageable, more solvable, and more changeable when they are not morally judged as unacceptable behavior.

What <u>Should</u> Be Accepted Because It <u>Can't</u> or <u>Shouldn't</u> Be Changed?

Are you obliged to accept some aspects of your partner? Does love create a moral imperative to accept some of your partner's features?

Some would say that to love, and certainly to marry, you must accept the essence of the other person. To pressure your partner to change some central characteristic would be asking your partner to be untrue to him- or herself. By choosing to love and marry this person, you have accepted who he or she is. You have forfeited the right to question your partner's central essence. You can push for change at the periphery, but not at the core.

A related notion is that people cannot change their basic essence even if they try to do so. Whether or not it is morally wrong for partners to press for change, it is futile to do so. People cannot alter what is at their core. Only the periphery is amenable to change.

We can call these two notions the "leopard argument": you shouldn't and can't ask the leopard to change his spots. It is wrong to ask. Even if you do ask, the leopard won't be able to change his spots.

Even if both partners accept this position, there is plenty of room to disagree about what is essence and what is not, about what is core and what is periphery. Denise may see Frank's inability to make affectionate gestures as just some learned behavior that he can change, while Frank may view his physical reticence as a central part of himself. Frank may view Denise's criticism as simply an annoying habit of hers, while she may view her discriminating high standards as an essential (and admirable) characteristic.

Sometimes such a disagreement may reflect genuine differences in how each views what is essential and what is not essential. At other times the issue can be raised simply to deflect a request for change. Like the leopard in the cartoon on the next page, one invokes the "essential characteristics" notion—You can't ask me to change who I am—as a way of thwarting any change at all.

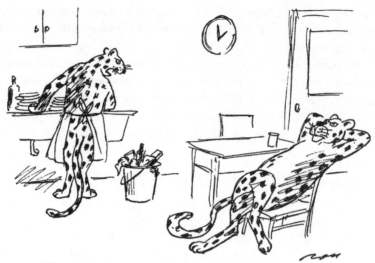

*"I'm not asking you to change your spots. I'm just
asking you to take out the garbage."*

Our core characteristics are certainly difficult to change. Indeed, many may be impossible to change. However, that doesn't mean that it is wrong to ask for change. Antonio has been a risk-taker all his life. He has always enjoyed challenging and dangerous sports, such as hang gliding and rock climbing. He chose a career on the police force partially because of the danger and thrill it provides, and he regularly volunteers for assignment to the most dangerous areas of the city. Boris was attracted to Antonio in part because he was so wild and reckless. Far from being something he wanted changed, he found Antonio's risk taking a source of excitement. He even joined Antonio in many of his risky leisure-time activities, such as fast motorcycle riding. But now that they have settled down and bought a house they're renovating, he fears for Antonio's life on and off the job. Antonio's partner was recently killed by a gang member, and Boris wants Antonio to seek a safe desk job with the police or change his occupation entirely. Boris also wants him to give up his dangerous hobbies.

Antonio may reasonably protest that Boris is asking him to change who he is. Boris has always known that he lives dangerously. How can he request that he change what is basic and essential about him? If he loves him, he must accept him as he is.

Boris may just as reasonably respond that he does love Antonio, but now they are at a different stage of life with different responsibilities. Their children need them both. Love for Boris and a commitment to their future together demand that he change.

Appeals to either acceptance or love are unlikely to solve Antonio and Boris's dilemma. Boris has the right to ask; Antonio has the right to refuse. This dilemma will challenge them and their relationship.

Although couples may disagree about whether a particular psychological characteristic is an unchangeable core feature of personality or merely an annoying habit, they are likely to agree that physical characteristics are largely unchangeable. Isn't it necessary to accept the physical characteristics of your partner because they cannot be changed? Even here the answer is not clearly a yes. First of all, some physical characteristics can be changed. While we can't change our age, we can try to lose the extra weight that we have gained with age. We can even treat the wrinkles that come with age, whether that be with makeup, skin medications, Botox, or plastic surgery. As medicine advances, what seemed to be unchangeable physical characteristics are being subjected regularly to change.

There is one final area in which one partner may argue that there is a moral obligation for acceptance. If partners have in good faith worked out an important agreement dealing with their differences, one may argue that they are both obligated to accept its terms unless both agree to change. Certainly, everyone would expect couples to honor their agreements with each other. However, changes may take place that make it difficult or impossible for one to follow through on an agreement. Mike and Beth handle their religious differences by pursuing their faiths separately. At the beginning of their marriage she attends mass at the Catholic church sporadically, while he attends the synagogue regularly. They agree even before their marriage that they will not raise their children as either Catholics or Jews. Rather, they will expose the children to both faiths and allow them to make their own choices. However, as their marriage progresses and they actually have children, Beth's religious faith deepens. She cannot bear the thought of her own children not being baptized. Mike points repeatedly to their agreement: "This is what we decided on; you must abide by it." Beth acknowledges that she made the agreement in good faith. However, she argues, the agreement was made years ago and now she has changed. She should not have to accept conditions of an old agreement that no longer works for her.

Obviously, there is no universal list of what should or must be accepted in relationships. Both partners can request or demand that the other accept certain aspects of themselves. Both can certainly refuse to make any changes in those characteristics for which they seek acceptance. However, whether the partner actually accepts those characteristics is another question entirely.

Demanding acceptance, like demanding change, can decrease the likelihood of its occurrence. Pressure, demands, and moral imperatives are barriers to acceptance just as they are barriers to change. In fact, they may even
be greater obstacles to acceptance than they are to change. While it is possible to make some changes on command, it is not possible to alter acceptance on command. Acceptance is in part an emotional reaction that is not
under voluntary control. One can no more create acceptance by demanding
it than one can create love by commanding it.

Acceptance and Change and Your Core Issue

In Parts I and II of this book, you identified a core issue in your relationship and conducted a DEEP analysis of that issue, targeting the Differences
between you and your partner, the Emotional reactions and associated sensitivities that make this such an important matter for you, the External
stressors that make handling it more complicated, and the Pattern of communication that you and your partner often get stuck in while trying to deal
with this issue. Let us consider each of these DEEP components and how
acceptance and change might be brought to bear on them.

Fundamental differences (or similarities) between partners do not
usually change very easily or quickly. They often result from the personality
makeup of each and are usually well stamped in by genes and experience. If
one is more extroverted and the other more introverted, then that difference
will not likely be erased soon. Likewise, if one is more a saver and the other
more a spender, if one is more planful and the other more spontaneous, or if
one is closer to his or her family of origin and the other more distant, these
differences probably preceded the relationship and may persist throughout
the relationship. It is not that these differences are unchangeable; it is just
that they are unlikely to change easily. Thus, for the Differences part of the
DEEP analysis, probably acceptance will be called for more than change.
That does not mean that change cannot be helpful in accommodating differences. An extrovert and an introvert may work out ways for the extrovert to satisfy his or her need for socialization without always involving the
introvert. But the differences themselves may need to be accepted.

The Emotional sensitivities that create the strong surface and hidden
emotions that people display in their core conflicts are also not easily subject to change. If one is sensitive to criticism, or feels abandoned easily,
or is anxious about being in control, he or she will not quickly "get over"
that sensitivity. Genetic tendencies and significant past experience have left
their mark on them, and these sensitivities are part of who they are. So

here too acceptance is more in order. This does not mean that change cannot help a couple accommodate or manage their sensitivities. For example, perhaps a partner of one who is sensitive to criticism learns when and how it is helpful to bring up their critical comments and, more important, when it is not helpful to do so. But the fundamental sensitivities are part of who the person is and are likely to change only gradually.

Unlike Differences and Emotional sensitivities, External stressors are not part of who we are. They are part of the environment in which we live. Often we have the ability to alter these stressors, such as not taking on a new project or deciding to spend less on recreation so we are not pushed to the limit financially. However, often it would be too costly to change a stressor, thus creating more stress overall for us. We could certainly quit a stressful job, but the consequences of that could be dire, leading to even more stress. We could move to a better neighborhood, but that might mean a longer and more stressful commute. Thus sometimes we can make changes in a stressor, but other times we may need to accept the stressor (at least for the time being) and can change only how we deal with it.

Our Patterns of communication are the area in which we have the most power to change. We can alter the way we talk with our partner, the way we deal with him or her about the issues that matter to us. Not that it is easy. Our personality differences and emotional sensitivities inform how we communicate. Yet all of us have talked in a reasonably constructive way about problems and all of us have talked about problems in ways that probably led to arguments and distance. So this is the area where change will be most prominent. Not that acceptance is not needed here also. It may be very helpful, for example, for a talker to realize and accept that his or her partner has less of an appetite for heavy-duty conversation or soul-revealing analysis. But helping you change the negative patterns of communication you identified in Chapter 6 will be a major goal of Part IV of this book.

RECAP

In this chapter we distinguished between acceptance and change. Change occurs when the perpetrator of some offensive behavior (or the partner who lacks some desired behavior) does something differently. A criticizer lowers the frequency or intensity of criticism; an unaffectionate partner becomes more affectionate. Acceptance takes place when the recipient of the offensive behavior or lack of behavior responds in a different way. The recipient of the criticism or the partner of an unaffectionate mate is less affected by the criticism or the lack of affection and is not so hurt by the offensive behavior (or lack of behavior). Problems in relationships can be solved, at least theoretically, by complete change on the part of the perpetrator, complete acceptance on the part of the recipient, or a combination of the two. The third solution, a combination of acceptance and change, is clearly the most viable path.

Certain behaviors, such as physical abuse, should never be accepted. Also, certain characteristics of the other, such as an unchangeable physical characteristic or a core personality characteristic, may need to be accepted. However, there are precious few universals that absolutely must be changed or must be accepted in all couples for a good relationship to exist. In fact, each of us must decide what is unacceptable to us in our partners and what we are unable or unwilling to change in ourselves (and thus may need to be accepted by our partners). The danger is that the list of what is unacceptable in our partners may grow too long and the list of what we are open to changing in ourselves may come up short.

When we consider the four aspects of the DEEP analysis of a core problem that we described in Part I, acceptance will be needed for fundamental differences between you and your partner as well as for the emotional reactions and sensitivities that each of you bring to the relationship. Some stressors can be changed, but others must simply be accepted; what can be changed is how you respond to them. The pattern of communication is the area where change will be needed most. Talking to your partner more constructively is something we all have the power to do.

In this book we focus first on promoting acceptance in relationships, not only because it is important in its own right but also because it can often lead to spontaneous change. When there is greater acceptance in a relationship, both partners will be less defensive and more open to hearing what the other needs and wants. Both may respond to those needs and wants simply because they care about the other.

Exercise: Change and Acceptance and Your Core Conflict

Think back over your core issue and your DEEP analysis of it and answer the following questions.

1. Is there anything that you are doing that is truly unacceptable behavior? If so, what is it and how can you change it?

_____

_____

2. Is there anything that your partner is doing that is truly unacceptable behavior? If so, what is it and how can you change it? (Note that we will return to unacceptable behavior in Chapter 15.)

_____

_____

_____

3. Is there anything that you have tried to change unsuccessfully and that would be better to accept, such as the way in which your partner is different from you or a sensitivity of your partner related to the core issue?

_____

_____

_____

Next Steps

In the next three chapters we will discuss ways in which you and your partner can promote acceptance in each other. Because acceptance is in part an emotional reaction not under voluntary control, we cannot provide recipes or formulas; we can only describe the kind of experiences that may promote acceptance and offer guidelines for generating those experiences in your relationships.

Promoting acceptance in relationships is a little like promoting trust. Exhortations and pleas, evidence and argument don't go very far. Steve entered a relationship with Joan bothered by questions about her trustworthiness, not because of anything Joan had done, but because his own history had engendered distrust: previous girlfriends had lied and cheated on him. How can Steve learn to trust Joan? It will do little good for Joan to command or demand trust; these actions would merely create resistance or, worse, suspicion in him. It might be useful at times for Joan to reassure Steve that she loves him, but he still might be wary because his other girlfriends had also professed their love. Joan could tell him of her history of honesty and monogamy in relationships; intellectually he might believe her, but emotionally he still may distrust her.

Experiences that demonstrate her faithfulness will help most. Situations like a party in which a man shows interest in her, a visit by her old boyfriend, and the development of a close relationship with a male colleague at work would challenge Steve's trust in Joan but also offer an opportunity for her honesty and faithfulness to be demonstrated and his trust to develop. If she is open and honest about these events, and if she maintains appropriate limits on all of these contacts, Steve's trust in Joan might grow—as might her confidence in his trust.

However, these situations could clearly challenge them both and exacerbate the trust problem. Because of his distrust, Steve could accuse Joan of having feelings about these men that she doesn't have. He could demand unreasonable limits on her behavior: that she refuse to meet with her old boyfriend, that she shun her colleague at work. In response, she could withhold information from him to prevent his unreasonable accusations and demands. Yet her lack of openness could fuel his distrust. She could rebel against his prohibitions about contact with these other men and provocatively increase her contact with them. She could show him that he can't control her, but in so doing increase his anxious and distrusting efforts to try to control her.

Thus the very occasions that offer the opportunity for trust to grow also generate the risk of trust deteriorating. How the couple handles these situations relevant to trust determines the experience they have of trust in their relationship. These experiences around trust influence the feelings and attitudes of trust, for good or bad.

As with trust, acceptance cannot be commanded or demanded. There is no recipe to make it happen, no formula to call it into being. Acceptance develops based on the particular experiences a couple has as they cope with their differences, their sensitivities, and their stressors. These characteristics of them and their life offer the opportunity for acceptance-enhancing experiences but also the risk of rejection-inducing experiences. For example, an evening in front of the television, in which Frank sits at one end of the sofa away from Denise and she feels unconnected and lonely, offers both of them an opportunity for either acceptance or rejection of the other. Depending on whether and how they discuss her desire for affection, they could on the one hand come to a greater understanding and appreciation of each other, perhaps even create greater intimacy between one another, or on the other hand get angry and grow more distant from each other. The very situations that may promote acceptance may also make matters worse. Conflict situations offer not only the risk of alienation but also the possibility of acceptance and intimacy. It all depends on how the discussion and the experience of it go. In the next three chapters, we will show you ways to turn potential conflict into greater acceptance and intimacy.

CHAPTER 8

A Story of Our Own

ACCEPTANCE THROUGH UNDERSTANDING

> To understand all is to forgive all—and to accept all.
> —VARIATION ON AN OLD ADAGE

> Narrative is radical, creating us at the moment it is being created.
> —TONI MORRISON, *Book of Nobel Lectures* (1995)

The definition of a problem contains the seeds of its solution. How we understand a problem determines the way we cope with it. As we have seen throughout this book, most of us try to resolve marital conflict by demanding an overhaul of our partners. Why? Because we have defined the problem in terms of the other person: *I have problems because of you. I have problems because of the way you are.*

We have also seen—many of us firsthand—that such solutions usually fall short and often even cause problems of their own. Defining relationship problems in terms of your partner can create destructive conflicts over who is bad or mad or inadequate, and thus over who should seek moral instruction, medical or psychological help, or remedial education. Even the ultimate solution to marital conflict, separation or divorce, often causes more problems than it solves—as many couples know.

Our goals in this book are twofold. We want to help couples deal with everyday relationship problems constructively, and we want to help couples deal with these relationship problems in ways that actively bring them closer together. The first goal is simply to manage a problem effectively; the second, more far-reaching goal is to create greater intimacy in the face of problems. To give you the greatest chance of devising solutions that work in achieving these goals, we want you to define the problem accurately. The method we have devised for doing so is to create a true and workable "story" about your problems.

In our couple counseling, we spend three or four sessions evaluating the problem and then provide couples with our feedback. An important part of this feedback is the story we tell about their problems, which must meet demanding criteria. First, the story must be true in the sense that it fits all the facts we have learned about the problem. Second, it must be unique in that it captures the particular experience of each partner and of his or her relationship. Third, it must be original and realistic. And fourth, it must be a story to which both can agree. This last criterion is the most difficult to meet. Usually a couple comes into treatment with different and incompatible stories about their problems. He sees the problem as resulting from something in her, her family, or her environment; she sees the problem as resulting from something in him, his family, or his environment. Our goal is to create a common story.

This problem story is essential because it provides the framework for our intervention efforts. It is the foundation for both acceptance and change by both partners. We know that couples spend time thinking about their problems and why they have them. We want them to incorporate a common story into their thinking.

You have already created a new story about the core problem in your relationship: your DEEP analysis. However, because the story is so new, it may not be fully developed and it may have some errors in it, some traces of the old story. In this chapter we will review that story, elaborate on it with an example, and be sure it has all the right ingredients.

What a Problem Story Should and Should Not Include

A good problem story is based on the analyses in Part II. It is the "anatomy of argument" for one unique couple. Like any good story, it emphasizes certain features and neglects others, as will be illustrated by three couples with common relationship problems. Chuck and Grace's problem is sex: they cannot agree on how and how often to have sex. Janice and Leif have a responsibility problem: they argue over who does what in the household. And Sal and Erik have an in-law problem: they argue about Sal's mother. Even though each couple has unique circumstances, their conflicts may sound familiar.

CORE ISSUE AND DESCRIPTION OF RECENT CONFLICT

Write down your core issue and briefly describe a recent conflict over this issue. For example, Chuck and Grace might write the following: Our core issue: conflicts over sex. Description of a recent conflict: Last Saturday night, Chuck wanted to have sex with Grace and wanted them to get in the mood by watching an X-rated movie he had recorded. Grace wasn't sure she was up for sex at all and certainly did not want to watch any X-rated movie.

Our core issue:

_____

Description of a recent conflict:

_____

_____

_____

DIFFERENCES RATHER THAN DEFECTS

A good problem story will emphasize *differences between* partners rather than *defects in* either of them. It focuses on incompatibilities between partners rather than faults in either partner. In our story of the sex problem, we would focus on the fact that Chuck has a different sex drive from Grace. He prefers frequent sex involving a great variety of positions, and he likes to begin lovemaking with Grace dressed provocatively in sexy underwear. Grace usually prefers physical affection to sex, feels uncomfortable in sexy underwear, and feels most interested in having sex after a romantic evening, with the lights off and in the missionary position.

It would be easy to find defects on either side of this story. We could label Chuck an oversexed husband who treats Grace like a sex object rather than a wife and lover; we could label Grace a sexually inhibited wife who is uncomfortable with her body in general and sexuality in particular. Instead our story will emphasize the simple differences in what Chuck and Grace find comfortable and pleasing in their sexual relationship.

In our story of the responsibility problem, we would focus on Janice's need for order in her environment and on her preference for equality between husbands and wives both inside and outside the home. Our story will acknowledge Leif's comfort with some level of disorder in people and things and his belief in equality in theory, if not according to the same exact standards held by Janice. We will resist the temptation to label Janice as compulsively neat and controlling or Leif as slovenly and passive–aggressive.

In developing a story about Sal and Erik's in-law problem, we will emphasize the difference in their attachment to their mothers rather than exploring whether Sal is a man who has "never cut the apron strings" from his mother or whether Erik is insecure and jealous of Sal's relationship with his mother.

But what if there really are defects in one or both members of the couple? Should we paper over these deficiencies by euphemistically calling them "simple differences" rather than facing them squarely? Shouldn't we make a clear distinction between what are defects and what are differences?

Except in the extreme, such distinctions are almost impossible to support, because all behavior falls somewhere along a continuum. Who is to say where "normal" differences end and pathological defects begin? Mental health professionals often cannot agree. Even if we had reliable data on the sexual responsiveness of women or the disorderliness of men, and even if we could prove that Grace was below average on the former and Leif was above average on the latter, any decision about a cut-off point for "defectiveness" would clearly be arbitrary.

And even if we could make reliable distinctions between differences and defects, what end would be served? A focus on defectiveness often leads to blame and accusation on the one hand and defensiveness on the other. As we have seen, this does not lead to solutions but often to reactive problems that are even more intense than the original problems.

Differences in Core Issue and Recent Conflict

Now that you've had a chance to think about your differences or similarities in more detail, write them out below. Describe them as fully as possible and detail the specific differences that generated your recent conflict, being careful to exclude any reference to deficits. For example, Chuck and Grace might write the following: General Differences: Chuck has a stronger sex drive than Grace and is more interested in adventurous sex, while Grace is more interested in romantic sex. Differences in the recent conflict: Chuck was interested in sex and wanted to use an X-rated movie to get them in the mood. Grace didn't want to watch any such movie and was unsure whether she was interested in sex. Refer back to the end of Chapter 6, where you first wrote out your DEEP analysis of your core conflict, for additional thoughts.

General differences in our core issue:

_____

_____

Specific differences in our recent conflict:

_____

_____

_____

EMOTIONAL REACTIONS RATHER THAN
PROVOCATIVE ACTIONS

In our stories about our problems, we are likely to focus on the violating behaviors that offend us, the provocative acts that upset us. Grace may focus on the aggressive way that Chuck grabs her. Janice may focus on the inconsiderate way in which Leif leaves his clothes scattered over their bedroom. Sal may focus on the coldness with which Erik responds to his mother.

If our partner does something that creates a strong negative reaction in us, we often assume our partner must *want* to create that reaction in us. Chuck often feels a mixture of anger and hurt because, in his view, Grace places artificial limitations on the sexual enjoyment they could both experience. Even on those occasions when they do have sexual relations, he feels limited in his sexual expression. Beyond his anger and frustration are feelings of hurt. It's obvious to him that Grace isn't satisfied sexually, and so he feels like a sexual failure. He feels emasculated by the whole situation; after all, a *real* man should be able to please his wife. So maybe Grace *wants* to emasculate him; maybe she is threatened by his masculinity and is trying to cut him down to size. Maybe unconsciously she wants him to be impotent!

For her part, Grace feels such pressure and dissatisfaction from Chuck that she questions her own sexuality. She vacillates between feeling angry at Chuck for his advances and feeling inadequate as a wife and lover. In her anger, she may think that only a porn star could satisfy Chuck. Yet she knows that she has always been shy and inhibited sexually. Unfortunately, her sexual relationship with Chuck is distorted by so much pressure that her inhibitions have increased, not decreased. So she starts thinking "Maybe he wants me to feel inadequate. Maybe he is taking out some kind of unconscious anger toward women on me."

Even if we don't assume that our own strong emotional reactions implicate unconscious, negative motives in our partner, there is another way that the emotional consequences of conflict can affect our stories about those conflicts. We may find, in the presence of our own strong negative emotion, evidence for an absence of strong positive emotion toward us in our partners. "If you are doing something that creates such a negative reaction in me, then certainly you couldn't care about my feelings. If you do things that hurt me, how can you possibly respect me? If you take actions that make me feel unloved, how can you really love me?"

Erik wants a closer relationship with Sal. Erik often feels neglected by Sal, particularly when he sees the amount of contact Sal has with his mother and senses the intimacy they must have together. He wonders whether Sal really loves him. In his anger, he accuses his partner of lack of love. In dramatic moments, he takes off his wedding ring and offers it to Sal with the challenge "Why don't you give it to your mother? She's really your spouse, not me!"

For his part, Sal feels hurt by and defensive about Erik's frequent attacks on his mother and his relationship with his mother. He tells Erik that he is not asking him to love his mother, only to accept her as she is, or at least not to attack her. Yet, much to his dismay, Erik can never seem to say a positive thing about his mother and highlights all of her shortcomings instead. Sal counters Erik's charge that he doesn't really love him with charges of his own: "How can you love me when you constantly attack someone who is so important to me?"

Not surprisingly, this focus on the violating behavior that offends us often leads to disagreement and argument. Chuck views his sexual advances toward Grace as simply showing a healthy sexual interest in her. In his view, she should be flattered rather than offended by his behavior. Leif regards Janice as compulsive rather than his own behavior as inconsiderate. Erik cannot imagine how he could respond differently to a mother who has fostered such an unhealthy dependency in her son. If we not only focus on the violating behavior but attribute it to unsavory motives in our partner or suggest it results from a lack of love for us, then the conflict will likely be more intense. Our analysis of the problem will make the problem greater.

To build a common story, it is better to focus less on the violating behavior and more on the vulnerability that the behavior triggers—less on the slight and more on the sensitivity, less on the arrow and more on the wound. However we might describe Chuck's sexual advances, to Grace they feel more like an assault than an invitation. They touch a sensitivity in her to being physically invaded. Janice feels anxious and out of control when her surroundings are in disarray. A sensitivity about control and disorder is triggered when there is clutter around her. Finally, Sal feels supremely protective of his widowed mother. As an only child, he knows she has no one else to care for her. He feels torn between his husband and his mother when Erik reacts to his mother in ways that don't seem friendly to him.

Emotional Reactions in Core Issue and Recent Conflict

Now write out the emotional reactions that each of you probably experiences, including both the observable surface emotions and hidden emotions. Make sure the focus is on each one's reactions rather than the other's actions or the reasons for those actions. Also note the specific reactions that each felt in the most recent example. For example, Chuck and Grace might write: Emotional reactions: Both tend to get irritated and angry. Underneath, Chuck tends to feel rejected and Grace tends to feel pressured. Specific emotional reactions in the recent conflict: Chuck felt some irritation but primarily disappointment. Grace felt surprised and even shocked by his suggestion of an X-rated film but eventually felt hopeless about ever being able to please him. Refer back to the end of Chapter 6, where you first wrote out your DEEP analysis of your core conflict, for additional thoughts.

Surface and hidden emotional reactions during our core issue (list first your own emotions and then your guess as to your partner's emotions):

_____

_____

_____

Surface and hidden emotional reactions during our recent conflict (list first your own emotions and then your guess as to your partner's emotions):

_____

_____

_____

EXTERNAL STRESSORS AND UNDERSTANDABLE REACTIONS RATHER THAN STRESSFUL OVERREACTIONS

If we include our partners' stress in our story of the problem, we may focus on their reactions to these stressors rather than the stressors themselves. After all, what we usually see in front of us are their reactions, such as when they come home worried, when they stay up late, or when they get preoccupied or irritable. We are often not privy to the particular circumstances that cause these reactions, such as the boss's demand for a work report by tomorrow or pressure from an aging parent for more time together. Thus we are likely to focus on their reactions and perhaps see them as not handling the stressor well or overreacting to the stressor. If we focus on these reactions, particularly if these reactions are less than stellar as reactions to stressors often are, then we are likely to trigger conflict and argument with our partners. They will see us as adding to their stressors rather than supporting them in coping with their stressors.

If we focus instead on the stressors themselves and try to understand the meaning of them for our partner, we may understand their responses better. Then we will naturally have more sympathy for them, but will also be in a better position to know how to help them or support them. For example, if Erik understood the sense of responsibility that Sal has toward his mother, his fear of her suffering, and his desire to be a good son, he might be more sympathetic to Sal when he gets anxious about upcoming surgery for his mother, even if it is minor surgery. Erik's comments about the surgery might come across as reassuring to Sal about the likely outcome rather than as dismissive of his concerns. Thus Erik might be able to help reduce his stress rather than redirect it toward an argument between them.

External Stressors in Core Issue and Recent Conflict

Now write out the external stressors that often affect your core issue and the specific stressors that affected the recent example. Be sure to focus on the external stressors and each of your understandable reactions rather than evaluating those reactions. For example, Chuck and Grace might write the following: External stressors that influence the core issue: Chuck finds sex a way to relax after a stressful day, while Grace has a difficult time relaxing and getting into sex when she has had a stressful day or is worried about tomorrow. External stressors in the recent conflict: Chuck was not stressed at all, was looking forward to making love to Grace, and alluded to that several times earlier in the evening. Grace felt pressure from Chuck's allusions to sex earlier in the evening; she enjoys making love most when it happens spontaneously. Refer back to the end of Chapter 6, where you first wrote out your DEEP analysis of your core conflict, for additional thoughts.

Typical external stressors and our understandable reactions that often affect our core issue:

_____

_____

_____

Specific external stressors and our understandable reactions that affected our recent conflict:

_____

_____

_____

PATTERN RATHER THAN PUNISHMENT; DESCRIPTION RATHER THAN EVALUATION

A good problem story includes a description of how each partner copes with the initial problem created by their differences, their sensitivities, and their stressful circumstances. How a couple tries to solve their problem is as important as its content. But the description of the coping process must focus on the prominent thoughts, feelings, and behaviors of each partner without judgments about whether the thoughts are distorted, the feelings overblown, or the behaviors inappropriate. Getting caught up in mutual evaluation as you construct your story will only distract you from your goal of trying to understand the problem.

One common way that a description of communication patterns can become evaluative is when partners incorporate punishment into their analysis. The reactions that each gets from the other as they cope with their problem can make them feel bad, as if they were being punished. They may assume that this is what the other intends. Chuck may feel he is being punished for his sexual interest by Grace's depriving him of satisfaction, while she may feel she is being punished for her reticence by pressure to engage in even more adventurous sexual activities. Janice may feel that Leif is punishing her by leaving his clothes a mess, while he may feel punished by her reactions when she finds something of his out of place. If they try to incorporate these presumed intentions of each other into their analysis, it will quickly become a source of argument rather than a basis for common understanding.

A good, nonjudgmental story captures the process by which Chuck and Grace try to deal with their sexual difficulty, but it does not condemn either one for the desperate measures they sometimes employ. There is a world of difference between saying "You are frigid" and saying "When I get frustrated, I accuse you of being frigid." Likewise, there is huge gap between saying "You try to punish me" versus "When we get into the heat of things, I start feeling that you are trying to punish me." The first is a judgment that will perpetuate the problem; the second is a descriptive account of the problem that may lead to understanding. Thus it is possible to have a non-judgmental description of the judgments partners make when attempting to cope with a problem.

A thorough description of the way a couple copes with a problem may include something on the development of that problem and the coping. The pattern of communication that occurs today was probably not what it was when the problem arose. Early on perhaps both members were more patient and tried to work it out but got frustrated as their attempts were unsuccessful. Maybe things changed for one or both that made the problem more difficult to solve. Consider, for example, Sal and Erik's efforts to deal with Sal's mother. Early on, Erik was eager to get along with Sal's mother and Sal tried to accommodate them both. Over time, however, Erik became less accommodating as he saw Sal responding to more demands by his mother while Sal became more frustrated as he experienced Erik's resistance. Also, Sal's mother developed more physical problems as she aged that made her more dependent on Sal, which increased both her demands on Sal and his desire to respond to those demands. Thus their pattern of communication got worse not only because of their repeated unsuccessful effort to deal with the problem but because the circumstances themselves changed.

Communication Patterns in Core Issue and Recent Conflict

Write a description of your pattern of communication, emphasizing what each of you think, feel, and do rather than evaluating those actions or attributing motives to them. For example, Chuck and Grace might write the following. The Pattern of communication in the core issue: Chuck often approaches Grace hoping for sexual contact but expecting a negative reaction from her. Grace often feels pressured for sex and then sometimes gives in to his requests but often resists. When she resists, they sometimes both withdraw tensely and at other times argue about sex, with each accusing the other of having sexual problems. Pattern of communication in the recent conflict: Chuck wanted to make love to Grace and tried to get her into the mood with suggestive comments and a proposal to watch an X-rated movie. Grace felt pressured by his comments and was upset by the notion of the movie. They argued briefly and then withdrew. Refer back to the end of Chapter 6, where you first wrote out your DEEP analysis of your core conflict, for additional thoughts.

The Pattern of communication typical during our core issue:

_____

_____

The Pattern of communication during our recent conflict:

_____

_____

_____

COMPLEX DILEMMAS RATHER THAN SIMPLE SOLUTIONS

A good conflict story stresses the complex dilemmas that long-standing problems present rather than offering simple solutions to them. Simple solutions usually derive from a limited understanding of the difficulties that a problem presents, often downplaying or even ignoring how one's own behavior contributes to that difficulty. These simple solutions focus on the obvious things that *your partner* can do to solve this problem. They are often solutions that further complicate the problems, cures that exacerbate the disease. Therefore, somewhat paradoxically, couples can resolve complex dilemmas more easily than they can implement simple solutions.

Leif's simple solution is "Look, I am cooperative and want to help. Ask me for help when you need it and ask me nicely, not in an irritated, angry way, and I will usually do what you want done." This simple solution ignores at least two major issues. Janice wants Leif to be a copartner, not just a helper. She wants him to notice when the children have needs, to notice when the house needs picking up, or the dishes need to be done, and then to take action. Instead, he withdraws into his own world, reading the paper or watching television, and she is left with the responsibility. When she gets overwhelmed with the household responsibilities and sees him "in his own world," she is too irritated to ask nicely and sweetly for his help.

Janice's simple solution to their problem is for Leif to "stand up and take an equal role in the family. Look around, see what needs to be done, and do it. Don't wait for me to tell you or for things to get out of hand. Just do it." Janice's simple solution also ignores some major facets of their problem. Leif has different standards for the household and for the kids than Janice has. For Leif to act on his own, the kids have to be louder and more boisterous and the household has to be in greater disarray than Janice can tolerate. So Janice wants Leif to take action according to her standards rather than according to his own, which would of course be much more difficult for Leif. Furthermore, when he does take action, whether it be with the kids or with the household, he often doesn't do it as well as Janice. She then criticizes him, which makes him feel that she won't be happy unless it is done her way. He reacts by withdrawing from household responsibilities altogether; he is not eager to take them on in the first place, especially if he gets criticized for his efforts.

Thus, the simple solutions proposed by each will not succeed. They lay full responsibility on the other, ignore each one's own role in the problem, and ignore the emotional barriers to their implementation. As Leif and Janice argue about these "simple solutions," they will likely create reactive problems that will, at the very least, complicate their initial problem. A story that describes their complex dilemma, rather than "obvious solutions" to it, may create more acceptance in each and possibly even more realistic opportunities for change.

A Sample Story

Up until now we have examined bits of conflict stories, snippets of each couple's struggle. Now we present one complete conflict story: Chuck and Grace's sexual difficulty.

The differences between Chuck and Grace's interest in sex and their ways of expressing it have multiple origins. In part they represent stereotypical sexual differences between males and females in America and thus may reflect the ways that boys and girls are socialized. In part they may represent biological differences between men and women. But their differences also reflect their own personal histories.

Grace came from a more religious home than Chuck, where modesty was the norm. She learned about sex from her parents, who made sure she heard it first from them so they could place sexual expression in the appropriate context of love. Prior to her relationship with Chuck, she had had only one sexual relationship, with a longtime boyfriend whom she considered marrying. Her sexual relationship with him was positive but very traditional. They made love in the dark, with him on top.

Chuck learned about sex on the streets from his friends. His father made a feeble effort to tell him about sex by leaving him a book and by inviting him to ask any questions "about men and women" he had. Chuck wasn't sure what his father was talking about and wasn't interested in pursuing it. When Chuck was older, his father advised him to "keep his pecker in his pocket." At that point his father had little credibility with Chuck. Chuck was sexually active during his late teens and early 20s. He had many different relationships, and sex was an important and enjoyable part of all of them.

Grace and Chuck met when they both were in their middle 20s. He was immediately attracted to her and pursued her energetically. She was flattered by his attentions but set firm boundaries about sexual contact. He respected her limits but was also challenged by them. As their relationship developed, Grace often found Chuck's intense interest in her a "turn-on" and his pursuit of sexual novelty provocative. He found excitement in the need to woo her constantly. Their differences sparked the sexual tension between them.

As time went on, his consistent sexual interest became less flattering, less exciting, and more clearly an annoyance to Grace. Her hesitancy and, at times, active resistance became less of a challenge to Chuck and more of a barrier to sexual satisfaction. Chuck's physical affection and loving attention to Grace, which had always served as an aphrodisiac to her, suffered from their sexual conflict and from the familiarity of daily contact. How could he be so attentive and loving to her when he felt so neglected sexually? To Grace, Chuck seemed less and less interested in loving her and more interested in merely using her for sexual pleasure. How could she be sexually responsive when she felt no love from him?

What were once his loving nudges and her demure limits became, over time, insistent pressures and bald refusals. Frustration at her lack of response and anticipation of a negative reaction robbed Chuck of the gentleness and charm with which he had often pursued her. The tension of his urgent demands hardened her into resistance.

What changed in them was not only the way they dealt with their differences but the very differences themselves. His demands dampened any spontaneous interest in sex Grace might have had. Her resistance to sex and the deprivation he experienced created greater, not less, desire in him. So now he wants sex more than ever and she wants it less than ever.

The sexual problems also created or accentuated vulnerabilities in each partner. Grace had never been completely confident in herself sexually. Now she felt even more anxiety about sexuality and, when she wasn't angry at Chuck, wondered what was wrong with her. Chuck had always taken pride in himself as a good lover. But he too, when he wasn't focused on Grace, began to wonder about himself. He certainly was not a good lover with Grace. So both became more sensitive about their own sexuality.

Stressful circumstances often exacerbated the problems that Chuck and Grace experienced. She was always more open to sex when she was fully relaxed, but with a full-time job and two small children she rarely found moments with no demands on her. Chuck had always found sexuality a release from stress and tension. The natural relaxation from orgasm was one thing he knew would reduce his stress. So his desire for sex often increased when he was under stress, while hers decreased when she was under stress. Yet they were often under stress at the same time.

Grace now feels a relentless pressure from Chuck to have sex. Even if he doesn't express it directly, the way he looks at her tells her he is thinking about having sex and wondering if now is the time. Even when she agrees to sex, she feels pressure to do it in ways that make her uncomfortable. It seems as if his own desires for sex carry the day. No allowance is made for her feelings. She wonders, "How can he care about me when he pushes his own sexual agenda and shows no consideration for my feelings?"

Grace's feeling of pressure about sex is real and intense. And furthermore, that feeling is grounded in reality: Chuck does "check her out" often in the hopes of finding interest or at least concession on her part for sex. During sex he often pushes for experimentation and variety. However, Chuck hardly ignores her feelings. He scrutinizes her so intensely because he is aware of her feelings and tries to gauge her emotional state before making any sexual moves. He rarely makes a sexual advance in which he is oblivious to her mood. In fact, his sensitivity to her moods in part creates the scrutiny that adds to the pressure she feels!

With a problem this large and consuming, they each think about it a lot. She wonders if he really loves her at all. He wonders if she secretly wants to emasculate him. As they share their individual ideas about the problem, these ideas become part of the problem. They argue not just over when and how to have sex but about why they are the way they are and about possible solutions to the problem. She accuses him of using her as a sex object. He accuses her of being frigid and compares her to other women. They generate angry, simple, and impossible solutions to the problem. He suggests that she "just do it," whether she feels like it or not. Then maybe she would get used to sex and become comfortable with it. She suggests he ignore his adolescent impulses and stop letting them control his life. Then maybe he could grow up and have an adult sexual relationship.

How can a story like this be helpful to a couple? Their problem seems so difficult, their pattern seems so entrenched, and they each seem so stuck that no solution seems possible. But if this story accurately defines their problem and truthfully describes the defeating ways that each tries to solve the problem, the story is right. And if the couple begins to understand their problem according to this story, they may be more accepting of each other's behavior in this situation. They may ease off on the accusation, blame, and defensiveness that made the initial problem a more serious reactive problem. They may be able to find some compassion for each other among the tatters of their sexual relationship. They may feel less alone in their experience of this hurtful problem because they find a fellow victim in, of all places, their partner. They may find emotional intimacy in their struggle together. And the intimate union of those who struggle together can be a mighty force against the biggest of problems.

RECAP

The first step toward solving a problem is to define it appropriately. A good definition of a relationship problem is a story about the problem on which both partners can agree. It is a story that incorporates the kind of analysis described in Part II but for a particular couple's unique problem. Like any good story, a story about a relationship problem emphasizes certain features over others. A good story is one that emphasizes differences between partners rather than deficits in either of them, that underscores vulnerabilities in each rather than violations by either, that highlights the stressors that each experiences and their understandable responses rather than the stressful overreactions that each may have, that focuses on description rather than evaluation of their efforts to cope, and that defines complex dilemmas rather than simple solutions to the problem. Such a story, which is a unique "anatomy of an argument" for one couple, gives each partner a rich understanding of the problem that provides a basis for both acceptance and change.

Exercise: What Simple Solutions Have You Tried?

You have completed most of the exercises in this chapter already, by writing out your DEEP analysis, being sure it doesn't include unhelpful elements, and using the DEEP analysis to look at a recent example of the conflict. A final brief exercise is to look at the simple solutions that both you and your partner have proposed but that have not worked, at least so far. It is helpful to know what doesn't work. However, as you achieve greater understanding and acceptance of your core problem and read later chapters on problem solving, you may be able to take some aspect of your simple solutions and incorporate them into a more workable resolution.

Simple solutions to the core issue that I have proposed (perhaps in the heat of conflict):

Simple solutions to the core issue that my partner has proposed (perhaps in the heat of conflict):

Next Steps

In this chapter, we focused on a DEEP and complex understanding of a problem by creating a story about the problem, a story that doesn't rely on simple one-sided solutions. Such an understanding can lead to greater acceptance and even subtle spontaneous change. At the very least such a story can lessen the likelihood that a reactive problem develops as a result of faulty dealing with the initial problem. However, there are other ways besides intellectual understanding to create acceptance, such as through sympathy and compassion, a topic to which we now turn.

CHAPTER 9

Walking in Your Partner's Shoes
ACCEPTANCE THROUGH COMPASSION

> ... the things that tormented me most were the
> very things that connected me with [others].
> —JAMES BALDWIN, *New York Times* (1964)

> Be me a little.
> —JOHN AJVIDE LINDQVIST,
> *Let the Right One In* (2008)

Sylvia and Gerard are in constant conflict over the level of closeness in their relationship. Sylvia feels she is not a priority in Gerard's life. He seems to get more excited about a possible promotion at work or a ski weekend with his friends than about being with her. For his part, Gerard sees Sylvia as constantly dissatisfied. He can never seem to do enough for her, as if he must constantly prove to her that he cares. The struggle of it all makes him wonder at times how much he really does care.

The problem over closeness has become an unbreachable wedge between them. Sylvia is easily angered by signs of Gerard's lack of commitment to her. If he gets heavily involved in work, or seems too excited about recreational events that don't involve her, or shows little interest in activity with her, her anger often reveals itself in sarcasm: "I hope it's not a burden for you to go with me." Or in provocative comparison: "You seem awfully happy about going out—a lot happier than I have seen you in a while." Or in outright accusation: "You don't make me a priority in your life. I am way down on the list." Gerard typically responds by defending himself, insisting that she *is* a priority for him, that he *does* want to be with her. However, when he gets completely frustrated with her, he may counterattack: "There is no pleasing you. You are so insecure, you need constant attention." At times Sylvia gets so worn out by the conflict and feels so hopeless about getting what she needs from Gerard that she shuts down. She stops blaming, but anger pervades her silence.

Can love, caring, or compassion ever break through the cloud of anger and distance that surrounds this couple? If you and your partner are stuck in a similar tornado of anger and hurt, it may seem impossible to extricate yourselves. But when your focus shifts from the offending actions of each of you to the emotional sensitivities that are bruised by these actions, you may come to a new understanding of each other—one that cuts angry arguments short and over time brings you closer together.

This is no simple task, of course. Anger is the most common surface emotion to erupt during conflict, and it tends to become a chronic state when we feel our needs are repeatedly thwarted, when we feel overwhelmed by constant demands, or when we feel slighted, discounted, or neglected day after day. Under those conditions we adopt the coping methods discussed in Chapter 6, which usually numb our compassion and blind us to what we need to stay focused on: the emotional sensitivities that get injured during this process. Whether we opt for the familiar trio of accusation, blame, and coercion; the evasive tactics of avoidance, minimization, and denial; or a more subtle strategy of putting up defensive barriers and striking back through passive resistance, we end up not being heard and not feeling safe in a relationship that should be a sanctuary for both of us. We get trapped in an emotional bind that erodes our love for and commitment to each other. We may wish for compassion, but our loved ones seem too alienated and angry themselves to give it.

The way to break this pattern of chronic anger, withdrawal, and defensiveness is for both partners to disclose aspects of themselves that they have never or rarely mentioned or to disclose these aspects in ways that they have never voiced them before. The revelation of the hidden emotions that we discussed in Chapter 4 is one important way to elicit empathy from the other and to alter the pattern of communication between you. But it isn't easy.

The Importance of the Unsaid

Much unhappiness has come into the world
because of bewilderment and things left unsaid.
—FYODOR DOSTOEVSKY

What we don't say is often more important than
what we do say.

Chronic conflict can leave you believing that you've already said everything that can be said on the subject of contention—and far too often at that. In fact, though, you and your partner probably have not revealed many of your important thoughts and feelings about the conflict. You may be only dimly aware of your feelings, or you may not feel safe disclosing them. Yet it is precisely these revelations that could alter the tone of the discussion and perhaps elicit empathy between you.

THE ANGER ITSELF MAY NOT BE DISCLOSED

As difficult as it may be to believe, considering the tone of your voices and your mutual accusations and defenses, you and your partner may not be expressing your anger directly. One of you may be caught up in laying blame, while the other is preoccupied with self-protection, rebuttal, and counterattack. One or both of you may be distant and resentful. Neither of you says outright, "I'm really angry at you right now."

Would such a disclosure help? Possibly not. One could respond to the other's disclosure competitively: "Well, you're not as angry as I am." Or sarcastically: "Well, isn't that too bad." Or dismissively: "So?"

There is certainly no automatic benefit from this or any similar statement, so why take the risk of merely escalating the argument? Because a direct statement of anger calls attention to what is probably the most important aspect of the discussion: its emotional underpinnings. This simple disclosure can be a first step away from futile debate over the evaluation of behavior and toward a potentially fruitful discussion of each one's emotional experience.

This first step is possible, however, only if the statement is made strictly to convey information about yourself, rather than information about your partner. If you say "I am really angry at you right now" as a cover for an attack, meaning "You made me angry because of all the horrible things you do," or as a challenge, meaning "I'm angry, and you better do something about it right now," you're not shifting the discussion from blame to personal disclosure. Even if you make the statement appropriately, with all the right intentions, your partner may believe, because of his or her own defensive state, that you are accusing or challenging.

Furthermore, it will probably take more than just a simple comment, no matter how pure, to keep the focus on your emotional experience and not get caught up with accusation and defensiveness. For an example, see the diagram on page 162. In the right boxes, Sylvia gets drawn into an argument with Gerard. In the left boxes, she avoids the temptation to attack his behavior or to defend her own. She keeps the focus on her emotional experience. Although there are no guarantees, her focus on her emotional experience may enable Gerard to listen to her and even share his own emotional experience.

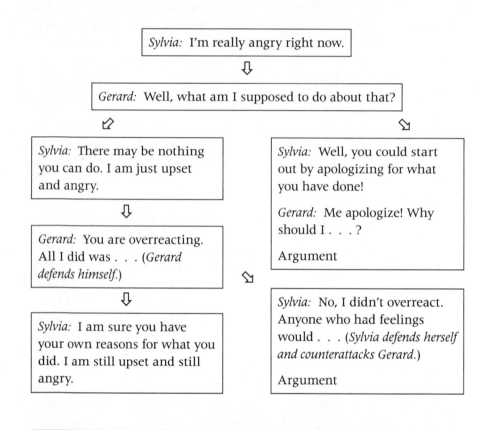

Tip 1: When you are upset, try to reveal your emotional state to your partner without blaming him or her for it. When your partner is upset, be curious about his or her emotional state.

URGES AND FEELINGS ARE ACTED UPON RATHER THAN VOICED

When Sylvia is frustrated by the lack of attention from Gerard and his apparent greater interest in his work and his hobbies, she accuses him of not loving her. Gerard responds by defending himself and asserting his love for her. He recounts evidence of his love—for example, that he has been sexually faithful to her, that he hasn't tried to leave the relationship. She often replies: "You list the things you haven't done that show love. Tell me anything you have done that shows love." Gerard will then try to list times he has attended to her, like when she was hospitalized with pneumonia. She then dismisses his evidence: "That was years ago" or "That is not love—any reasonably responsible person would have helped."

In fact, Sylvia is so angry at Gerard's neglect that she is unlikely to be swayed by any factual evidence he can muster. It is as if she is saying "I am angry, so I am going to prosecute you for lack of love." And he is saying in response "I'm threatened by your upset, so I'll try to calm you with terse, dismissive recitations of fact."

If Gerard were aware of what was going on with himself emotionally at the moment and could genuinely articulate it, he would say something like "Right now I'm feeling attacked by you and feel like I need to defend myself. And when I'm focused on defending myself, it's hard for me to feel love, even though I know I *do* love you."

Such a disclosure might be scary for Gerard to make. He would fear an even stronger reaction from Sylvia: "See? There—you finally admitted it. You don't love me." And he might be drawn into an even bigger defense: "I just said 'right now.' I didn't mean I don't *ever* love you." On the other hand, Gerard's disclosure might stop the frustrating charade they go through in which Sylvia tries to generate love through angry accusations about its absence and Gerard tries to prove his love with a defensive listing of facts.

If Sylvia were aware of what was going on with herself emotionally at the moment and could genuinely articulate it, she would say something like "I'm so angry at you right now that I'm not open to hearing you. I just want to attack you." Such a message would be difficult for Sylvia to make because Gerard could easily use it against her. "See, you admitted it. You don't care about whether I love you or not—you just want to attack me." However, her disclosure could prevent his fruitless efforts to prove himself to her. And it might make him listen to her.

These kinds of communications are certainly difficult, sometimes even impossible, during conflict. But they can take you another small step away from your vicious cycle of argument because you are saying what you feel like doing, such as attacking or defending, rather than actually doing it. They express the urge in place of the action.

> **Tip 2:** When you are emotionally upset, try saying what you feel like doing rather than actually doing it. When your partner is upset, try to discern what he or she is feeling that may be driving your partner's upsetting actions.

CRUCIAL BACKGROUND INFORMATION MAY BE LEFT OUT

Arguments can become so habitual and reactions so immediate that partners play their parts with little knowledge of what set them off. They may not even notice important conditions that set off a particular discussion and make it different from previous ones. Or if they do notice, they may be hesitant to disclose those conditions.

For example, Sylvia is concerned about some lumps she has felt in her breast. She tried to get Gerard to feel them, but he made only a half-hearted attempt, saying "I'm no doctor." He told her to see her doctor, which he often says in response to her (admittedly) many physical complaints. At this point, his message to "see your doctor" seems dismissive, a cover for "Don't bother me about it."

Sylvia's concern is great enough that she does make an appointment with her doctor. She lets Gerard know of the appointment in advance—to which he responds with an unconvincing "That's good." Angry that Gerard shows so little interest in her concerns, Sylvia is dimly aware that her notification of the appointment is in part a test: Will he remember her appointment and comment on it?

Sylvia has a fitful night's sleep before her appointment. That morning she awakes worried, she feels her breast, and she detects what clearly seems to be a lump. She goes into the kitchen and finds Gerard, as usual, with his head in the newspaper, eating his breakfast. He barely acknowledges her entry into the kitchen.

Her fear over her appointment turns to anger at Gerard. She sarcastically voices the observation: "That must be a fascinating article in the paper."

He replies defensively: "I said hello."

"Oh, was that hello? I thought it was some bodily noise."

Gerard assumes that this is the same old conflict: "Come off it, Sylvia. Can't a guy read the paper in peace?"

Sylvia has an urge to blurt out something about her appointment but doesn't, for fear he will dismiss her concerns. Then if her "lumps" prove to be nonsignificant, he would gloat about being right and lecture her again about not getting so worked up. The angry part of her hopes that the doctor will find something serious so she can use it against his dismissal and lack of concern for her.

Gerard leaves Sylvia that day irritated by what he labels her "weird moodiness." He wonders in passing if she is premenstrual. She leaves that day in a mix of anger at Gerard and fear about what the doctor might find.

The crucial piece of information that would have made the morning understandable—her worry about her upcoming visit to the doctor—was never a point of discussion. Gerard forgot it. Sylvia never brought it up, partly for fear of his likely dismissal of her concerns and partly in anger, to save as a later weapon against him.

Even if Sylvia did mention her appointment, she might have done it in such a blaming way that Gerard would get caught up in defending himself rather than in hearing her concerns. Even if she were not blaming, Gerard might have been defensive rather than responsive to her. Yet her mentioning that day's appointment and her feelings about it might have served to refocus their discussion. It could have led to some genuine support from Gerard. Not mentioning it at all robbed them of that opportunity.

> **Tip 3:** If you are upset, give your partner enough background information to make your emotions understandable. If your partner is upset, inquire about factors that may have triggered the emotion.

SOFT EMOTIONS MAY REMAIN HIDDEN

When things happen to us that we don't like, we experience hard emotions such as anger, irritation, impatience, resentment, frustration, and disgust. These emotions, and their accompanying hard thoughts, express a strong self that says in no uncertain terms "I'm upset with the world" and "I'm not going to take this anymore." These are often the surface emotions and thoughts that we readily reveal. Expression of them is beneficial because it often provides a release for some of the negativity we feel and because it establishes our boundaries with others. Unfortunately, it also often invites a response in kind: anger may elicit anger and resentment. This cycle not only can lead to escalation but also may actually discourage the love and compassion whose absence evoked the hard emotions in the first place.

Soft emotions, in contrast, reveal a vulnerable self experiencing inward anguish. Hurt, guilt, sadness, disappointment, and fear all signal a pain inside. They reveal a wounded self rather than an assertive self. They are often accompanied by softer thoughts that express doubt and uncertainty. These are the hidden emotions and thoughts that we usually keep to ourselves.

Any significant negative experience in relationships is likely to lead to both hard and soft feelings and both hard and soft thoughts. If my partner ignores me at a party, I may feel anger at the neglect, but I also may feel hurt and insecure. I may wonder "How can you treat me this way?," but I may also feel hurt that my partner didn't find me more interesting. If I end up doing most of the housework, I may resent the injustice of it all but also feel devalued as a partner because my role is to "just do the housework." I may decide not to be manipulated into being a housekeeper but also wonder about my value.

The expression of soft emotions such as hurt and fear can often trigger caring and concern in your partner. When we see others in pain, particularly others we care about, we naturally feel compassion for them. We want to comfort and protect them. We forget about our own needs and reach out to them. Unfortunately, soft emotions and soft thoughts usually go unexpressed in conflict. Often they are attempted but sabotaged by the atmosphere of hard emotion around them. One may voice "I feel hurt by you," but the manner in which the admission is delivered and the emphasis on the "by you" at the end make it more an accusation than an expression of pain. Even the simple statement "I felt hurt" can be expressed more in anger than in pain.

A genuine expression of soft emotion, a voicing that you are lonely or hurt or disappointed or feel neglected or abandoned, is difficult because it opens you up. It presents you as vulnerable and defenseless. It may feel uncomfortable to do in any circumstance and impossible to do when you are angry.

Gerard and Sylvia rarely give voice to their hidden emotions surrounding their conflict over closeness—for the very good reasons of self-protection. Exposure of these feelings might make them more vulnerable to each other and more open to attack. Yet exposure of these feelings might elicit compassion and caring for each other. In voicing these feelings, they might be able to listen to each other's pain without assigning responsibility for that pain. They might experience connection and closeness with each other in the joint realization of how distant they are and how much it hurts. The problem could bring them together. Paradoxically they could experience closeness from a compassionate sharing of their feelings of distance from each other.

Tip 4: When you are upset, try revealing the soft emotions that may exist alongside the hard emotions you experience. If your partner is upset, see if you can discern what softer emotions he or she may also be feeling.

THE OTHER SIDE MAY NEVER BE DISCLOSED

In an enduring conflict, each partner stakes out a position, argues that position, defends that position, and becomes more and more entrenched in that position. Sylvia's position is that Gerard doesn't express enough love and affection for her. Gerard's position is that Sylvia demands more than any reasonable man could give. In their regular conflicts over this issue of closeness, neither backs off or acknowledges any validity in the other's position.

In Sylvia and Gerard's conflict, as in most conflicts between couples, there is some truth in each person's position, and there are no clear external standards for judgment. Logically, then, each must question his or her own position at times. Sylvia must wonder if she is asking too much of Gerard or if she is too needy or oversensitive. Similarly, Gerard must wonder at times if he is selfish or ungenerous or unloving. Both are reluctant to express such doubt about themselves because these disclosures of doubt could easily be used against them.

Yet expression of these doubts would acknowledge the validity of each person's position. Questioning their own position or admitting to the truth in the other's view, if made genuinely, without either false modesty or pretentious nobility, might elevate both Sylvia and Gerard from the struggle over who is right and who is wrong. Then they might be able to join one another in the realization that both are right and both are wrong. Relieved of the burden of defending themselves or attacking the other, they might be able to struggle more successfully with their difficult problem. They might even feel closer together as two human beings who both have limitations.

> **Tip 5:** If you can genuinely do so, acknowledge the validity in your partner's position without abandoning your own position. Know that your partner at times may question his or her own position and sense the validity in yours.

ANTICIPATIONS MAY NOT BE SHARED

Even when couples are *not* in the middle of conflict, they may anticipate future conflict. Having been through certain arguments so often in the past, they know the kinds of events that provoke them. These "preliminary events" take place, and couples anticipate, often accurately, that conflict will soon follow. They may be reluctant to share their anticipations for fear that the very act of sharing will hasten the conflict. Yet, without some intervening communication, the anticipated conflict may proceed inexorably.

On their way to a skiing weekend, Sylvia gets concerned that Gerard, who is a better skier than she, will abandon her on the slopes or will devote so much attention to skiing that their relationship will get short shrift. She remembers one ski weekend a year ago when he got up early to get on the slopes before the crowds arrived, skied all day, and then made noises about going night skiing. At that point she blew up and threatened to go home by herself. He didn't go night skiing, but he might as well have; they had a horrible evening together.

If Sylvia tries to express her concerns with an irritable and challenging "I hope you don't turn this weekend into the fiasco we had last year," Gerard is likely to respond negatively. He may defend himself: "All I wanted to do was try a little night skiing, and you went ballistic." Or he might counterattack: "There you go again. We're not even in the mountains, and you're already anticipating the worst."

Even if Sylvia tries to express her concern in a nonattacking way, such as by saying "I'm worried that we're going to get into a struggle about skiing," Gerard may hear her concern as an attack. He may respond with an irritable "You just can't leave things alone, can you? Always have to worry about things going wrong. Maybe that's what makes them go wrong."

If it were Gerard rather than Sylvia who voiced concerns about the weekend, we could easily imagine a similar scenario. He might express his concerns in an accusatory way ("I hope you don't go ballistic this year about skiing") that leads to counteraccusations by her. Or he might express his concerns more cooperatively ("I hope we can cooperate on skiing this year"), but she might hear them as accusations, leading to an identical outcome. With such risks involved in an anticipatory discussion, both might choose to avoid a discussion and simply hope for the best.

A history of struggle inevitably leads to emotional anticipations. If Gerard and Sylvia have had difficulty coordinating their needs on skiing trips or on vacations in general, they are going to have anticipatory thoughts and feelings about the upcoming weekend. They can avoid an open discussion of their anticipations, but they can't avoid having anticipations. If those anticipations are strong, it may even be difficult to keep them from slipping into a conversation. Sylvia's seemingly innocent comment that she wants to relax and "sleep in" may be a "trial balloon" to test whether Gerard plans to hit the slopes at first light, or it may be heard by him as such a test. Gerard's seemingly innocent comment that skiing conditions are supposed to be great this weekend may be a test of Sylvia's possible reaction to his skiing as much as possible. Even Sylvia's casual comment that she hopes they have a great weekend may carry a subtext of "You better shape up and watch it" or be heard by Gerard as such.

If Gerard and Sylvia could openly disclose their concerns about the upcoming weekend without sparking a conflict, they might feel some relief in their joint apprehension. Having their concerns validated might ease those concerns.

Sylvia: I'm a little worried about this weekend.

Gerard: You mean about us.

Sylvia: Yeah.

Gerard: We don't have a great record when it comes to ski weekends, do we?

Sylvia: (laughing ruefully) No, we don't.

A discussion about the upcoming weekend could do more than simply relieve their concerns. They might be able to discuss how to manage the weekend so both get their needs met. They could make sure they have time together as well as time apart for Gerard to challenge himself on the expert slopes. It is possible for Gerard and Sylvia to have both a close relationship and good skiing, but it might take some communication and cooperative effort. Avoidance of discussion leaves a lot to chance.

Tip 6: Try sharing your anticipatory concern with your partner before you approach a challenging event. See if the two of you can acknowledge the difficulty you have had in the past and possibly plan for a better event.

Recovery from Conflict

In the heat of conflict, we often feel so angry or defensive that we are unable or unwilling to disclose the kinds of information just discussed, information that offers the possibility of understanding and intimacy even in the face of conflict. Even if we are able to disclose this information and follow the preceding tips, our partners may not be responsive to it. Therefore, despite our best efforts to alter the course of our conflicts, argumentative patterns are likely to be repeated at times. Progress toward intimacy can be slow despite your commitment to inject acceptance and compassion into arguments.

For this reason, learning how to recover from conflict may be just as important as altering the course of conflict. Barring divorce, all couples recover, to some extent, from their conflicts and resume their normal behavior toward one another. But for days after a conflict partners may withdraw from each other, they may be curt with each other, or they may avoid conversation entirely. If you can short-circuit this process, if you can learn to recover more quickly and with less emotional hangover, you can lessen the total stress of conflict. Furthermore, you are more likely to achieve understanding and intimacy after a conflict than during it.

In the recovery from conflict, as during conflict itself, compassionate understanding of each other is key, but how can that happen? Let's consider one extended conflict between Sylvia and Gerard and then see what they might have done to recover from the conflict. One Friday morning, just as he is about to leave for work, Gerard tells Sylvia that he is going to go on a camping trip the next day with his friend Daren and will be back Sunday afternoon. She reacts angrily because she thought they were going to spend Saturday together. She asks, "Why didn't you tell me sooner?" He replies defensively that they had no plans for Saturday and that no matter when he told her of the camping trip, she would have gotten angry. He leaves for work, and she is furious. As he rushes out, she accuses him of being a coward, afraid of any confrontation with her. He accuses her of overreacting to everything in life and suggests that she is mentally unstable.

Later that day, hoping she has calmed down, Gerard phones Sylvia and tries to be friendly and chatty. He is met with cold nonresponsiveness. Frustrated, he ends the conversation. He tries again for reconciliation after work. He greets her happily and proposes dinner and a movie. She refuses unless he gives her an apology. He resists: "I won't apologize for going camping with my best friend." She replies angrily: "You don't have to apologize for going camping. What you owe me an apology for is for not letting me know until the last minute—and for being such a chicken shit, not telling me until you have to leave for work so you don't have to deal with me and my reactions." Gerard bristles at the accusation, and they argue unproductively, first about whether he should apologize and then about camping and when he should tell her about a planned trip. Finally they set the argument aside and go out to dinner, where their interaction is tense but civil, warming up only a little over the evening.

The next morning as she lies in bed, Gerard kisses Sylvia good-bye. She tells him to be careful but to have a good time. He hears the genuine concern in her voice and tries to reassure her by reminding her when he will be back and saying he will miss her. She doesn't really believe him—he enjoys camping and his friend too much to miss her—but she accepts the warmth with which the comment was given.

Gerard has a great time camping with his friend. The day is beautiful, and the hike is invigorating. He and Daren exchange jokes, argue politics, bring each other up to date on their lives, drink too much beer in the evening, and genuinely forget all their troubles. Saturday doesn't go as well for Sylvia. She tries to make arrangements with some friends, but they are busy. She does some housework but gets resentful because she is at home working while Gerard is out having fun. Later in the evening she tries shopping and a movie, and while both are distracting, she feels lonely. On Sunday, she makes a valiant effort to put aside her resentment and disappointment. She looks forward to Gerard's arrival and wants their reunion to go well.

On Sunday they greet each other happily with a big hug and a kiss. Gerard is relieved that she is happy to see him since he wasn't sure what kind of mood she would be in on his return. Still glowing from the pleasant trip with his friend, he launches into a description of his trip. As he goes over some of the details of the trip and his conversations with Daren, he notices her interest flagging. He asks how her weekend was. She replies, "Not that great!" He offers a perfunctory "That's too bad." Then he describes how tired he is from the trip and goes into the bedroom for a nap.

When he wakes from his nap, Sylvia is angry. He shakes his head and utters a disgusted "What is it now?"

"You just don't get it, do you?" she asks accusatorily.

"No, I don't," he says, with a clear message that he doesn't really want to get it. She storms off into their bedroom. On other occasions he would have followed her, trying to find out what was wrong. Just waking from his nap and worn out by the continuous conflict, he feels no urge to do that now. They spend the rest of the evening in cold distance from each other. They go to sleep without the usual goodnight kiss. The next morning and evening they begin to warm up to each other again, but the whole experience has deepened their negative convictions about each other. She feels more strongly validated in her view: "He just doesn't want to understand me or connect with me." He feels more convinced in his: "She is just like a baby—getting upset if she doesn't get the right kind of attention when she wants it."

Any attempt by Gerard and Sylvia to recover from this incident by talking about it with each other would be risky. They might relive the incident rather than learn from it. Discussion could easily deteriorate into the blame, defensiveness, and withdrawal that characterized the incident itself. This is particularly likely if they focus on the egregious acts by the other and treat them out of context. Gerard could talk about how she called him a "coward" and a "chicken shit"; she could mention his comment suggesting she was mentally unstable. However, it is possible to discuss a conflict in ways that speed recovery from it.

To recover from conflict and have a beneficial postconflict discussion, both partners have to be ready to "get back to normal." Often partners recover at different rates, with one partner initiating recovery when the other partner is not ready, so efforts by one are met with a negative response, setting that one back in his or her desire to recover and perhaps reigniting the conflict. So both partners being in a positive or at least neutral, let's-put-this-behind-us state of mind is a necessary condition for recovery. But what do they actually do to ensure recovery? They can of course act like nothing happened and ignore the conflict, relieved that they are now on a more positive course. But if they wanted to learn from the conflict, what would they talk about?

THE BUILDUP BEFORE THE CONFLICT

One topic that would be productive to discuss and that might aid in their recovery from the conflict would be what went on with each prior to the conflict. Gerard had actually been thinking about a trip with Daren for some time, had discussed it with him 2 weeks earlier, and had finalized it on Tuesday. He had gone to some pain to pick a weekend that would not interfere with any of his and Sylvia's plans. He did not let her in on any of his thinking or planning because he was apprehensive about her reaction; she often got upset when he planned something without her. Once he had finalized the plans with Daren, he knew he had to let her know. But Tuesday night he had to work late. On Wednesday and Thursday they were having such a pleasant time together that he did not want to spoil it by bringing up the trip with his friend. He hoped that the positive experiences might buffer a negative reaction. The buildup of anticipation in him about telling her got so great that he did want an easy escape—so he told her Friday morning because he couldn't in good conscience delay any longer and because he would have to leave for work immediately. Her reaction validated his fears: no strategy of disclosure would work with her.

Sylvia had been feeling good about the relationship. She and Gerard had been talking a lot, sharing their experience with each other, but also being playful. They had made love during the week—on Wednesday night—which was unusual for them. Sylvia was looking forward to the weekend because they had no plans; they could just "hang out." Maybe go out for a good dinner and a movie. Maybe play some tennis. Maybe shop together. When Gerard brought up his plans for the weekend on Friday morning, she was crushed and furious. She was upset about his camping plans and angry at the way he had handled them. Why couldn't he let her know what was going on with him? The experience validated her suspicions that he could not be trusted, that she could never know what he had up his sleeve.

A discussion of the events and emotions that led up to the conflict might bridge the emotional difficulties that separate them. As Sylvia learned more about Gerard's efforts to fit his plans into their schedule, of his apprehension about her reactions, and of his search for an opportune time to reveal his plans to her, she might empathize with his dilemma. Similarly, if Gerard learned more about Sylvia's experience—her growing closeness with him during the week, her hopes for the weekend, and then her disappointment and consequent distrust of him—he might feel compassion for her plight.

If Gerard and Sylvia could voice what they had experienced prior to the conflict and if they could empathize with each other's dilemma, they would feel closer to each other in spite of—or perhaps even because of—their conflict. Such a discussion might also be a first step toward change. Even though one productive discussion is unlikely to create dramatic change, Gerard might move a step toward greater disclosure to Sylvia the next time. And although Sylvia may never greet with joy the possibility of Gerard spending a weekend camping without her, she may be more open to hearing his ideas and plans.

Tip 7: To recover from a conflict, try revealing to your partner what was going on with you prior to the conflict. Try to find out what was going on with your partner right before the conflict.

ATTEMPTS AT RECONCILIATION

A second area of potentially productive discussion after a conflict is partners' attempts to reconcile. Sometimes a discussion of recovery and reconciliation is a way to facilitate that recovery and reconciliation. In the conflict between Sylvia and Gerard, each made efforts to reconcile after their initial blowup on Friday morning. Gerard called Sylvia later in the day and tried to be friendly and chatty. Although that effort was unsuccessful, he tried again that evening, but to no avail. After coming home from the camping trip, he also tried to be friendly, and he shared with Sylvia some of the interesting details of his trip. But that too was unsuccessful. Not surprisingly, Gerard became frustrated when his repeated genuine efforts to reconcile led nowhere.

Sylvia also tried to reconcile. On Friday evening, she thought she could reconcile if Gerard would simply apologize. It seemed so clear-cut that he had done something—giving her very late notice of his weekend plans—that was at the very least inconsiderate. Why couldn't he give her a genuine apology? She would not hold a grudge; she could be forgiving. But she would like some acknowledgment of what really happened: that he had failed to consider her feelings. The fact that he refused to apologize not only foiled her attempt at reconciliation but also reignited the conflict.

Although it would pose dangers of initiating a conflict itself, a discussion about these failed attempts at reconciliation could lead to important new understandings between Gerard and Sylvia. Gerard's efforts to reconcile by being friendly and chatty don't work for Sylvia because she sees them as his attempt to avoid dealing with the conflict they have just had. It comes across to her as his effort to duck responsibility for the problem and pretend it doesn't exist. But even if he did not do something that to her seemed to be so patently wrong, she cannot suddenly switch gears from being upset to being friendly and chatty with him. She wants some acknowledgment of the conflict and her hurt feelings before moving on. In the worst of scenarios, Gerard chides her for "holding on to her feelings," which just upsets her more.

Gerard also has a difficult time responding to Sylvia's efforts at reconciliation. Her demands for an apology hardly motivate him to apologize; instead, they create resistance and counterattack. Even when he has done something that he knows was not right—not telling her earlier about the camping trip—the intense anger and demanding tone in Sylvia's voice make a genuine apology impossible for him. He knows that his neglect came not from lack of concern for her feelings; in fact, he put off telling her precisely because he was so aware of her feelings. He doesn't like being the focus of her blame and accusation but, apart from that, he also genuinely hates to see her upset for any reason, both of which led to his avoidance. Furthermore, he believes with some justification that whenever he announced his plans, her reaction would have been negative.

A discussion about these efforts to reconcile and how they went awry might enable them both to see that each was taking action, however misdirected, to get past the conflict. It might enable them to empathize with the other's frustration. More important, it might help Gerard realize the futility of his efforts to reconcile by putting on a happy face or help Sylvia realize the futility of demanding apologies. Neither is likely to be able to change his or her behavior dramatically or suddenly. But Gerard may be more likely to listen to Sylvia's concerns rather than meet her unhappiness with unwanted cheer. And Sylvia may be less likely to demand apologies, which must be given freely if they are to be genuine.

> **Tip 8:** To recover from a conflict, try revealing to your partner your ways of attempting to reconcile or recover. Try to learn how your partner may have been trying to reconcile or recover with you. See if you can understand why your genuine efforts went awry.

THE DANGEROUS AREA OF PAIN

A third area of potential discussion, but a very dangerous one, is injury to one or both. During an argument people often make exaggerated claims and dramatic accusations. While these are hardly pleasant, they may not really injure. When there is injury, when one person's accusation hits a sensitive spot in the other, discussion can both facilitate recovery from the conflict and promote greater closeness. For example, Sylvia's comments that Gerard is a coward and a chicken shit and Gerard's claim that Sylvia is a mental case could be just part of their repertoire of conflict, but these comments might hit a vulnerable spot for one or both. If, for example, Sylvia is sensitive about suggestions that she is not mentally stable, then Gerard's accusation deserves follow-up. If their conversation about this accusation led to some disclosure about how painful it was to her and he could find a way to genuinely apologize for his comment, she may not only recover from the conflict more easily but also experience Gerard's concern for her feelings, an issue that triggered the argument in the first place. Thus their recovery from conflict would address the central issue of their conflict.

You and your partner need to know what jabs truly hit below the belt for each other. Often threats to leave the relationship or statements about not loving the partner are poison arrows that inflict painful wounds. Specific accusations may touch a sensitive spot. A discussion, after an argument, of these below-the-belt jabs risks generating a new conflict of its own. But if partners understand the pain they create in each other and experience some compassion for that pain, there is hope for recovery, future restraint, and even greater closeness after a conflict.

> **Tip 9:** To recover from a conflict, see if you can learn from your partner whether something you said or did was really hurtful to him or her. Try to understand why it was hurtful, and if you can, apologize for what you did. Reveal to your partner, but not in a tit-for-tat way, any injury that you may have experienced from the conflict. Help your partner learn more about your sensitive areas.

THE POSITIVES

A final area of discussion that can aid in recovery, and that is least likely to backfire, is a focus on the positive. Even in a painful struggle, such as the one that Sylvia and Gerard had about his camping trip, each partner often takes actions that deescalate the conflict or that communicate concern or caring. The morning that Gerard left for camping, Sylvia told him to be careful and have a good time. The sincerity he felt in her comment made it easier for him to enjoy his trip without guilt about her. He tried to return her warmth, and even though she didn't literally believe what he said (that he would miss her), she accepted it with the intent with which it was given. Also, when he returned from the trip, they were happy to see each other. The hug and kiss felt good to both. Any attention that a couple can give to their positive actions, any word of acknowledgment or appreciation, may help them recover from a conflict that was too filled with negative actions.

> **Tip 10:** To recover from a conflict, acknowledge any positive action of your partner's that was helpful to you.

RECAP

When all is said, it is rarely done. It is not even all said.
                    —VARIATION ON AN OLD ADAGE

Because arguments are repetitive, couples may assume that they have said everything relevant about a particular conflict. Thus they may feel that their partners just haven't heard them or just haven't responded to what they have said. In this chapter we have discussed many things that are left unsaid in ongoing conflicts. Partners may not disclose their genuine, immediate feelings, even their anger. They may leave out important background information about what led to their feelings. They may express only the "hard" surface thoughts and emotions they experience and not the hidden, softer ones. Stuck in a particular position, they may never express the other side of that position, which they may fear is true. They may not fully disclose their anticipations about future conflict.

Disclosing this unspoken information is indeed risky. The information can be conveyed in accusatory ways or heard as accusatory so that it leads to further conflict. But these disclosures offer important information about the sensitivities of the other. The ensuing discussion could alter the course of their argument and lead to an empathic connection between the two. It could promote compassion in each for the other, a response that each needs. It could move the couple to accept each other's different behaviors and experiences rather than battle over them. Although the stakes are high for failure, these kinds of discussions can bring couples closer together in spite of their differences. Therefore, this chapter offered six tips for revealing this often unspoken information and for discerning that information in your partner:

1. Reveal your emotional state and be curious about your partner's.
2. Reveal your urges to take negative actions rather than taking them; try to discern the urges that may drive your partner's negative actions.
3. Reveal enough background information to make your emotions understandable; try to find out what led to your partner's emotions.
4. Reveal the softer emotions that may exist alongside your hard ones; try to discern your partner's softer emotions.
5. Acknowledge the validity in your partner's position and know that he or she may sense some validity in yours as well.
6. Try sharing your anticipatory concerns before a challenging event as you also try to discern your partner's concerns about that event.

Often couples are too angry and defensive to disclose their vulnerable side to their partner during conflict. Their arguments take their usual course. But then they are confronted with recovery from the conflict. Unless the conflicts lead to divorce, couples eventually return to their normal way of dealing with one another. How can they recover from conflict more quickly and with less emotional hangover?

After a conflict, both partners are often less angry and more open to the other's experience. Sometimes couples can recover more quickly and more fully if they can discuss the conflict without reengaging in it, but only if both are ready to engage in such a conciliatory discussion. The chapter gave four tips for such conciliatory discussions:

1. Reveal to your partner what was going on internally with you prior to the conflict, but also learn what was going on internally for your partner.
2. Reveal your efforts at reconciliation and learn your partner's efforts for the same.

3. Inquire whether something you said or did was really hurtful to your partner during the conflict; reveal to your partner any injuries you experienced.
4. Acknowledge any positive action of your partner's that was helpful to you.

Some couples experience their moments of greatest intimacy after conflict. They heal each other's wounds with love. They demonstrate that conflicts don't just alienate; they can also unite.

Exercise: What You Would Say If You Said the Unsaid

One of my former colleagues used to give the following advice about relationship conflict: "When in trouble, self-disclose on the double!" He was suggesting that self-disclosure of what we have called hidden emotions and thoughts can often alter the conflict you find yourselves in or can help you recover from an immediately preceding conflict. Of course, to do that, you have to be fully aware of those feelings and thoughts, and you have to be willing to express them. So our advice is "realize and reveal!"

Let's look at a specific example of how that might be done. Call to mind your last heated conflict about your core issue. Once you have remembered it clearly, consider the following topics, see if you can recall what you felt or might have felt, and jot down some ideas for what you could have revealed.

PRIOR TO THE CONFLICT

Concerns/fears in anticipation of the conflict that might have been shared:

_____

_____

_____

DURING THE CONFLICT

Feelings or urges that you acted on but didn't reveal:

_____

_____

_____

Important background information you may not have mentioned:

_____

_____

_____

Soft, hidden emotions that you weren't completely aware of or that you were hesitant to mention:

_____

_____

_____

Any validity in your partner's position:

_____

_____

_____

RECOVERY FROM THE CONFLICT

Attempts at reconciliation that you attempted or noticed your partner attempting:

_____

_____

_____

Particularly painful things that you or your partner may have said that really hurt each other:

_____

_____

_____

Positive efforts at reconciliation that you attempted or noticed that your partner attempted:

_____

Next Steps

Emotional acceptance cannot be mandated, but it can be fostered. In the last chapter we saw how acceptance can be fostered through a true understanding of the problem, what we called a common "story" about the problem that both endorse. Then, in this chapter, we saw how acceptance can be fostered by compassion, an empathic connection to the distress your partner feels without denying or abandoning your own distress. Empathy is most important when emotional sensitivities in you and your partner are essential parts of your conflict. In the next chapter we will explore a final and very different way for fostering acceptance, one that works well for the differences between the two of you that create conflict.

CHAPTER 10

Getting Some Perspective on the Conflict

ACCEPTANCE THROUGH TOLERANT DISTANCE

> Emotion recollected in tranquillity. . . .
> —WILLIAM WORDSWORTH,
> "LETTER TO LADY BEAUMONT" (1807)

If compassion is the best response to a loved one's emotional sensitivities, then tolerance is the optimal attitude toward problematic differences (or similarities). When our sensitivities cause conflict, empathy may prevent an escalation of argument or foster recovery from it. We may find greater emotional closeness as we accept each other's weaknesses. But when emotional soft spots are not the issue, a little distance and objectivity can remove the barbs that make our differences sting.

When both of you remove yourselves from the fray, you become more like observers and less like combatants. Distance allows you to view your struggles from a similar vantage point, to see your conflicts more clearly, and to accept each other's role in them. This emotional distance and the acceptance that goes with it may not solve the initial problem, but it often heads off associated reactive problems.

It is easy to see why tolerant distance rather than compassion is the best way to handle incompatibilities that differences may create. In a case of "pure" incompatibilities, there is nothing to be compassionate about, except the struggle that the incompatibility entails. If you and your partner can never agree on whether the house is too warm or too cold or if you differ on whether to go to bed late or early, it is unlikely that either of you feels vulnerable about your position. The incompatibility does not, by itself, raise primitive fears or threaten self-esteem. Thus there may be little or no need for empathy.

Our most important struggles, however, are *not* likely to center on pure incompatibilities. In most cases, our sensitivities combine with our incompatibilities to produce emotional volatility. In these cases, the approaches discussed in the previous chapter are appropriate. However, the ways of seeking a joint, tolerant distance, which we describe in this chapter, can be helpful for incompatibilities even when they are powered by vulnerabilities. For most of us, getting some distance from our conflicts through a broader perspective, objective observation, or humor is helpful even when the problem taps deep and sensitive emotions. We may take our conflicts less personally, deal with them more reasonably, and recover from them more rapidly.

However, for some couples, emotional distance may be part of the problem and therefore not a solution to the problem. For example, a husband may use his excellent sense of humor to avoid dealing with difficult issues. His humor may serve to distract his wife from her concerns with him. If it is hard for her to articulate her concerns in the first place, his efforts may be successful. As another example, both members of a couple may be adept at objectivity, observation, and analysis but use these skills to avoid taking a stand on issues. Afraid to confront each other with their different needs and desires, they keep such a distance from the issues that they are unable to resolve them. In these cases, we would not want to encourage emotional distance.

The "story of your problem"—your DEEP analysis of your core issue, if it accurately captures the difficulties you face, your struggle over these difficulties, and the emotional consequences of that struggle—offers guidance as to the appropriate antidote for your difficulties. It can help you sort out what may resolve your conflicts and what will merely perpetuate them. We will discuss this notion more fully in Part IV of this book.

For most of us, who aren't prone to avoid issues through distancing, tolerant distance can be very helpful. Consider Eleanor and Terry. Eleanor is more emotionally expressive than Terry; when she feels upset about something or happy about something, she lets everyone know it. Terry, on the other hand, is more comfortable with understatement than exaggeration. He often finds Eleanor's expressive style irritating; in public he is frequently embarrassed by the attention her expression provokes. In extreme cases, he is overwhelmed by what he sees as her unnecessary hysteria. Eleanor is frustrated since, as she sees it, her own husband won't listen with concern to her troubles; instead, he discounts them. Their incompatibility about emotional expression is fueled by Eleanor's sensitivity about being heard and Terry's about being "put upon" emotionally.

To get emotional distance from a problem about strong emotion, and to be united in their distance, will be a challenge for Terry and Eleanor. But such distance, like compassion, can prevent conflict or facilitate recovery from conflict and foster acceptance of the characteristics that lead to conflict.

Treating the Problem as an "It" Rather Than a "You"

Partners often experience their problems as "things *you* do to me" rather than as "difficulties *we* have." To move from this first position, seeing problems as a "you," to the second position, seeing problems as an "it" or a "them," is a major leap forward. It transfers the fault from one or the other to outside both. How can couples make this experiential leap?

BROADENING THE CONTEXT

Because our partners' differences hurt and annoy us, it seems as if that is their intent. Terry believes Eleanor's emotional expression is intended to get his attention or upset him just because that is the effect her expression has on him. Eleanor believes Terry is trying to exclude her from his inner life because his lack of emotional expression does have that result. Neither can see that the other's behavior is her or his style of emotional expression because they are too close to the immediate conflict.

Of course, there is a little truth in each one's views of the other. Anticipating that Terry may discount her feelings, Eleanor exaggerates her feelings or expresses them more stridently than she would otherwise. And Terry does sometimes avoid telling Eleanor about his feelings because he's concerned about how she might react to them. These behaviors confirm their mutual suspicions of deliberate intent, so they hold fast to their views.

When you are too close to a conflict, a partial truth may obscure the larger truth. In the case of Eleanor and Terry, the larger truth is that their different manners of emotional expression come naturally to each of them. Eleanor's style of emotional expression is primarily Eleanor, rather than a manipulative means of provoking Terry into responsiveness. And Terry's limited expression of emotion is primarily Terry, rather than a conscious attempt to exclude Eleanor from his inner life.

By putting their differences in a larger context, couples are better able to see the larger truth that much of their behavior toward each other is not a deliberate offense but a product of many factors over which they have little control, including their genetic heritage and their upbringing. If Terry viewed Eleanor's greater emotional expressiveness as typical of women and Eleanor viewed Terry's emphasis on action over emotion as typical of men, neither would view the other's behavior as so personal. Books on gender differences sell in great numbers because they make it easier for men and women to understand and accept behavior that they often find baffling in each other. If Terry were much older than Eleanor, their differences in emotional expression could be viewed as a product of the social mores of the times in which they grew up. If they came from different cultural backgrounds that put different emphases on emotional expression, they could attribute their differences to their cultural heritage.

Perhaps the most effective way to gain emotional distance from differences is to view them in their historical context. Partners who have a sense of how each other was raised or the role each played in his or her family of origin may view their differences more charitably. For whatever reason, Eleanor's family was emotionally expressive. During one of his first visits with her family, Terry observed an argument among Eleanor and her mother and father that both amused and frightened him. He worried that her family was at risk of splitting apart even as he was amused by the strong feelings about what to him was nothing. In contrast, Eleanor finds Terry's family nice and polite but surprising in their careful avoidance of controversy. She wonders why they don't "engage their issues." If Terry and Eleanor viewed their own differences in the light of their divergent family experiences, their differences would make perfect sense.

Seeing your differences in the context of gender, age, culture, or personal history eliminates some of the blame and fault finding. You are not "bad" or "wrong" for being the way you are. You are simply the natural product of your gender, age, culture, and personal history. Without blame and fault finding, your problems are less likely to escalate or polarize or lead to alienation. In short, they are more acceptable.

> **Tip 1:** Try to understand your differences in the light of the differences in your backgrounds, including the cultural experiences associated with your age, gender, ethnic identity, and family history.

OBSERVING RATHER THAN PARTICIPATING IN THE INTERPERSONAL DANCE

Trying to discuss your problems puts you in danger of reliving them. Rather than probing your difficulties, you end up reproducing them. When Eleanor and Terry try to discuss their differences in emotional expression, Eleanor is liable to get emotional and Terry is liable to discount her concerns. They reveal the same pattern in their discussion of the problem as they do in the problem itself.

Even if you don't re-create the problem, you may create another reactive problem. If you were trying to talk with your partner about the fact that the two of you have not made love in a while, your discussion could easily deteriorate into blame and defense. Now, in addition to the sexual neglect and deprivation you feel, you have a problem of argument and anger.

If you can step back and observe your own interactions, you can describe what goes on between you rather than each championing a particular position. You can identify the pattern of interaction that occurs between the two of you rather than perpetuate that pattern. You can describe your problems rather than reenact them.

Observation requires distance. You and your partner must step back emotionally or physically if you are to focus on what is occurring. If a soldier is asked to report on a battle, he must temporarily put down his gun, move to a different vantage point, put on his binoculars, and focus not on aiming at a particular target but on looking more broadly at the field of conflict. A soldier cannot be a good warrior and a good observer at the same time. The demands of battle preclude observation, and the demands of observation preclude attack.

What should you be observing once you're able to step back from your conflict? You can scrutinize your coping processes. How does each of you deal with whatever differences or sensitivities were triggered? You can look at the sequence of communication as you try to solve the initial problem. The key is to describe what goes on rather than judge what goes on.

For Terry and Eleanor, the conflictual sequence typically starts with an event that upsets Eleanor, such as a problem at work or an interaction with a friend. She voices her concerns to Terry, who responds by minimizing them. These comments upset Eleanor, who then expresses her concerns more vociferously. Then Terry, upset at the way Eleanor handles her concerns, remarks on Eleanor's emotional reactivity. These comments, which Eleanor feels are unsupportive at best and critical at worst, further upset Eleanor. An argument ensues, with both eventually withdrawing in anger. After some time during which they maintain emotional distance, they gradually get together again.

This bare-bones analysis could be fleshed out with a description of the triggers for each person's emotional reaction and a description of the emotional reactions themselves. The initial trigger for Eleanor is a disappointing or frustrating event that takes place in her world apart from Terry.

Of course, she can also be disappointed or frustrated by Terry, but when a problem starts with her and Terry, the dance is somewhat different. She talks to Terry about her problems with the world because he is the one to whom she feels closest. The emotional trigger for Terry is seeing Eleanor upset: he gets upset by her upset. In his view, she frets about every little thing that happens to her. He responds by trying to show Eleanor that she has no basis for being upset. His comments serve as a second emotional trigger for her: not only does she have to deal with the event in the real world that upset her, but now she also has to deal with Terry's dismissal of her feelings and his not-so-subtle criticism that she is too reactive to her world. Now Eleanor has to face both the issue in the outside world that originally upset her and an interpersonal struggle with Terry. Of course, Eleanor's increased upset feelings serve as a second emotional trigger for Terry. So now the two are off and running. The initial problem that bothered Eleanor has been replaced by a far more serious reactive problem between Eleanor and Terry.

One way to detach yourself from your emotions is to examine them logically, almost like a scientist would study them. Even the simple act of rating your emotional intensity on a 10-point scale, in which 1 refers to no emotional arousal and 10 refers to the greatest emotional arousal you have ever experienced, can help you get some valuable perspective on a conflict because it requires you to back away from the emotion you are feeling now and look at it in comparison to other emotional experiences. This "backing away" helps you distance yourself from the emotion, and the ratings may shed light on it. For example, the level of emotion Eleanor experiences about events she wants to discuss with Terry is usually about a 5. Of course, there are those rare occasions when she gets really upset by something, but mostly her emotional reactions to daily disappointments are in the middle of her emotional range. However, if the event Eleanor experienced happened to Terry, he would respond with only a 2. In contrast, Terry's emotional reaction to Eleanor's emotional reaction is usually higher in his range, about 6. So he can handle daily frustrations with less emotion than Eleanor, but he can't handle Eleanor's emotion about those daily events without getting emotional himself. When Terry reacts to Eleanor with a 6, she reacts to him with an 8. This in turn leads to about an 8 emotional reaction in him. So the emotional intensity goes from 2 to 8 for him and from 5 to 8 for her in short order. Their interaction has amplified the emotional intensity caused by whatever event Eleanor originally experienced. If they were mindful of this process and could observe it while it was happening without judging it, that escalating intensity could be reduced.

> **Tip 2:** In mindfulness training, the acronym STOP is often used to instruct people how to separate briefly from immersion in their daily activities and become more mindful of what they are doing: **S** stands for "**S**top what you are doing," **T** stands for "**T**ake a deep breath," **O** stands for "**O**bserve what is going on," and **P** stands for "**P**roceed with what you were doing." Try using a slightly different version of STOP when you get into a difficult situation with your partner: **S**top what you are doing, **T**ake a deep breath, **O**bserve the interaction between the two of you, and **P**roceed differently with the interaction. Below we will show you some ways to proceed differently.

CREATING A NAME TO BLAME

There is often value in naming a problem in relationships. The name creates some emotional distance, suggesting that the problem is an "it out there" rather than "a you/me in here." Thus you can talk about the problem, the "thing" you two get into, rather than creating a problem through your analysis of it.

You can name both the role you each play in the conflict and your communication together. For example, a possible name for Eleanor's role is "volcano" since her emotional eruptions strike Terry as unpredictable and disruptive. At times they feel that way to Eleanor too. A good name for Terry's role would be "muffler," since his efforts are aimed at muffling the emotional intensity that Eleanor both feels and expresses. Although these mixed metaphors might not fit the canons of ideal English expression, they express the futility of their positions. There is no effective muffler for a volcano.

Be aware, though, that selecting names for the roles you each play can backfire. Names chosen to ridicule or blame will not distance you from the conflict but rather further it. A safer route is to name only the pattern of communication that generates toxic solutions. Unfortunately, our language doesn't provide many terms to describe a process between two people, so creativity will be required. But it will be worth the effort since names that describe a process cannot be used as easily against each other. Eleanor and Terry originally chose "emotional amplification and escalation," or "EAE," to describe the way their emotions built up during communication, but they eventually settled on "MAD" for "mutual amplification and destruction" because it was more creative, it acknowledged the contributions of each, and they liked the irony of its similarity to the cold war policy of "mutual assured destruction."

Having a name for your conflicts can enable you to talk about them without reliving them because it describes your dance without condemning either of you. You can use these names to avoid or limit the enactment of your conflicts. When Terry says to Eleanor, "I feel a MAD coming on," he often deters or lessens their conflict. When Eleanor asks Terry, "Are we fully into MAD yet?" she sometimes facilitates an exit from their conflict.

> **Tip 3:** After stopping, taking a deep breath, and observing your interaction, try to proceed differently by labeling the pattern of interaction between the two of you. Even simple phrases such as "I think we are getting into it again" or "Here we go with our usual dance" can often be helpful. If you have previously agreed on a term to describe your pattern of interaction, invoking that term can be most helpful.

LAUGHING AT OURSELVES

Humor can create emotional distance by providing comic relief and facilitating a quick change of perspective. Exaggeration, self-deprecation, and gentle sarcasm can short-circuit automatic retorts and give you both a chance to handle the situation better than you might have without the humor. Eleanor might say, "I am really upset about this—and I know you will want to hear all about it." Or Terry might comment, "Oh, tell me all about it—you know how I love to hear the ins and outs of your emotional upheaval." These comments might work as long as they are not made with such sarcasm that they could be interpreted as criticism.

Conflict in couples has provided rich material for comics and cartoonists because intimate arguments are often filled with paradox, contradiction, and absurdity. If you catch a revealing glimpse of this absurdity, even if you never share it or laugh at it together, the intensity of your conflict may diminish. If Terry notices the contradiction in his getting upset about Eleanor's getting upset, or if Eleanor observes the absurdity in their efforts to quell each other's emotional arousal by getting more aroused themselves, both may find themselves a bit removed from the conflict.

Anyone who has ever tried to relay a funny story or joke knows the difficulty of importing humor. It is even more difficult to offer any advice about humor in the context of conflict. But when partners can laugh—or even smile—at their predicament, they have achieved some healing distance from their conflict. Even a sense that "We'll laugh at this someday" can dampen the passion of the moment.

> **Tip 4:** Try injecting humor into your interaction as a means of lessening the tension. Be aware, though, that laughing at yourself, such as with a self-deprecating comment, is more likely to succeed than poking fun at your partner, no matter how gentle the poke.

Reality Check: When Is Distance Achievable?

Achieving the kind of intellectual distance and detachment we have been discussing is rarely possible in the heat of battle. There may be times when you can momentarily take an observer's stance during conflict. Like the soldier mentioned earlier, you may put down your weapon temporarily to get a better view of the battle. Even these brief attempts to observe rather than participate can dampen the current conflagration. However, it's unrealistic to expect ourselves to talk about an "it" when we have just been stung by a "you." The ability to create emotional distance and the benefit from it usually comes well before the battle or well after it.

If we see an argument coming enough in advance, our ability to anticipate its sequence can sometimes lessen the pain it causes even if it can't prevent the argument entirely. For example, Eleanor might worry aloud that she will get only a small bonus at work this year and remark, "And if I don't get a decent bonus, after all my work, I will probably have an emotional meltdown—which I am sure you will enjoy." Or if Eleanor is worrying about her bonus, Terry might comment, "Well, even if you don't get a decent bonus, I'll be able to share in your pain!" Such comments might bring a rueful smile to one or both and protect against a blowup if Eleanor does not get what she wants.

Even the act of describing an oncoming pattern of conflict may prevent or alter its occurrence. The husband in the cartoon on page 190 describes a potential sequence of argument with his wife rather than engaging in that argument. His pithy description may minimize their conflict.

Perhaps the biggest benefit of emotional distance accrues after a conflict. Establishing some distance is another way to facilitate the recovery from conflict that we discussed in Chapter 9. Let's assume that Eleanor does get a meager bonus, and she and Terry play out their usual pattern of emotional escalation. After they have calmed somewhat, humor might help them recover. Terry might poke fun at himself: "I have been considering a career change. Maybe I should become a therapist—since I'm so good at handling other people's emotional problems." Or Eleanor might acknowledge their predicament: "I think you got smothered in the ash of my vol-

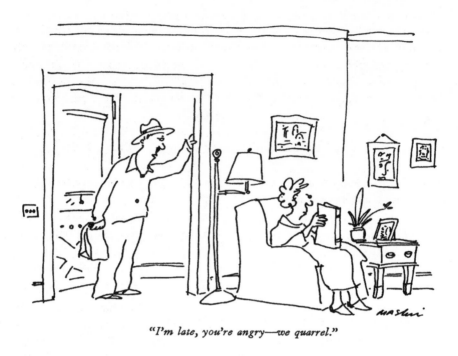

"I'm late, you're angry—we quarrel."

cano." With these comments Terry and Eleanor make fun of themselves and acknowledge, with humor, their role in their struggle. These comments then aid in their recovery from that struggle.

> **Tip 5:** Try making a light comment when you see the two of you getting into a conflict or after the two of you have weathered a conflict, as a means of lessening the tension between you. Again, a comment at your own expense is more likely to be successful than one at your partner's expense.

Finding the Blessing in the Curse

In Chapter 3 we discussed confusing differences, those complex differences with our partners that arouse mixed feelings. Sometimes we want our partners to be different; at other times we like and support the way they are. In the heat of conflict, the negative characteristics of our partners may stand out so dramatically and may be broadcast so powerfully that we fail to see the larger context in which they appear. However, if we are able to distance ourselves from the conflict, we may get some perspective on our partners' characteristics. We may see the positive features and the attractive pull of our partners' negative characteristics. This "understanding from a distance" may help us recover more quickly from conflict and perhaps even avoid some future conflict.

Terry is often so focused on Eleanor's negative emotional reactivity that he is not aware of the pull of her emotions for him. Early in their relationship he found her broad emotional range exciting. It added color to his life. Her energy, excitement, and enthusiasm appealed to him. Even her negative emotional reactions were often engaging for him; he felt good when he could comfort her in her upset state.

For her part, Eleanor found Terry's emotional stability comforting. He was so logical and organized and reasonable that he could help her with many of the problems she faced. There was a synergy between their characteristics. Her emotionality added excitement to his life, and his stability provided an anchor for hers. Despite their conflict, they have learned from each other. His connection with her has added emotional depth to him; her connection with him has provided much needed structure in her life. Typically, their struggles over her emotional reactivity eclipse the positive characteristics that each brings to the battle. However, when either becomes even dimly aware of the complex exchange they have made—a measure of emotion for an equal measure of stability—they may shake their heads with a mixture of frustration and appreciation. And they may feel greater acceptance of the differences between them and struggle less over those differences.

Even when the negative characteristics of our partners don't have an obvious attractive side, they may force us to confront some of our own negative characteristics. Because Terry was not used to strong emotion and was somewhat intimidated by it, he often avoided confrontation with others. He chose to evade rather than to risk a showdown; he opted for the white lie rather than the bald truth. With Eleanor, however, his strategy of avoidance didn't work. Her "in your face" emotional reactions forced confrontation. The struggle with her drove Terry to take a stand on issues. Although Terry will never relish open confrontation, now he is less intimidated by strong emotion at work or other settings. And he has Eleanor to thank for it.

Eleanor's emotional reactivity seemed to have only two positions: on and off. There seemed to be surprisingly few degrees of intensity to her emotional reactions. Some trivial negative event could arouse almost as much feeling as a truly important event. In her struggles with Terry, he derided her for getting "upset over nothing." He sometimes refused to listen to her emotions. Although his actions provoked additional distress in her at the time, their cumulative impact was not all bad. Eleanor learned to choose what she needed to tell Terry and what she didn't need to tell him. Although she is disappointed that she cannot share more of her emotional life with Terry, she has learned to define what is and what is not important. Eleanor will always have something of an all-or-nothing emotional system, but she has learned to handle her emotions when they are "on" and to make some choices about what she wishes to share. Terry has been her reluctant teacher and she his resistant student.

The grudging respect that each has gained for what the other brings to the relationship has taken some of the edge off the struggles that Terry and Eleanor have over emotionality. They still get into their arguments, but these arguments are somewhat lighter, less painful, and easier to recover from.

> **Tip 6:** After the heat of battle, consider the positive benefits that your partner's negative characteristics have provided for you. A consideration of these mixed blessings may ease your discomfort with your partner.

It's Not as Bad as It Seems

Couples conflict consists largely of significant reactions to trivial events. Although there are high crimes in relationships, most of the struggles are over misdemeanors. Some of us may betray, deceive, or otherwise violate our partners, but usually the struggle is over lesser matters.

To an outsider, it may seem unreasonable that such trivial events raise such strong emotions. An objective observer might view Eleanor's emotional reaction to her frustrations at work as excessive, Terry's reaction to Eleanor's attempt to tell him about it as an overreaction, Eleanor's subsequent response as exaggerated, and Terry's subsequent response as almost hysterical.

An objective observer of Terry and Eleanor's interaction might try to explain to them the unreasonableness of their reactions. This observer might try to use logic to convince both that their emotional responses are inflated. Reason, however, is impotent in the face of strong emotion. Someone who is phobic about flying will be unaffected by statistics on the safety of airline travel. Someone who lives in terror of snakes won't make distinctions between those that are poisonous and those that are not.

Psychologists have developed powerful ways to desensitize strong emotions, particularly fear. They gradually expose the person to the feared object but in a safe and supportive environment. As people experience their feared object at a comfortable distance, they may be able to tolerate closer and closer contact until their fear eventually subsides. Likewise, we can gradually expose our partners to pieces of our behavior that cause emotional distress in them. If we know the triggers that set them off, we can create a situation in which those triggers are less likely to get activated. For example, Eleanor might approach Terry with the comment "I want to share some emotional stress in my life. Are you in an okay position to listen?" With this remark, Eleanor shows that she understands what triggers emotional reactions in Terry, she warns him of what she wants to do, and in so doing, she may enable him to handle her emotional distress without himself getting so distressed. Of course, a comment like this requires some perspective by Eleanor. If she is too distraught, she will just unload on Terry without any warning. Also, Terry may not be in a position to listen to her even if she does approach him with sensitivity to his possible reactions. She may have to accept no for an answer sometimes.

For his part, Terry could warn Eleanor of a potential trigger for her if he voiced his intent before his action. For example, he might say, "I have this urge to talk to you about your reaction and explain to you that the problem is not a big one, but I don't know if you are open to that. I don't want you to feel discounted or criticized." Such a comment would indicate considerable awareness and restraint by Terry. Depending on his own emotional state, he might simply be unable to say something like this, mean it, and accept the possibility that Eleanor might not be open to hearing him. However, on those occasions when he could make such a comment, it might enable Eleanor to listen to him.

> **Tip 7:** Try checking with your partner before you expose him or her to something that may trigger your partner's sensitivities. Your respectful consideration of those sensitivities may enable your partner to respond more positively to what you have to do or say.

On Your Own—But with a Little Help from Your Friends

Intellectually, we can probably all endorse the notion that our partners cannot meet all of our needs or fulfill all of our desires. We know that there are differences for which accommodation or compromise is no solution. For some of our needs and desires, we don't expect or seek fulfillment from our partners. Particularly if our partners have never met our needs in a particular area, we may have no difficulty going elsewhere. Or if our desires seem like a "male thing" or a "female thing," we may find it easy to get satisfaction with a friend of our own gender. Terry has no problem going to football games with his friends without Eleanor as she has no problems shopping with her friends without Terry.

If a need or desire is intense and personal, however, it may not be easy to fulfill outside of the relationship. Also, if the need has historically been satisfied inside the relationship, a partner may understandably expect continued satisfaction at home. Early in their relationship Terry was happy to comfort Eleanor when she got upset, but the frequency and intensity of her emotional reactions have since discouraged Terry's responsiveness. Eleanor still believes that in marriage you should be able to share your troubles, no matter what they are, with your partner. Terry also endorsed that ideal once upon a time.

Eleanor does have several friends who serve as emotional supports for her. Often they are better help for her than Terry. But if Eleanor has to go to them too often, she gets upset at Terry for not being there for her. And she feels more distant from him because he is not part of her emotional life. Yet the reality is that Terry is not able to listen to her distress as much as she would like him to. At times, she will be distressed and he will be unavailable. She will be alone in her upset. For Eleanor to seek comfort from her friends can be a solution, but only a partial one, for their incompatibility.

Although friends offer solutions to some incompatibilities, seeking their help and counsel has risks. It's very easy to try to turn friends into allies against our partners, which only hurts our own relationship, as was discussed in Chapter 6. Friends help most when they can meet some of our needs without joining in the conflict we have with our partner over those needs. Then these friends enable us to accept our partners and their limited ability to meet all of our needs.

> **Tip 8:** Try using your friends to meet some of the needs that your partner has difficulty meeting, as long as your partner is okay with that and your friends don't become allies against your partner.

RECAP

Because their conflicts are so painful, couples would like to exorcise them from their lives. They want to obliterate the repetitious quarreling and make it go away, right now. Certainly Terry and Eleanor would like to surgically remove their repeated trauma of Eleanor's upset, Terry's reaction at her upset, and Eleanor's further upset. In this chapter we have provided no remedies to exorcise conflict. Rather, we have shown ways to tame conflict, to domesticate it rather than demolish it. We have shown that it is possible for couples to accept conflict and live with it.

In dealing with any problem, the first step is to identify it properly. When partners identify the problem as being one or the other, their efforts to solve the problem will often make it worse. If couples can treat the problem as an "it" that they both face, they may be able to view their differences in a more dispassionate way. They may see their differences in the larger context of their gender, their age, their culture, or their personal history. They may be able to observe the sequence of what happens between them and discuss that sequence from a mutual vantage point. They may be able to identify the roles that each plays and to see their struggle in a larger, even at times humorous, perspective. Thanks to this larger perspective, they may see the blessing in the curse: the advantages as well as the disadvantages their partners' characteristics provide them. They may be able to tolerate the negative side of those characteristics, with perhaps a little help from their friends. We provided the following eight tips to help you achieve these goals.

1. Try to understand the differences between you and your partner in the light of your backgrounds, including the cultural experiences associated with your age, gender, ethnic identity, and family history.
2. When you get into a difficult situation with your partner, STOP: Stop what you are doing, Take a deep breath, Observe the interaction between the two of you, and Proceed differently with the interaction as indicated in the next three tips.
3. Try labeling the pattern of interaction between the two of you, particularly if you have mutually agreed on a good descriptive term.
4. Try injecting humor into your interaction as a means of lessening the tension. Be aware, though, that laughing at yourself, such as with a self-deprecating comment, is more likely to succeed than poking fun at your partner, no matter how gentle the poke.
5. Try making a light comment when you see the two of you getting into a conflict or after the two of you have weathered a conflict, as a means of lessening the tension between you.
6. After the heat of battle, consider the positive benefits that your partner's negative characteristics have provided for you.

7. Try checking with your partner before you expose him or her to something that may trigger your partner's sensitivities.

8. Try using your friends to meet some of the needs that your partner has difficulty meeting, as long as your partner is okay with that and your friends don't become allies against your partner.

It is almost impossible to maintain a tolerant distance and implement the relevant tips in the heat of the battle. During an actual argument each member will experience the problem as a "you," not an "it." However, taking this larger perspective before a battle may ease the conflict; taking it afterward may facilitate a quicker and easier recovery from conflict.

If couples cannot exorcise their demons, maybe they can tame them.

Exercise: Preparing for Tolerant Distance

To better prepare you for the inevitable conflicts you will have with your partner, we want you to review some aspects of your core conflict and consider possible ways to implement the tips above. Then you may be able to lessen your conflict by distancing somewhat from it.

Consider your core conflict and your DEEP analysis of it. How are the central differences or similarities that give rise to this conflict related to your age, gender, cultural background, or specific personal histories? Jot down a couple of ideas about what may have given rise to these differences.

_____

_____

_____

Describe some of the positive features of those differences (or similarities). How are they helpful to you or the relationship even though they are also problematic?

_____

_____

_____

Recall the last conflict you and your partner had over your core issue (which you considered in the last chapter). Presumably it involved some variation of the pattern of interaction you identified in your DEEP analysis.

Describe the sequence of that specific interaction as if you were an objective observer (i.e., without blaming either of you). Then try to come up with a humorous name to describe that general pattern of interaction.

_____

_____

_____

Still considering that last conflict, what comment could you have made early on in the conflict or before the conflict got heated that might have altered the course of the discussion? What comments could you have made afterward that might have facilitated recovery from the conflict?

_____

_____

_____

Considering the core conflict as a whole, are there any desires/needs related to that conflict that you could satisfy elsewhere that wouldn't escalate the problem? If so, describe them.

_____

_____

_____

Next Steps

In Part III of the book, we first reviewed the differences between acceptance and change and considered what things in the relationship should be accepted and what should be changed. There were precious few, albeit very important, things that should be changed universally, such as violence, or accepted universally, such as a partner's basic essence or personality. Other things that should be accepted or changed are individual matters, with the caveat that what we think should be changed in our partners or accepted in ourselves usually make up prohibitively long lists. We then reviewed ways of fostering acceptance, since it cannot be commanded or forced. Having an objective and joint story about the problem is the first step. Fostering empathy for each other's emotional sensitivities that are triggered in conflict is a second step. Finally, developing a tolerant distance for the differences that engender conflict is a third step. We offered concrete tips for moving toward an empathic connection with your partner and developing more tolerant distance before, during, and after a conflict.

These strategies for fostering acceptance often create greater emotional closeness in the relationship. Furthermore, they can bring about spontaneous change, as each partner usually loves and wants to please the other. A person who feels more accepted and less pressured will often try to improve the relationship on his or her own. However, sometimes change is needed and is not forthcoming. So in our next section, Part IV, we will explore ways of bringing about constructive change in relationships.

PART IV

Deliberate Change through Acceptance

CHAPTER 11

The Dilemmas of Deliberate Change

There is nothing permanent except change.
—HERACLITUS, QUOTED IN DIOGENES
LAERTIUS, *Lives of the Eminent Philosophers*,
TRANSLATED BY ROBERT HICKS (1925)

If we want things to stay as they are, things
will have to change.
—GIUSEPPE DI LAMPEDUSA,
The Leopard (1957)

As many old sayings tell us, there is nothing as certain as change. It is not a question of whether we and our relationships *will* change but of *how* they will change. In fact, keeping things the way they are often takes considerably more effort than changing them. If you doubt this, try keeping your new car or new house in the same condition it was in when you bought it.

One kind of change is the slow, imperceptible modification that comes inevitably with time. In relationships, such changes can be either good or bad. Time and experience may mellow us. Issues that seemed very important to us early in the relationship may seem less so later. But sometimes our experience makes things more difficult. We become more sensitive and irritated by our partners. We become less tolerant. We become less appreciative of the good things our partner does. We become better and better at being worse and worse.

Another kind of change is more sudden, usually brought about by circumstance. Negative events that affect our relationships may happen unexpectedly, such as losing a job, getting injured, or developing a serious medical problem. Or positive events may affect our relationship just as suddenly, such as getting a promotion that requires a move or becoming pregnant after several unsuccessful attempts. Whether the changes brought by time and circumstance are sudden or gradual, they often affect our relationships in unplanned ways. If an accident has occurred, not only did we not know we were going to get injured, but we had no idea how dramatically it would affect the division of labor in the relationship. While we may have strived for the job promotion that meant the family moved, we may not have anticipated the disruption to our circle of family and friends and how that would affect our relationship.

In contrast to these changes, another kind of change that can occur in relationships is deliberate change. We want our partners to change in specific ways. We want them to act and to be different so that our relationships can be different. Sometimes we want these deliberate changes from the very beginning of the relationship when we notice something aversive in our partner. More often, the inevitable changes that time and circumstance bring to our partners and our relationships make us seek deliberate change.

From Acceptance to Change

Part III of this book focused on acceptance as an alternative to deliberate change. When you give up the effort to change your partner and instead accept him and his behavior toward you, he often makes spontaneous changes in the direction that you originally wanted. Relieved of the pressure to defend himself but with an experience of the emotional impact of his behavior on you, he may make accommodations for you on his own. Similarly, when you experience acceptance from him, you may make spontaneous changes in the direction that he desires. In the best of cases, these mutual changes promote further accommodation to each other.

While that is the ideal scenario and often occurs in relationships, it doesn't always work that way. Acceptance doesn't always lead to spontaneous changes. Nor does it always lead to greater intimacy. Even when it does, these changes may not be enough. Sometimes we want and need deliberate change.

Our first impulse is usually to seek immediate and dramatic change.

The Showdown: Immediate and Dramatic Change

> It is only in romances that people undergo a
> sudden metamorphosis.
> —ISADORA DUNCAN, *My Life* (1942)

We may fantasize about an overnight transformation in our partners. We may wish for a single confrontation, where we drop any pretense that all is well, where we no longer spare our partners' feelings. Instead, we point out bluntly and forcefully how their misguided actions and neglectful inactions have caused not only our suffering but their own suffering as well. We point out their limitations and their inadequacies. We provide elaborate and detailed examples, which have been preserved carefully in our memory, that illustrate their deficiencies. They may battle our logic, but it is a battle of the defeated. Inside, they know the validity of our claims. They soon abandon any defense and acknowledge the truth in what we are saying. They summon the strength and courage to make the changes we enumerated. The next day, all is different in the relationship. A transformation has occurred. There is a sea change in their behavior and attitude. We are happier, and they are happier too. Ultimately, they are grateful to us for making change happen. And we live happily ever after.

As we saw in Part I of this book, most of our efforts to change our partners—and thus our relationships—are driven by this fantasy. And most of these efforts are unsuccessful. Yet we often persist in this tack. And when repeated confrontation brings no change, we may threaten our partners, implicitly or overtly, with negative consequences. At one extreme are destructive threats, which not only destroy mutual trust and respect but may end in violence (which is never acceptable and is discussed in more depth in Part V). At the other extreme are empty threats. We may warn of unforgiving anger, unbridgeable distance, or relationship breaches such as infidelity, separation, or divorce. Because these threats are never carried out, our partners eventually recognize them as cries of "Wolf!" and tune them—and us—out.

Most threats are ineffectual at best, destructive at worst. But the most powerful threat—the *ultimatum*—has the potential to alter the course of a relationship dramatically and positively—as long as it meets certain crucial criteria. When these criteria are not met, the ultimatum's potential for inflicting damage is as great as its potential for evoking change.

Betsy and Frank had dated for a year before they started seriously discussing marriage. In those early discussions Frank professed his love for Betsy but insisted that he was not ready for the binding commitment of marriage. In his eyes, marriage was a prelude to having children, and although he wanted children eventually, he knew he wasn't ready yet. Betsy expressed some urgency to "get on with their relationship." She was not ready for children either, but at age 31 she wanted the assurance of a commitment to marriage and the goal of children in the future. Over the next 6 months they had a series of discussions about marriage that frustrated both of them. Betsy grew more and more doubtful about Frank's attachment to her and his willingness or ability to commit to marriage. Frank grew more and more uncomfortable with the increasing pressure he felt. Betsy began indicating to Frank, at first indirectly and then directly, that she would break up with him if he was unwilling to marry her. At first Frank advised her not to give him an ultimatum. When pressured, he called her bluff. Betsy left, vowing never to see him again.

Because they missed each other terribly, they got together again, but it wasn't long before the old problem arose once more. Betsy insisted again that they either marry or break up; Frank tried to talk her out of her ultimatum. She ended the relationship a second time, but this time with greater conviction, knowing that a reconciliation without marriage would only prolong her pain. Although she talked to Frank on occasion, she refused to see him. Her actions thrust Frank into a major reevaluation of his life. He feared the loss of someone who had become the central figure in his life. He ultimately decided to marry Betsy.

Betsy insisted on a marriage in the near future, to which Frank at that point agreed. Despite some conflict about the marriage ceremony itself and some adjustment after the marriage, Frank and Betsy got along well. Because their relationship was essentially a good one, and because they cared about each other so deeply, their marriage was a solid connection between the two. Years later, they looked back with amusement at Betsy's ultimatum. Frank appreciated the strength Betsy had shown in insisting that their relationship move on. Betsy appreciated the fact that when push came to shove, Frank had been there for her.

Frank and Betsy's experience represents the best-case scenario for ultimatums. Their outcome was positive because Betsy's ultimatum met five crucial conditions.

First, Betsy's threat was real. As much as she loved Frank, she had made a decision to break up with him if he didn't marry her, and he eventually realized she was serious. Second, Betsy's ultimatum centered on a single decision: that Frank marry her. Her ultimatum did not demand unspecified changes or some indeterminate amount of change. Instead the ultimatum forced him to make a crucial choice. Third, Betsy's ultimatum demanded the change within a short time frame. She insisted that they set a date immediately and that the date be within 9 months. She did not demand repeated actions over some undetermined but long period of time. Fourth, Frank did not lose his sense of independence or autonomy by acquiescing to her ultimatum. Because of the nature of their relationship and the way she delivered the ultimatum, Frank knew that Betsy was not simply making a power move to exert control over him. He knew her decision to give him an ultimatum was a tortured one for her and made in part out of desperation. Even though he didn't want to, part of him also believed that it was time for them to make a choice about marriage. Finally, the decision that the ultimatum demanded was something that set into motion a whole series of additional positive changes (rather than something Frank had to "grin and bear"). By getting married, Betsy and Frank changed their status with friends and family, had greater daily contact, and were legally entwined, among other things. For the most part, the two experienced these changes as positive.

When all of these five conditions don't exist, ultimatums usually fail. If you're not serious in your ultimatum, you will communicate ambivalence and probably not get an answer. If you demand something nonspecific and vague, it will be impossible to tell whether the demand is met. If Betsy had insisted that Frank show her more consideration or more respect or more love, Frank would not know exactly what he was supposed to do and when he had done it. Likewise, requiring change in an indeterminate time frame makes it impossible to tell when the demand has been met. If your partner perceives your ultimatum as primarily an attempt at control, your partner may reflexively reject it. Compliance would mean not only giving up something but also giving in to someone. Frank could have rejected Betsy's ultimatum because he couldn't stand her telling him what to do—even if he would have eventually chosen on his own to marry her. Even if Frank had succumbed to Betsy's ultimatum, the resentment he might have felt after being forced to marry her might have contaminated their marriage from its beginning. Finally, if compliance with an ultimatum doesn't have the prospect of creating additional positive changes, that ultimatum and compliance with it will be a mistake. Betsy made the astute judgment that Frank's doubts indicated real but temporary anxiety on his part but did not reflect serious inadequacies in Frank or in their relationship. She believed that after marriage his doubts would fade as they enjoyed their life together. Frank eventually came to the same conclusion. Fortunately their judgments were right. If they had been wrong, they would have married only to face the difficulties for which Frank's reluctance had been a warning sign.

Even if you meet these five conditions, your partner may refuse to comply, or the decision to acquiesce may not have the anticipated positive effects. Ultimatums are high-risk ventures and should be your last-ditch effort at change. Yet many couples owe their satisfaction, even their very relationships, to a well-placed ultimatum to have a child, to enter couple therapy, to get married, to seek treatment for alcohol abuse—or else. However, for many more couples, failed and abandoned ultimatums litter the battlegrounds of their relationship.

Tip 1: Use ultimatums rarely if at all, and only in the rare circumstance when there is a major relationship violation, a major decision, or a major personal problem. Then use them only when you are serious about following through, when you are asking for a specific change within a particular time frame, when the change is likely to bring future positive changes, and when you can do it without creating such resistance in your partner that he or she will refuse simply to save face.

Everyday Change

Fortunately, ultimatums are usually considered—by all but the most histrionic—only in the rare circumstances where a major, seemingly intractable, problem is encountered. Most of the change we seek in our relationships, and most of the change we will get in our relationships, is gradual change in everyday behavior.

The gradual changes we want often seem simple and direct to us: Do more of the housework. Spend more time with the kids. Don't be so critical. Pay more attention when I talk to you. Be more ambitious at work. Put more energy into our relationship.

At times these deliberate changes come relatively easily. Our partners try to do what we want; we try to do what they want. At other times the changes are much more difficult. Why?

WHEN DELIBERATE CHANGE IS RELATIVELY EASY

Specific versus General Changes

A specific change can be made more easily than a general change. If Caitlin requests that Luke "put more energy into the relationship," and he is motivated to comply, he may make heroic efforts but fail to give her what she wants because he isn't sure what that is. If what she wants is for him to do more things like plan their recreational events, she'll have more success if she specifically asks him to do just that.

Asking your partner to comply with your requests for general change requires your partner to do two things: translate your general request into specific changes and then make those specific changes. The first step— translation of a general request into specific changes—can be difficult if you do not have a lot of awareness of what your partner really wants. Chances are that, since you're reading this book, you tend to think a lot about your relationship, your partner, and the impact your behaviors have on your partner and the relationship. However, your partner may not have the same level of awareness. If not, making specific rather than general requests is going to be especially important.

Turning a general request into a specific request is complicated because any single request, however accurate, may not be sufficient to satisfy the general request. Caitlin would feel better if Luke did more of the planning of their recreational events, but that alone might not be sufficient to satisfy her desire that he put "more energy into the relationship," because there are many other ways in which he still seems unenergetic. Furthermore, if he invested more energy in general into the relationship, then the fact that he never made the plans for their Saturday nights would not bother her. Thus, there are a variety of ways that Luke could put more energy into their relationship; several changes are needed to satisfy Caitlin, but no particular change is mandatory.

Despite this complexity, Caitlin will be more successful in getting Luke to change if she lists the specific things she wants him to do. If he knows concretely what she wants, he is more likely to act on at least some of her requests.

Taking Action versus Restraining Action

It is easier to change by doing something positive than to change by stopping something negative. It is normally easier to do more of something good than to do less of something bad. Therefore, when possible, a change should be phrased in terms of what you want rather than in terms of what you don't want. It is easier to "vacuum every Saturday" than to "stop waiting until I tell you it's time to vacuum." It is easier to "initiate sex with me occasionally" than to "stop being so passive in sex." In each case, the listener will hear a positive request for action rather than a combination of criticism and a request to stop some action.

Although this admonition to phrase requests in a positive way is useful, it can sometimes miss the boat. Luke complains that Caitlin is "too negative," and he would feel better if she were not so critical of him. She could change more easily by doing something active for Luke, such as being more complimentary of him, than by holding back her criticism. Yet this would not satisfy Luke. Yes, he could always use a few more compliments, but she is already generous with her praise. What bothers him is her criticism, and it would still bother him even if she gave a stronger dose of praise. So even though it is easier for Caitlin to increase a behavior than to decrease it, the change that Luke really wants from Caitlin is less criticism.

However, most often the changes we want from our partners are specific, positive actions on their part. In our frustration with them, we may focus on what they shouldn't do. But what we really want is for them to take some concrete actions. For example, Caitlin may chide Luke for being lazy and urge him to stop "pampering himself." However, what she may really want is for him to do specific things like getting up with the kids on a weekend and giving her a chance to sleep in. He is more likely to do what she wants if she makes the direct request for the action she wants rather than requesting he not do the actions that she doesn't want.

Changing How You Are with Me versus Changing How You Are with the World

There are two kinds of changes we can seek in our partners: a change in how they treat us or communicate with us and a change in how they are with the rest of the world. An example of the first is Caitlin's request that Luke "pay more attention to me," while an example of the second is her request that he "be more ambitious at work." Certainly, some requests for change, such as "be more open and communicative," can cover how our partners are with us *and* with the rest of the world. However, this distinction is important for at least two reasons. First, we have more legitimacy when we request changes in how our partners treat us. When our concerns are directed at how our partners talk to us or play with us or work with us, it is clearly "our business." Caitlin certainly has a right to discuss, for example, whether Luke is attentive to her or not. However, if we want our partners to behave differently at work or with their friends or with their family, they can argue that these areas are "none of our business." Although we have joint control with our partners over what happens when we are together, they have primary control over what they do with their lives apart from us. If Caitlin wants Luke to be more ambitious at work, he can insist that it is his job, not hers.

Not only do we have more legitimacy but we also have more power to create changes in our partners when the changes concern their behavior toward us. We can observe their actions and directly influence them by what we say and do. Caitlin can usually tell, for example, whether Luke is paying attention to her, and then she can say something about it. However, when we request changes in how our partners deal with the rest of the world, we are not a party to the actions that concern us. We cannot observe their actions or directly influence them. Caitlin cannot, for example, directly observe how ambitious Luke is at work; nor can she intervene directly to encourage him to be more ambitious. Because of this important distinction, we should try to separate our requests for change into those that have to do with our partners' behavior toward us and those that have to do with our partners' behavior toward the rest of the world. If we want our partners to be more open and communicative in general, we might separate our request to be more open and communicative with us from our request that they be more open and communicative with the world. And we might deal with the request that they be open and communicative with us first. It is easier to foster change in how our partners deal with us than in how they deal with the world apart from us.

Change Supported by Circumstances versus Change through Sheer Willpower

One of the easiest ways to foster change is to shift the circumstances in ways that may facilitate change. For example, Caitlin feels that she can never get a break from her kids when she is at home with them. Even though Luke is "officially" responsible for them on Saturday mornings, they continue to come to her with their problems rather than go to him. Indeed, knowing that she is always there as his "backup," Luke tends to slack off on his supervision. Thus Caitlin has difficulty being "off duty" even when Luke is supposedly "on duty." The quickest and easiest solution to this problem is to change the circumstances. If he takes the kids out, then she truly is free at home; similarly, if she leaves the house, then she is also truly free. In each of these cases, the kids must bring their problems to and seek attention from Luke, and he must supervise them. The circumstances allow no other option.

Similarly a husband who wants his wife to join him in an activity that she really doesn't enjoy may be more successful if he orchestrates social circumstances that would support the activity. A bike ride, for example, may be more appealing to his nonathletic wife if it included his wife's good friend or ended at a destination that she wanted to visit.

Studies of couples have consistently shown that wives do more housework and child care than husbands even when both work full-time outside the home. But when husbands and wives work different shifts, and the husbands are home with their kids while their wives are at work, husbands do much more child care and housework than they would otherwise. Circumstances encourage—in fact literally force—the changes the wives may have desired when they worked the same shifts as their husbands.

Tip 2: To bring about change in your partner, request specific rather than general changes. Be sure your request is that he or she take particular positive actions rather than stopping certain negative actions. Focus primarily if not exclusively on changes in how your partner acts with you rather than in how he or she acts with the world (work, family, and friends) when you are not present. When possible, try to arrange circumstances that support the change you are requesting.

WHEN CHANGE IS DIFFICULT

Most of us find that making deliberate change is difficult even when we ourselves want that change. At the beginning of each year, millions of Americans make a decision to lose weight and get more exercise. Some of those millions actually sign up for programs to help them reach these goals. All too often, however, a few days, weeks, or months later the desire for change has vanished and old habits return in full force. Appealing food and soft couches are formidable, attractive alternatives to diet and exercise, so it's easy to understand why we often fail to make the weight and exercise changes we desire. With relationships, we have to deal not only with attractive alternatives to change but also with conflicting desires about change. It is often our partners, not ourselves, who are invested in our changing. Furthermore, there are other complexities about the nature of interpersonal change that complicate our efforts.

"I Want You to Change YOU"

Perhaps the most important reason that change is difficult in interpersonal relationships is that it touches on incompatibilities between partners or on emotional sensitivities in one or both of them. To make a change may threaten a fundamental characteristic of the other. For example, Luke wishes that Caitlin would take life easier, not worry about so many things, and just "go with the flow." His mantra to her is "Don't sweat the small stuff." And although at times Caitlin agrees that she should take life easier, she has a difficult time doing so. She is not by nature easygoing. And, for her part, she wants Luke to take life more seriously and to be more ambitious. In fact, they are fundamentally different in their approach to life, and their requests for change in each other run up against these basic differences.

Emotional sensitivities can also get in the way of change. Luke wants to spend more time with Caitlin. He likes to hang around with her, even when she is working on a project at home. But Caitlin's sense of freedom and independence is abridged when he is around her all the time. He cannot understand why she does not want to be around her husband more and is hurt by what he perceives as her disinterest in him. She cannot understand why he invades her space so much and often feels uncomfortable, even irritated, with Luke's hovering presence.

Requests for change will often center on incompatibilities and vulnerabilities. These are the areas that create pain for each individual, so these are the areas in which partners will often make their change requests. If one partner is vulnerable about issues of approval, he or she may request that the other be more complimentary and less critical, while the other may respond with requests to be "less sensitive" or more "thick-skinned." These will not be easy changes to make.

"I Want You to Want To"

With many changes we seek in our partners, such as wanting them to do more of the housework or wanting them to take the kids to soccer practice, there is little concern with how they feel when they are doing what we want. Of course, we would prefer them to feel happy with what they are doing. And it would create a problem if they felt resentful. But our concern is with their behavior, not with their emotional state. Our message is: Just do it!

There are other times when the changes we seek in our partners prove more complex. We want behavior change, but we also want attitude change. We are concerned not just with what they do but also with their motives for doing it and their emotional state while they are doing it. Luke may want Caitlin to be more verbally demonstrative with him. He would like it if she complimented him more often and if she expressed her love to him more frequently and more fervently. Certainly, it is within Caitlin's power to perform more of these affectionate acts. But if she forced herself to perform them, it would not be satisfying either for her or for Luke. He might accuse her of "just going through the motions." Although Luke would like more verbal affection, he also wants the motivation and attitude that usually accompany it. He wants her *to want* to do it.

Caitlin would like Luke to earn more money at his job. But apart from this concrete change, she would like him to be more ambitious in general. She wants him to be more achievement-oriented. Although he can and does listen to her dreams for a better financial future, what she really wants is for him to share her passion for that future. She wants him to get ahead, but, more than that, she wants him *to want* to get ahead.

Requests for change such as these present a difficult dilemma for couples. Making changes in behavior is quite challenging in and of itself. When we ask for change, our partners must hear our request for change, respect it, endorse it, remember it, and support it. If we ask for a change in attitude, motivation, or emotion in addition to a change in behavior, our partners are faced with a much more difficult task. Not only must they change something that is under their control—their behavior—but they must change something that is not directly under their control: their desires and emotions. They can control what they do but not what they *want* to do.

"Handle Your Emotional Distress Differently"

We often want our partners to act differently when they are experiencing strong emotions. We may want them to refrain from offensive actions or engage in desirable actions when they are upset. Luke wants Caitlin to stop being so critical because he believes she searches for someone to blame every time she is upset. Caitlin wants Luke to be more expressive because she thinks he goes off into a corner when he is upset and reveals little of what is troubling him.

The difficulties we have in making deliberate changes while emotionally at ease are magnified when we are emotionally aroused. When emotions are high, we repeat well-worn behavior patterns and are less flexible. Even if we can see alternatives to our old patterns, we may be unable to alter our behavior in the moment.

Often we want our partners to do more than change the way they act when upset; sometimes we really want them not to be so upset. Our message, stripped of any euphemistic and self-justifying wrapping, is simply "Don't be so emotional." Their emotions upset ours, so we insist that they throttle theirs. Of course, telling your partner that the circumstances at hand are not worth getting upset over only makes him or her feel invalidated and thus upsets your partner even more.

"I Won't Allow the Changes I Need"

Don't call a man honest just because he never had
the chance to steal.
                    —YIDDISH PROVERB

Ernie does not trust Josh for good reason. Early in their relationship, Ernie discovered that Josh was still seeing his old boyfriend secretly. He knows Josh's style with men is to be flirtatious and provocative, and he also knows that Josh doesn't exactly proclaim to the world that he is in an exclusive relationship. Ernie has dealt with this problem by keeping a watchful eye over Josh. In fact, he is convinced that it is his vigilance that keeps Josh faithful. If he let up, Josh might wander. In fact, the only way he could be assured that Josh is trustworthy would be for him to relax his vigilance and discover that Josh remains faithful to him. But Ernie is afraid, with some justification, to engage in the actions that could lead to a trusting relationship.

Similarly, Gayle worries that Leo is not careful enough with their active, adventuresome toddler, Donny. Because Leo is not nearly as worried or as vigilant as she is, Gayle is hesitant to turn over full parenting responsibilities to him. Even when Leo is supposedly "in charge" of Donny, Gayle keeps a cocked ear and a watchful eye. She overrules Leo when he is watching their son, and she may criticize Leo for his lack of concern. Except for occasional angry efforts to show Gayle he is responsible, Leo is actually becoming less watchful of Donny *because* Gayle is always there to back him up. And even though Gayle needs Leo to take charge sometimes so she can have a break from Donny, she fears allowing Leo full responsibility because she doesn't want to risk an accident. So Gayle wants Leo to be in charge but won't allow it. But Leo won't insist on truly being in charge either.

> **Tip 3:** Change is going to be difficult if not impossible for your partner if the change you request is contrary to a central feature of who your partner is or is tied up with strong emotional sensitivities in him or her. Change will also be extremely hard if it is not just a change in behavior that you request but a change in attitude or a change in emotional reactivity, or if you undermine that change because of your own concerns. Being aware of these difficulties with change may mitigate your frustration with your partner or may allow a more nuanced and constructive discussion of those changes with your partner.

Why You Should Change

When the change we've requested is difficult, our partners may question why they should change, or they may ignore or resist our requests. Even if they acknowledge the validity of our requests, they may not follow through with change. In response, we may try to justify our requests by proving why they *ought* to change. However, some types of justifications may be more effective than others in creating the change we want.

"OTHERS DO IT"

One way we can justify the need for change is to point to other partners, such as other husbands or other wives, who do what we want our partners to do: "Ben takes a lot of responsibility for their kids." "Most of the other wives go to this party." This strategy can easily degenerate into arguments about whether in fact the other partner in question does what is claimed. "I don't think Ben does that much with his kids. He makes a show of it in the presence of others, but. . . ." Or our partners can provide counterexamples: "But look at Joey and Mike. They are so busy with work they hardly know who their kids are." Or other features of the comparison spouse can be called into question. "So you really want to be married to a nerd like Ben?" What began as an effort to justify a request for change can become a fruitless argument about friends and acquaintances.

Social psychologists write about two kinds of comparisons: upward social comparisons, in which we compare ourselves to people who are better than we are by some criterion, and downward social comparisons, in which we compare ourselves to people who are worse than we are by some criterion. With most characteristics, it is possible to make either upward or downward social comparisons. So if you try to justify your demand that your partner do more by saying "You don't do as much as Joe," he can easily counter with "But I do more than Harry." And both kinds of comparisons are complicated by the fact that we rarely know exactly how much either Joe or Harry actually does. Again, the attempt to justify the original request is futile and may end in a whole new argument.

"I DO IT FOR YOU!"

We can make a more compelling case for change through appeals to fairness or equality. "I do it for you, so why can't you do it for me?" Or "I don't treat you like that, so you shouldn't treat me like that."

During the difficult days of the Constitutional Convention in this country, Benjamin Franklin served as an excellent moderator, using his humor and wisdom to help resolve disputes. At one point during a struggle between representatives from large and small states, he told a story of how a rooster was trying to negotiate barnyard rules with a horse. The rooster proposed what seemed to him a reasonable plan: if the horse would not step on his feet, then he would not step on the horse's feet! The horse failed to see the wisdom in the rooster's proposal, since it didn't bother the horse how much the rooster stepped on his feet.

Similarly, proposals for change based on fairness and equality fail to consider the fact that partners are different and that the same act involves different levels of "psychic energy" or "psychic pain" when it is done by two different people. It is fundamentally a more difficult task for Caitlin to express her love for Luke than for Luke to express his love for Caitlin. Similarly, it is much easier for Caitlin to get up early on a Saturday morning and accomplish some household task than it is for Luke.

When we don't accept the truth that the same act is different when done by different people, we can create a new conflict on top of the original one.

"LOOK AT ALL I'VE DONE FOR YOU!"

We can also justify our requests by pointing out that we've tried to make our partners happy by changing in ways that they seemed to want; now it is our turn to get the changes we want. In this justification for change, there is an implicit assumption of inequality and debt. We have given more than they, so they owe us something.

Although it may be believed fervently, this assumption is often false. Psychologists have discovered an "egocentric bias" when two people in a relationship are asked to estimate their own contribution to some joint activity like child care: their individual, reported percentages add up to more than 100% because they both give themselves more relative credit than the other does. A husband and wife may both agree that she does more child care than he does, but he estimates that he does 40% while she estimates that she does 75%! Psychologists theorize that this bias occurs because each of us has more information about our own contributions than we have about our partners' contributions, so we give more weight to our own contributions.

With or without egocentric bias, there are bound to be real inequalities in your relationship. But the fact that inequality exists does not necessarily justify your demanding that it be rectified. Your partner can rightfully argue that he or she was unaware of any reciprocal agreement for change. If a husband proposes that his wife should meet his social needs because he has adapted so much to her desires to live near her parents, she may reply: "I didn't remember agreeing to a trade-off here! You drew up a plan without getting my consent to it." So, whether there is a skewed perception of inequity in your relationship or actual inequity, you're unlikely to encourage change in your partner by trying to prove you are a victim of your partner's unfairness.

"I REALLY NEED YOU TO CHANGE"

In contrast to the other justifications we've seen so far, the simplest and in some ways the most compelling justification for change is based on our own desire: "I want you to change" or "It is important to me that you change." There is little room for argument with this honest approach because we know what we want and what is important to us. Such a message does not ensure change, but it clarifies the reason for it: the change would please me.

However, some of us don't feel entitled to request change from our partners. "Just because it would please me" doesn't seem like a sufficient justification. So we may add weight to our requests by amplifying an "I want" into an "I need." Needs sound more urgent than wants. Satisfying needs ensures survival, while satisfying wants only ensures pleasure or contentment. Therefore, if we phrase our requests as needs, we communicate that somehow our survival depends on our partners' changing.

We may also buttress our request for change with an appeal to our partners' love for us. "If you really loved me, you would make the changes I need." "If you really care, you would do this." But this tactic can easily backfire. Our partners may respond: "If you really loved me, you would accept me as I am." Or they may in turn appeal to our love to push for the changes *they* desire.

Whatever methods we use to justify the changes we request—appeals to love, to fairness, to equity—these justifications often lead to a struggle over change. Our partners experience our efforts as pressure for them to change, and paradoxically, the greater the pressure they feel to change, the more they may resist change. We may demand of them: You must change. I cannot survive without change. You owe me change, and if you loved me, you would change. In response, they may defend themselves, counter with demands of their own, or ultimately refuse to discuss our requests further.

Tip 4: Requests for change that come with arguments that others do it, that I have done it for you, that you owe it to me, or that I have to have it, are paradoxically more likely to lead to argument rather than the desired change. Simple requests for a specific change, unencumbered with justification and argument, are more likely to be responded to positively. Most likely your partner does want to please you; simply requesting what would please you is the best way to ask for change.

RECAP

Change is an inexorable force. Inevitably, we change, our partners change, and our relationships change. But these changes do not necessarily move in the direction we want. What we want is deliberate change in particular areas of concern. Sometimes we want big changes immediately and confront our partners to get what we want. On rare occasions, dramatic, positive change is possible from a showdown, an ultimatum, but only when you ask for a specific change such as a decision within a particular time frame, when the change is likely to bring about future positive changes, and when you can make the request without creating so much resistance in your partner that he or she refuses. Rarely do we request change under these conditions. Furthermore, what we often want is not a single decision or a single action but ordinary, everyday changes in what our partner does or says to us.

Sometimes everyday change is easy. We ask our partners to take some specific actions in our relationship, rather than asking them to change something general or asking them not to do something, and events conspire to support those actions. However, most often the changes we request are not easy for our partners to make. Our requests strike at the core of incompatibilities or vulnerabilities that divide us. Changes in these areas are always complicated. Furthermore, we may request change not only in our partners' behavior but also in their emotional state. We may want them to feel more passion for us or want them not to be upset when they get upset. Although they have control over their behavior, they have little direct control over how they feel. Therefore, compliance with our requests is difficult.

If our partners don't make the everyday changes we seek, we may try to justify those changes to them. We may point to how other spouses are, we may appeal to fairness or to love, or we may tout our extensive change on their behalf to justify our requests and inspire compliance. These efforts often backfire. Rather than prove the need for them to change, our efforts only generate a struggle about change. We press for the changes, and they resist them.

The chapter offered four tips for making change:

1. Use ultimatums only in the rare circumstance when there is a major relationship violation, a major decision, or a major personal problem. Then use them only when you are serious about following through, when you are asking for a specific change within a particular time frame, when the change is likely to bring future positive

changes, and when you can do it without creating such resistance in your partner that he or she will refuse simply to save face.

2. To bring about change in your partner, request specific rather than general changes. Be sure your request is that he or she take particular positive actions rather than stopping certain negative actions. Focus primarily if not exclusively on changes in how your partner acts with you rather than in how he or she acts with the world (work, family, and friends) when you are not present. When possible, try to arrange circumstances that support the change you are requesting.

3. Be aware of difficult areas of change, such as requests that seek change in a central feature of who your partner is or that are tied up with strong emotional sensitivities in him or her, requests for change in attitude or a change in emotional reactivity, or requests for change that you may undermine because of your own concerns.

4. Make simple requests for a specific change, unencumbered with justification and argument about what your partner should change.

Exercise: Facilitating Change in Both You and Your Partner

This exercise is designed to prepare you for making changes in your relationship. As always, start by considering your core conflict and your DEEP analysis of it.

Is there something you would like from your partner or that your partner would like from you that does not involve complicated incompatibilities or vulnerabilities?

1. Changes I would like from my partner that seem clear-cut and simple:

_____

_____

_____

Is there anything about the way you could reframe your change requests to make them more successful? For example, can you make them more specific, make them things to do (not things NOT to do), or change the circumstances of the change so that it's easier or less aversive?

_____

_____

_____

Try asking your partner directly and specifically for those changes and try to alter circumstances to support those changes. Don't try to justify the changes by framing them as an urgent need, by using comparisons to others, or by making appeals to fairness or love. Simply indicate how those changes would make your life easier or more satisfying.

2. Changes I could make for my partner that my partner wants and that are relatively clear-cut and simple:

_____

_____

_____

Try offering to try to make these changes for your partner.

Also consider the more difficult changes you would like from your partner. Do some of the changes you want from your partner invoke incompatibilities and vulnerabilities? Are you seeking a change in the emotions and attitudes that your partner experiences as well as a change in his or her behavior?

3. Some changes that I would like from my partner that will be very difficult for my partner to make:

_____

_____

_____

Are you engaging in any efforts to create change that backfires, decreasing the chances that your partner will do what you wish (such as justifying your request, pointing out what other partners do, making appeals to love or fairness)?

4. Actions of mine that get in the way of change rather than facilitating that change:

_____

_____

_____

Next Steps

In our first chapter on change, we considered different types of change and some difficulties with bringing about change, but focusing on simple change that you may be able to bring about without many complications. In the next chapter we will consider making change that is more complicated but still possible if you approach it wisely and mindfully.

CHAPTER 12

Deliberate Change through Mindfulness

CUSTOM-FITTING CHANGE TO SUIT YOUR RELATIONSHIP

> Sometimes just acknowledging what's actually going on instead of what "should" be happening is all that is needed to transform our experience.
> —MARK WILLIAMS, JOHN TEASDALE, ZINDEL SEGAL, AND JON KABAT-ZINN, *The Mindful Way through Depression* (2007)

> The best way out is always through.
> —ROBERT FROST, *A Servant to Servants* (1914)

> In mindfulness, acceptance always comes first, change comes after.
> —SHAMASH ALIDINA, *Mindfulness for Dummies* (2010)

Sal and Hava were locked in a pattern of distance and criticism. Distressed at what she felt was Sal's abdication of any responsibility in the family—he rarely helped with child care or housework—Hava criticized him relentlessly. From Sal's point of view, nothing he could do would please Hava. So why bother to do anything, except tune her out?

In my (A. C.) initial work with this couple, I established some reasonable, positive goals for therapy, to which both agreed: Sal would become more involved in the household, and Hava would provide more acknowledgment and appreciation for Sal's efforts. As my first intervention with them,

I asked Hava to keep track of her daily expressions of acknowledgment or appreciation for Sal's efforts and Sal to keep track of his daily efforts to participate more in the household.

At the beginning of the next session, I asked for their records. Hava had hers ready at the top of her purse and produced it proudly. She had carefully made a calendar of the days of the week and faithfully recorded every instance of Sal's actions on behalf of the family and her corresponding communication of appreciation or acknowledgment. Sal, it turned out, had forgotten to do the assignment until late in the week and then only when Hava reminded him. He tried to keep track mentally of what he had done and later to write it down. Hava noted that he had not written it down until they were in the waiting room before the appointment.

As I read over the very sketchy and hurried notes that Sal had made, Hava looked at me with the confidence of a prosecuting attorney who has just handed the jury the smoking gun. Then she launched into her husband: he could not even do therapy right. His behavior in here was a perfect example of his behavior at home: too little, too late. Sal shook his head and tuned her out.

My therapeutic effort to change their behavior had simply given them a new occasion to exhibit the same old behavior. My assignment had given Sal a new opportunity to fail and Hava a new opportunity to criticize him. They were using my assignment to engage in exactly the same pattern that my assignment had tried to end!

The kind of experience I had with Hava and Sal is just one way my therapeutic efforts sometimes backfire. Sometimes couples use the positive action I suggest to justify their existing behavior. Let's say that, as one positive step toward resolving conflicts between a critical husband and a withdrawn wife, I urge the couple to express their feelings to each other. The following week the husband harangues his wife over some misdeed of hers. In the next session, he justifies his criticism of her by saying "I was just expressing my feelings, like you said."

Sometimes I offer partners a crutch to help them communicate, and they end up hitting each other over the head with it. The critical husband may use my suggestion to express feelings as another opportunity to attack his wife: "You never express your feelings! How can you expect me to respond to you when you don't even do a simple thing like that, which the doctor here recommends?"

Attempts at change, I have learned, often lead instead to more of the same. As a therapist I've allowed this to happen by failing to anticipate the interplay between my intervention and the vicious cycles of interaction in which the couple is stuck. You can avoid the same trap by looking honestly at the steps you're taking to try to elicit change and anticipating, based on your story, how your own partner is likely to react.

When Old Patterns Come Dressed in New Clothing

Chan has a stronger sex drive than Gwen and has pushed for more frequent and diverse sexual contact. In response to Gwen's resistance, Chan makes vague threats about the viability of their marriage and hints about "looking elsewhere." Although disturbed by these threats, Gwen often challenges them: "If you think threats are a sexual turn-on, you have a lot to learn about women."

Chan doesn't really want to leave Gwen or to threaten their relationship further by having an affair, so he decides to try to make some positive changes on his own. Knowing how pressured Gwen feels by him, he decides to pull back, to give her "more room sexually," as she has often requested. That would certainly be a change, and a difficult one for him to make. Maybe it would help.

Chan tells Gwen: "Look, I'm not going to push you sexually anymore. If there is going to be any sex, you'll have to initiate it. I'll just wait and see how this works."

Although his actions may have seemed like a major change to Chan, their impact on Gwen was the same as that of his old behavior. "I'll just wait and see how this works" felt like another form of pressure to her, and the comment came with a veiled but vague threat that he might take more drastic measures if Gwen didn't start initiating sex right away. His comment that "If there is going to be any sex, you'll have to initiate it" was made with resentment and anger. Despite Chan's genuine efforts to do something constructive, his actions were merely variations on his theme of pressure and threat.

To an outsider, a couple's efforts to change can be amusing because they are so transparently "more of the same." A husband who wants more say in his marriage pleads with his wife to let him make more of the decisions. A wife who realizes the truth in her husband's complaints that he takes most of the responsibility for housework asks him to remind her when things need to be done. They, however, are so mired in their vicious cycles of interaction that they don't see any irony in their efforts.

Realistically, of course, the husband who wants more power may need his wife's assistance in becoming more assertive and the nondomestic wife may need some gentle reminding as she takes on more responsibility for the housework. If they can recognize the irony in their requests, convey this irony to their partners, and their partners can hear these requests with accepting compassion, the changes they desire are more likely to occur.

When "More of the Same" Becomes "Worse of the Same"

When a tolerant understanding of each other is missing, efforts to change can exacerbate an existing conflict by escalating a negative pattern of communication. The couple gets better and better at being worse and worse.

When Allie feels that June has set herself up as her superior and evaluated her performance as both wife and mother, Allie withdraws from June verbally and emotionally, which upsets June. After one particularly painful incident where June critiqued her behavior toward their daughter, Allie withdrew in hurt and anger and started brooding over how unfair it was that June criticized her but never turned her forever pointed finger at herself. Allie decided to teach June a lesson and refused to talk to June at all. In that Allie had never before *completely* refused to talk to her, Allie's response to June was new and different, but it was hardly a change in the pattern. Instead it was an intensification of the old pattern.

There is a mythical Danish village whose people are known for their goodness and tenacity on the one hand and their ignorance and stupidity on the other. Many wonderful stories are told about this group. In one particularly relevant story, some members of the group dig a well so they can have easy access to fresh water. Although the well is successful, the well-digging project leaves behind an ugly pile of dirt. Wanting their project to be aesthetically pleasing as well as functionally successful, the villagers decide to get rid of the pile of dirt. They dig an appropriately sized hole and put the dirt from the well in the hole. Of course, what remains is the new dirt that was left over from digging the new hole. They dig another hole for that dirt but are faced with the same problem. Once more they repeat their efforts, to no avail. How can they get rid of the remaining ugly pile of dirt? They consult their wise leader, who listens to their story carefully. He goes to the site of the dirt and studies the situation. Then he spends valuable time alone thinking about the problem. Finally, he announces the solution, which the whole village agrees is brilliant. The village will dig a huge hole, which is big enough to hold all the dirt!

Deliberate Change Starts with Mindfulness

So, how can you create deliberate change in your relationship without its backfiring or even making things worse? To make genuine change in your relationship, you must be aware of what is going on in your relationship. If you don't know your own story—the vulnerabilities and incompatibilities that have contributed to your conflicts and how the two of you have developed certain patterns, even vicious cycles, of interaction in a vain effort to solve your problem—you can simply make things worse. You can fool yourself into thinking that you are doing something positive when you are not. But knowledge of your story, while a great place to start, is only the beginning. You need to follow that with greater mindfulness, which is in-the-moment attention to what is happening in your relationship and a nonjudgmental awareness of those happenings. When you are not engaged in an evaluation of your experience, you are more open to that experience and more able to be guided by it, as we will illustrate below.

IN-THE-MOMENT AWARENESS

In Part II of this book you developed a DEEP understanding of a major relationship problem. In Chapter 8, you turned that analysis into a true and workable story about your problem. The construction of that story should have helped you develop a general awareness of your problem, which could enlighten your efforts to solve it. However, a broad awareness of your story may not be enough to help you make change. Unless you understand how your general story plays itself out in particular incidents, you will not see how your efforts at change are likely to be, and produce, more of the same. In Chapter 8 you also applied your knowledge of your general story to an analysis of a particular recent incident. Now we will show you how awareness of the here-and-now, a sense of what is going on emotionally right now in this particular discussion with your partner, greater relationship mindfulness, can foster genuine change.

One Saturday morning as Norman is putting away the breakfast dishes, Cheri asks in a nice voice, "Do you know when you'll be done with the garage?" Norman replies with annoyance, "I'll be done when I'm done." Cheri walks away without a word. About 15 minutes later, Cheri approaches Norman again and asks politely, "Want to do our run now?" Norman looks at her incredulously and replies, "Not really." Cheri says sarcastically, "You're certainly in a great mood today," and storms out of the room. Norman follows her and tries to apologize: "Don't get so upset. I just didn't feel like a run. Maybe we can do it later." Cheri locks the bedroom door from the inside. Norman yells in at her, "Damn it, I hate it when you do this."

To become more aware of what went on emotionally in this brief encounter, let's first consider the "general story" of this problem for Cheri and Norman. Cheri is far more invested than Norman in organization and order. She feels most comfortable when things are put away where they belong. Although Norman has no objection to order in their household and even finds it helpful, disorder doesn't bother him as long as he can "kick back" in his easy chair and read. For him, rarely is the goal of a well-organized closet or shelves or drawers—or even an organized counter—worth the effort required to achieve it. So Norman's motivation for order is rarely enough to spur him into action. In contrast, Cheri often will put forth energy to keep the counter neat, to see to it clothes are in their proper place, and so on. Yet she doesn't feel like she should have to do all the work while Norman sits and reads. What particularly upsets her is getting stuck with sorting and organizing his stuff. So Cheri resorts to encouragement, reminders, and prompts as a way of getting Norman more involved in keeping the house in order. Norman has grown sensitive to these gentle suggestions. He doesn't want to be "managed"; nor does Cheri want to be a nag. Yet without some intervention on her part, Norman won't take much action. As with the garage, which he promised he would clean up.

To see how this general story plays out in this particular incident of the garage, we have to take a look not only at the words and actions of Cheri and Norman but also at the emotional communication that was part of those words and actions.

Words Spoken or Actions Taken	Emotional Message
CHERI: (*nicely*) Do you know when you'll be done with the garage?	I want to remind you to work on the garage, but I don't want to cause an argument, so I am asking nicely.
NORMAN: I'll be done when I'm done.	I don't like to be nagged, even when you try to camouflage it with a nice exterior.
(*Cheri walks away.*)	Gosh, I try to be nice to you and you get irritated.
CHERI: (*politely*) Want to do our run now?	I don't want us to fight today. I am trying to be conciliatory by suggesting that we do something we both enjoy. But my patience has its limits.

Words Spoken or Actions Taken	Emotional Message
NORMAN: (*incredulously*) Not really.	You nag me, which I hate, and then come in and act like nothing has gone on and we should just go on a run together. I don't get it.
CHERI: (*sarcastically*) You're certainly in a great mood today. (*She storms out.*)	I try to be nice to you, and it just doesn't work. I'm angry. I'm done with you.
NORMAN: (*follows her*) Don't get so upset. I just didn't feel like a run. Maybe we can do it later.	Oops! Now she's really upset. I hate that. I'll take back what I said. I'll do anything to appease her if she just won't go off in such an angry fit.
(*Cheri locks the bedroom door from the inside.*)	I'm really angry. This is over for me.
NORMAN: (*yelling in at her*) Damn it, I hate it when you do this.	The day is ruined. There is no way I can pull her back. I'm angry and upset.

When you are aware of the emotional messages in a conversation, you have the option of openly expressing these messages. For example, Cheri might have opened the discussion by saying "I don't want to be a nag or create an unpleasant scene between us, but I'm eager to have the garage cleaned." Or Norman might have said, no matter how Cheri started the discussion, "It bothers me when you remind me about something I've agreed to do." Because these comments are more direct and open, they have a better chance of success.

Awareness of emotional messages also allows each of you to acknowledge the other's reactions. Instead of proposing a run, Cheri might have said, "I bet you're annoyed that I mentioned the garage." If Cheri had proposed a run, as in the original exchange, Norman might have said, "I know you're trying to be nice and smooth over any tension between us by suggesting a run, but I just don't feel like it." This acknowledgment of what the other is experiencing can often prevent emotional escalation.

Third, awareness allows for the possibility of positive actions by either party. Knowing that Cheri was concerned about the garage yet not wanting to fuel an argument, Norman might have offered her a time line for completion. With the knowledge that Norman was upset about her mention of the garage, Cheri might have delayed her request for a run. Either of these actions might have prevented the emotional distress that followed.

Let's look at another example of the benefits of in-the-moment awareness in a conversation that took place between Chan and Gwen one Saturday evening when they had no plans.

Chan looks through the cable TV guide and suggests a movie to watch. He reads the short description and notes, "I've heard it's supposed to be kind of sexy."

There is a long pause from Gwen. "It doesn't sound that interesting."

Chan replies with some disappointment in his voice, "Well, there's nothing much else on."

Gwen says, "You can watch it. I have reading I'd like to do."

"I was hoping we could do something together," Chan replies.

"We'll both be in the family room. Maybe I'll see if it's interesting."

Chan says "Great" sarcastically and leaves the room.

Gwen calls after him, "So if we can't do exactly what you want, you're not happy?" Chan doesn't bother to reply.

We already know the general story of Chan and Gwen's issue with sex. Let's see how this conversation sent emotional messages that both failed to hear or respond to directly.

Words Spoken or Actions Taken	Emotional Message
CHAN: (reading the description of the movie) I've heard it's supposed to be kind of sexy.	I hope this movie will put you in a sexy mood and we can make love.
GWEN: It doesn't sound that interesting to me.	I'm feeling pressure to have sex. I don't want you to get your hopes up.
CHAN: (with disappointment) Well, there's nothing much else on.	I am disappointed. I wasn't insisting on sex, just hoping it might happen.
GWEN: You can watch it. I have reading I'd like to do.	I don't want you to be disappointed, but I don't want to feel pressured.
CHAN: I was hoping we could do something together.	I can't believe you won't even allow us the possibility of sexual intimacy.
GWEN: We'll both be in the family room. Maybe I'll see if it's interesting.	Okay. I'll allow for that possibility. But it's just a possibility.

Words Spoken or Actions Taken	Emotional Message
CHAN: (*sarcastically*) Great.	I'm getting upset. Let's forget the whole thing.
GWEN: So if we can't do exactly what you want, then you're not happy?	I'm angry. I offer you the possibility, and you reject it.

If Chan and Gwen were more aware of what was going on between them, they might be more open with their own emotional messages. For example, Chan might have opened the discussion by saying "The movie is supposed to be sexy. Maybe it can put us in the mood. ..." Even if Chan had opened the conversation as he did, Gwen might have said, "When you describe a movie as sexy, I feel you're telling me you want us to make love afterward, and then I feel pressure and I start resisting that pressure."

Awareness would also enable them to acknowledge each other's reactions. At some point in the conversation, Chan might acknowledge that "I bet you feel pressure for sex when I propose a sexy movie." Or Gwen might acknowledge, "I think you're disappointed that I may be rejecting any possibility of sex tonight."

Awareness also opens the possibility for positive actions. Chan might decide not to comment on the movie's sexiness, knowing the effect that might have on Gwen. Or Gwen might make a humorous comment: "I'll watch the movie with you, but I'm going to keep my chastity belt handy."

Thus awareness of emotions makes it possible for *either* partner to acknowledge his or her own feelings *or* the other's feelings *or* to take actions that can change the course of their discussion. None of these alternative actions are foolproof ways of avoiding an ugly conflict, yet they often promote more constructive communication.

All of our examples of alternative actions that could avert conflict focused on the early stages of the discussion. Once emotions run high, partners may be too upset to be aware of the struggle going on between them. Or, even if aware, they may be too angry to take any constructive action. Once Cheri locked herself in the bedroom, both she and Norman were too upset to be aware of what had led to their struggle, to be aware of what positive actions could lead them out of it, or even to be receptive to any positive actions by the other. They simply needed distance from each other to calm down.

To be fully aware, moment-to-moment, of what is going on emotionally during a discussion with your partner, even during the early stages of such a discussion, is an ideal goal. Typically, people have only limited awareness of their own emotions and even less awareness of their partners' emotions. Judgment often clouds our awareness of our own emotions. If Cheri is upset at herself for being upset with Norman (he really hasn't had a chance to clean the garage yet) or if Norman is upset at being upset by Cheri's inquiry (she was just asking nicely), then they are less likely to be aware of their emotions and less able to describe them. Judgment also clouds our awareness of our partners when we are judgmental of them. If Chan and Gwen both judge the other's sexual feelings as deviant and distorted, they will be less aware of the variation in those feelings and of the struggles the other actually experiences. Neither will be open to hearing what the other is going through. We on the outside may see the emotional interplay between Cheri and Norman and the unspoken sexual dialogue between Chan and Gwen, but it is much more difficult for them to see it as it is happening. Any increment in their awareness of their "general story" and how it plays out in a particular incident provides them with more options to alter their usual pattern.

Tip 1: When you and your partner start getting tense with each other, START a different communication between the two of you: **S**top what you are doing for the moment, **T**ake a deep breath, **A**ttend to what is going on with you emotionally in the moment, **R**eveal your emotional state to your partner, and **T**ake an interest in what is going on emotionally with your partner. When you voice what is going on emotionally with you, it is okay if you are only vaguely aware of the emotion or uncertain of what triggered it. A comment such as "I am beginning to feel tense but am not sure why" may alter a potential conflict because it shifts attention away from the content of the discussion to the emotional underpinnings, which could easily derail a constructive discussion of that content. A good way to take an interest in your partner's emotional state is to gently ask what he or she is experiencing at the moment or to express curiosity about what your partner is experiencing at the moment. If you think you know what your partner may be feeling, express it only tentatively as your partner is the final authority on what he or she is feeling. This effort to stop the course of what typically happens and START a new and better direction may interrupt a frustrating pattern of interaction and lead to a more constructive interaction.

HINDSIGHT AWARENESS

There are serious limits to the moment-to-moment awareness of Cheri and Norman and of Chan and Gwen, as well as of our own. Often in the midst of discussion, we have only limited awareness of what is happening with us and our partners emotionally. Fortunately, awareness does not have to occur "in the moment" to be helpful. A retrospective awareness can aid us as well. Hindsight awareness may not be able to prevent a conflict from happening or even interrupt its course, but it can enable you to accept the conflict and recover from it more quickly. To illustrate, let's pick up Cheri and Norman's conflict where we left off.

Cheri is now locked in the bedroom, angry and replaying in her head the scene she has just had with Norman. *I have no impact on him,* she thinks. *I try to be nice to him, I approach him kindly and ask him a simple question about the garage, and he rejects me. Like a fool, I hang in there, try to be nice, invite him for a run, and he rejects me again. When am I going to learn? He has* no *consideration for my feelings. The only effect I can have with him is when I really blow up; that gets his attention. So I have to be furious to get a response from my husband. Is this any kind of marriage?*

Norman also fumes over the conflict they have just had. *What's with her? She nags me again, and then she can't stand it that I'm annoyed. I turn her down for a run, and she acts like I've committed murder. Now she's the one who acts hurt and angry. But she started it all!*

Thoughts and feelings like these will make it difficult for Norman and Cheri to recover from this conflict. Any discussion based on these internal experiences will further inflame their argument. If at some point after the conflict they became aware, even in hindsight, of what really happened between them, they might recover more easily and quickly. For example, if Norman realized that his procrastination created a problem for Cheri, or that her manner of asking and her proposal of a run were genuine efforts to be positive, or that he was being overly sensitive to reminders, then he might be more accepting of her behavior and of his own. Similarly, if Cheri realized that her reminders presented a problem for Norman, even when masked in kindness, or that she had difficulty tolerating rejection from him, or that he had difficulty with her emotional distress, she also might be more accepting of him and of herself. An awareness of any of these features of the conflict might have eased a return to normalcy by them both. Cheri might get over her anger and come out of the bedroom sooner with this hindsight awareness. Similarly, Norman might get over his anger sooner and initiate some reconciliation between them.

A few specific guidelines might help in achieving hindsight awareness. First, we (and our partners) are probably more blaming than we (or they) realize. During arguments, even during the most civil arguments, we may say things that reflect negatively on the other. Without ever calling each other names or engaging in character assassination or even raising our voices, we can manage to convey plenty of accusation and blame. Consider a conflict between a husband and wife about whether to visit her parents on the weekend. During the course of the discussion the husband might say, "Do we have to visit them again?"—implying that his wife already pushes them to visit more often than is reasonable. He might ask, "Can't you manage without seeing them one weekend?"—implying that his wife is too dependent on her parents and can hardly survive psychologically without constant contact with them. She might be stung by these remarks, yet he may be unaware of how subtly aggressive they were. Similarly, she might ask during the discussion, "Can't we do what I want to do for at least one weekend?"—implying that he selfishly determines what they do and never accommodates her needs. In addition, she might offer during the discussion, "I'm sure it will require a little unselfishness on your part to go"—implying that he is very selfish and would have difficulty being even a little selfless. As with the husband's comments, these comments by his wife may hurt and anger him, but she may be relatively unaware of their accusatory power.

A second guideline for hindsight awareness is to remember that our partners have their own side of the story, their own experience in the conflict, and *it is a legitimate one*. Most of us could agree that each person in a conflict has his or her own take on it, but how can it be a legitimate position if it is diametrically opposed to ours? And how can it be a legitimate position on those occasions when they are clearly in the wrong? Won't their version simply be an excuse for their failure to do what was right?

Let's consider an example in which one person is clearly in the wrong: Sterling did nothing for Joyce's birthday—no card, no gift, no acknowledgment, nothing. By most of our standards for thoughtfulness, consideration, and love between spouses, we would judge that Sterling had done wrong. Joyce's hurt and anger are justified. In fact, she is so hurt and angry that she really doesn't want to hear anything from him, because any explanation he might have would seem like an excuse.

But there is a story behind Sterling's failure to acknowledge Joyce's birthday, and it is important for Joyce to be aware of it. Consider some of the various possibilities:

1. Sterling makes very little of events such as birthdays, anniversaries, and the like. He has never been very good at remembering

them. He doesn't get upset if others forget his birthday (he often doesn't remember himself), and so he can't understand why Joyce makes such a big deal about it. He is not fully aware that even though birthdays don't mean much to him, they are important to Joyce.

2. Sterling was very aware of Joyce's birthday. Yet he is furious at her for several things she has done to him. He deliberately avoided any action on her birthday because he wanted to hurt her as she had hurt him.

3. Joyce's birthdays have been controversial for a long time. Sterling feels that no matter what he does, it is not good enough for Joyce. The card he picks is funny rather than romantic. The gift he buys is too practical. He is not clever enough to surprise her. Nothing he does seems good enough. Sterling was aware of her birthday, didn't feel right about buying her a romantic gift and card, knew she would resent anything less, and didn't know how to resolve the problem. He avoided dealing with her birthday and got caught up with work right before it and genuinely forgot about it. Maybe at some level he was saying, if you don't like what I do for you, maybe I will do nothing for you.

Each of these stories is very different. None portrays Sterling in a positive light, but they all show the human side of his error. Each makes his action understandable, if not acceptable. Both Joyce and Sterling need to be able to understand his side as well as hers so they can deal with the problem effectively. Of course, the first challenge will be for Sterling to voice his thoughts and feelings without seeming like he's making an excuse or transferring blame to Joyce.

A third guideline for hindsight awareness follows from the second. If our partners' message does not make sense to us, if their story seems unconvincing, then we probably are lacking awareness of what is really going on with them. Maybe they have not been able to articulate their position. Maybe the message became too clouded with blame and accusation or with defensiveness. But whatever the reason, we are missing a major piece in the puzzle.

Carlisle has been without work for 3 months, ever since his company closed down. Because he has been unable to find a job, he, Janie, and their two teenage daughters have survived on Janie's income. Janie does not understand why he has not been more aggressive in pursuing a job. It seems as if she is more concerned about his getting a job than he is. Does he want to be dependent on her? Does he lack the drive to get out there and fight for a job? She has begun to lose respect for him. She just doesn't understand what is going on.

For his part, Carlisle sees Janie not as an ally in his job search but as an adversary. She seems so cold and angry with him. She tries to control him. She comes home and demands an account of his performance. She feels the television to see if it is warm. She wants to know how many calls he has made—a tally of his activities. Now he often refuses to answer her. Why should he have to answer to her? What is going on with her?

Because neither is aware of what is going on with the other, Carlisle and Janie have distanced themselves from each other. They are struggling individually with strong emotions, but they struggle in isolation. In this difficult situation, both lack the support of the person who cares for them the most.

What would each ideally convey to the other, even if they could not completely articulate it? What does each need to be aware of in the other?

Janie's message would be: I'm frustrated that you haven't found a job. That's probably obvious to you. But more than that, I'm anxious that you won't get a job. I fear for our financial future. I'm worried that we'll have to survive on my income alone. Then there will be no way for us to all fly back east and visit my parents, no way for us to pay for college for the girls. I'm not even sure we could continue to keep the house. In the face of these powerful and realistic fears, I need to see that you are concerned. I need reassurance that you also feel some urgency about the situation. When I don't get any information about what you're considering in terms of a job and what you've done, I get suspicious. I fear that you don't care about it. That you've done nothing. And then I go into my controlling mode—checking up on you, interrogating you about what you have done. I need information to calm my fears, and I'm not getting that from you.

Carlisle's message would be: Getting laid off and trying to find a new job is the most difficult crisis I have faced in a long time. I have lost confidence in myself, and I don't think I have all the technological skills I need to make it in a new job. I have to struggle with myself every day to motivate myself to take some action. I definitely avoid action because I don't feel up to it, because I anticipate another failure. And if I can motivate myself, I must also struggle with the various employment bureaus and personnel officers and counselors. And if that's not enough, I also have to struggle with you. I hate it when you check up on me, when you interrogate me about what I've done, when I see disgust all over your face. It makes me feel worse about myself.

In the heat of their struggle, Carlisle and Janie would both be unable to articulate their positions as clearly as we have laid them out. Nor could they fully understand each other's position in the midst of their conflict. However, any communication that either could make that approximated his or her position, even if made after a struggle—a hindsight communication—would be helpful because it might increase awareness of their predicament. Even without communication, each might be able to achieve some increment in hindsight awareness simply by thinking through the problem alone.

There are at least two advantages of any gains in hindsight awareness by either Janie or Carlisle. First, as we've been discussing, it may lessen their interpersonal struggle. Janie might be less cold or angry with Carlisle and might not monitor him so closely. And, if Carlisle came to view Janie's behaviors as resulting from fear rather than disgust with him, he may be more likely to open up about his own fears. However, there may be a second benefit: hindsight awareness could also help Carlisle find a job. If Janie understood what Carlisle was experiencing, she might be able to encourage or support him in ways that really did motivate him. If Carlisle understood what Janie was experiencing, he might feel some strength, even be empowered, if he could assure her that her financial fears would not be realized. He might make a stronger, more consistent effort to find work. He might be more forgiving of her efforts to control the situation.

> **Tip 2:** After a difficult interaction with your partner, consider the possibility that you have been more blaming during the discussion than you realize. Remind yourself that your partner has a legitimate and understandable position, even if he or she did something wrong. Try to understand that position as then you will be more likely to accept the conflict that arose, recover from it, and move on. That understanding will also make for a better discussion if the two of you revisit the conflict or meet it again in the future.

RECAP

Efforts to change a relationship, whether by an outside therapist or by ourselves, may have unintended consequences. Instead of creating change, our efforts may simply be more of the same. In fact, we can create a situation that is a worse version of the same old problem. To prevent our well-intentioned efforts from falling into these traps, we need awareness of what is going on between us. A good starting point is awareness of the story of our problem, elaborated in Chapter 8. Then we can see how the general story of our problem plays itself out in everyday interactions; we become mindful of the emotional communication during our discussions with each other. This awareness shows us options for altering the course of our conflicts as they're occurring, sometimes preventing them or at least minimizing their impact and facilitating recovery from them. Although such in-the-moment awareness is often difficult to achieve, a hindsight awareness of what went on between us can also help by facilitating acceptance of an argument, a quicker recovery from that argument, and motivation to pursue a more productive discussion.

The chapter offered two tips, one for in-the-moment awareness and one for hindsight awareness.

1. Early on in a conflict, as you are just getting tense, START a different communication between the two of you: **S**top what you are doing for the moment, **T**ake a deep breath, **A**ttend to what is going on with you emotionally in the moment, **R**eveal your emotional state to your partner, and **T**ake an interest in what is going on emotionally with your partner.

2. After a difficult interaction with your partner, realize that you have been more blaming during the discussion than you realize. Remind yourself that your partner has a legitimate and understandable position. Try to understand that position as it may help you recover and deal with this conflict in the future.

Exercise: Increasing Your Own Awareness

It's easier to start with hindsight awareness than with in-the-moment awareness. Look back at a recent argument about your central conflict. Can you see how the general story of your problem played itself out in this particular argument?

- How were you more blaming than you may have realized at the time? What did you say that your partner may have experienced as blaming?

  _____

  _____

  _____

- What were the main messages that each of you was unable to get across to the other? What was the message that you were trying to get across that your partner may not have heard?

  _____

  _____

  _____

- What was the message that your partner was trying to get across that you might not have heard?

  _____

  _____

  _____

Now consider the same conflict.

- If you had had greater in-the-moment awareness, what might you have said early on in the conflict that would have been a more direct expression of what you were feeling and that might have altered the course of the interaction?

  _____

  _____

  _____

- What might you have said that would have acknowledged what your partner was feeling or that might have shown your interest in what was going on with your partner?

  _____

  _____

  _____

Next Steps

We have now discussed two ways of bringing about change. In the previous chapter we considered simple and direct requests for change that can sometimes be successful. In this chapter, we considered making changes in your interaction with each other through greater awareness of that interaction. In the next chapter, we consider further ways of changing your communication with your partner by looking at guidelines for good communication skills, guidelines that you may have heard about. We will discuss those guidelines but also conditions when those guidelines can be helpful and when they may be harmful.

CHAPTER 13

Deliberate Change through Communication

TAKING GOOD ADVICE
ABOUT TALKING AND LISTENING
WITH A MINDFUL GRAIN OF SALT

> The single biggest problem with communication is the illusion that it has taken place.
> —GEORGE BERNARD SHAW

What is it about enduring love that makes communication between partners so difficult?

As we've seen, love makes us especially vulnerable to hurt and anger. The lack of interest or disagreement that we view philosophically from a friend or coworker cannot be sloughed off so easily when it involves our partners. When our incompatibilities and vulnerabilities are triggered, our emotional reactions often impede productive communication between us. We can be too angry to communicate constructively. Even then, however, communication usually does not break down completely: we can still talk to our partners about topics other than the conflict subject. Sometimes, however, a conflict may gradually spread until even everyday communication becomes difficult.

The legions of advice givers for couples—those mental health professionals or clergy or television "relationship experts" or bartenders or friends who claim some special knowledge about love—are well aware that communication is at the heart of many of our problems. So they have formulated a wealth of advice for expressing our complaints, airing our feelings, and eliciting the changes we want in our loved ones and our relationships.

We will now examine some of those rules, with the goal not only of promoting them but also of exposing their limits and inadequacies. Knowing the "rules of good communication" can be instructive, especially if you know when they often don't work but also when they do.

"Apple Pie" Advice

Much of what passes for advice about communication and love is a bit like politicians' support of motherhood and apple pie. You wouldn't argue with the admonition to love your partner any more than you'd claim that motherhood and apple pie are un-American. You wouldn't disagree in theory with the advice to honor, respect, cherish, support, or love your partner for what he or she is. But these nice sentiments don't get you closer to the transformed relationship you desire any more than espousing the wholesomeness of Mom and apple pie tells voters what a politician will do once she or he is elected to office.

Advice that encourages some general, admirable state such as love or respect is well intended but oversimplified in the extreme. When our relationships are going well, it may be easy to be respectful or supportive or loving without even trying. When the relationship is not going well, we may not have a clue as to how to achieve those states.

Even advice that is more specific can be impossible to follow. The common suggestion to say something nice to your partner every day tells you exactly what to do—say you love your partner or give your partner a compliment daily—but discounts the role of your feelings in this communication. It's no problem to say "I love you" when you feel loving or to say "You look gorgeous" when you feel attracted to your partner, but what about the times you don't feel that way? Is it really a good idea to say something to your partner that you don't mean?

Another common kind of advice explicitly addresses feelings but assumes they are completely under our control. Consider the oft-repeated advice not to go to bed angry with each other, not to be angry at the same time, or to be optimistic and cheerful with your partner. When you are feeling angry or pessimistic, it may not be possible to cut off your anger on command, much less transform it into optimism and good cheer.

Our society generally recognizes the distinction between feelings and thoughts on the one hand and behavior on the other, so it seems odd that those giving advice on interpersonal relationships often don't. Our customs and laws hold us responsible for what we do but not for what we think or feel—and for good reason. Our feelings and thoughts are private, they are not harmful to others unless they lead to particular harmful actions, and, most important, we can't control them as easily as we can control our behavior. Sometimes we can use distraction or reason to alter our feelings somewhat, especially if those feelings are not intense. We can also try to prevent certain feelings or thoughts by avoiding their predictable triggers. But generally our thoughts and especially feelings come unbidden.

Advice that exhorts us to have certain feelings or ban certain thoughts fails to consider the elementary distinction between what we do and what we think and feel. Therefore, it's generally not very useful.

When Good Advice Is Bad for Your Relationship

Obviously, lots of good advice doesn't fall into either of the traps just discussed. The advice to "apologize when you make a mistake that affects your partner" is certainly specific and is directed at behavior rather than at emotions. It is also good advice. Relationships would do better overall if partners were more willing to apologize for their mistakes.

However, even good advice can be bad when it ignores the emotional context. Jamal may be angry with Letitia and demand an apology, which she gives knowing that she made an error but still feeling resentful of Jamal's angry demand. Her ungracious apology leaves them both dissatisfied. Even if Letitia was able to provide a genuine apology, Jamal might be too angry to accept it, might continue to rail against her, and might anger her in turn.

Good advice can also fail because it ignores the larger relationship context in which behavior, even "good" behavior, occurs. Evan generally uses apologies as part of an appeasement strategy, apologizing quickly to avoid Steven's anger and further discussion of the topic. As a result, Steven only ends up annoyed by Evan's frequent apologies. For Jamal and Letitia as well as Evan and Steven, what sounds like "good advice" is actually bad for them and leads to a toxic solution.

Unfortunately, this problem is compounded because we are often attracted to "good advice" that is bad for us. Advice that fits in with what we normally do is likely to appeal to us. Evan likes the advice to apologize because that is his normal tendency. And he pushes that "good advice" on Steven. Steven likes the advice to "speak your feelings" because that is his natural tendency. But often, as with Evan and Steven, the advice we heed is not the advice we need.

Armed with your DEEP understanding as well as in-the-moment and hindsight awareness, you can discriminate good advice from bad advice for your particular problem. If Evan and Steven understood that blame on Steven's part and appeasement on Evan's, including his apologies, were part of their problematic pattern of interaction, their toxic solutions, they would know that this otherwise good advice for Steven to "speak his mind" and for Evan to "be willing to apologize" could simply further their problem.

The rest of this chapter will review common advice for achieving good communication that may be helpful for you. Knowing the benefits, the risks, and the difficulties of implementing particular advice on how to communicate will enable you to approach change in the context of acceptance. It will enable you to evaluate advice mindfully, based on your understanding of your particular problem and your observation of your ongoing pattern of interaction. Finally, it will enable you to understand that any advice may backfire, even if it is implemented correctly, and prepare you to accept and learn from those situations in which it does backfire. Sometimes we learn as much from our failures as from our successes.

Guidance for Talking with Your Partner

There are several pieces of communication advice that may be helpful to your relationship—when taken with a mindful grain of salt.

PICK A TIME AND PLACE TO TALK THAT WORKS FOR BOTH OF YOU

Probably most discussions about relationship issues occur when triggered by some provocative incident. When these discussions occur in this way at the "scene of the crime," it is not surprising that they often go poorly. One or both partners are upset, and they are likely to exchange accusations and defenses. They may get some benefit from venting their frustrations, and the discussion certainly underscores what one or both don't like. However, they are unlikely to have a productive, meaningful, and satisfying discussion. To have such a discussion, the time should be one where both partners are emotionally calm and receptive to the other; the place should be one where both feel comfortable. Let's consider an example of how Oliver and Suzanne use this advice by invoking their understanding and acceptance of their way of handling conflict.

After an unpleasant argument about their plans for the weekend, Oliver and Suzanne go to their separate corners and busy themselves with their Saturday morning tasks. Oliver hates the tense silence that comes after any argument with Suzanne and wants to explain his position about the weekend, which he believes she distorted. He approaches Suzanne, proposes kissing and making up and then starting over with their discussion of the weekend plans. He suggests that they have the whole weekend ahead of them and can still enjoy most of it. Suzanne only feels annoyed by his proposal. She takes longer to recover from conflict than Oliver, and right now she has no interest in making up.

At this point, both are in danger of creating a reactive problem that is more serious than the initial problem of their disagreement about the weekend. If they follow their usual form, Suzanne will rebuff Oliver's overture with a dismissive wave of her hand, Oliver will get angry again and criticize Suzanne's unresponsiveness to his "positive gesture," she will question the honesty of his gesture, and they will end up arguing about the way they recover from arguments more vehemently than they disagreed initially about their weekend plans.

However, they don't follow their usual form. Both are mindful of the DEEP understanding of their conflicts and have come to accept their pattern of recovery from conflict. Both know that a conversation has to be held at a time and place that works for both. Suzanne takes a deep breath and, harnessing her in-the-moment awareness, quells her impulse to reject Oliver's overture without a word of explanation or, worse, with an accusatory comment, such as "You always want to talk at the worst times." Instead she says honestly and directly, "I'm not there yet, Oliver."

Even though she didn't "kiss and make up" and discuss what he wanted, Suzanne's comment explains her action. For Oliver, it is worlds different from simply waving him off. The "there yet" also implies that she will get to a place of reconciliation in due time. Therefore, her comment plus his own in-the-moment awareness that his well-meaning overture could lead them into deeper conflict helped him back off. He said, "OK, I'm ready to talk when you are." Then he let Suzanne be.

With the pressure to make up relieved, Suzanne actually recovered more quickly from her distress than she otherwise would have. She later joined Oliver in the kitchen and helped him with the dishes. He made no demand for a kiss to mark their reconciliation but accepted her way of easing back into a connection with him. They resumed the discussion about their weekend plans, the discussion went much better, and they ended up having a good weekend together.

Oliver and Suzanne were able to follow the advice to pick a time and place that works for them both because they did so thoughtfully—by understanding and accepting their pattern of interaction. Suzanne has come to understand that Oliver gets anxious when there is emotional distance between them, tries to bridge that distance with efforts to make up and talk, and then gets furious when those overtures are rejected. Her accep-tance of Oliver's way of handling conflict and her ability to hold on to that acceptance in the moment enabled her to tell him "I'm not there yet" rather than wordlessly dismiss his attempt.

Similarly, through hindsight awareness, Oliver has come to accept that his efforts at reconciliation only put pressure on Suzanne and make it more difficult for her to reconnect with him. This acceptance enables him to let her come back to him at her own pace and in her own way. Their combined approach, their mutual awareness, understanding, and acceptance of how they handle conflict differently, enabled them not only to follow some good advice but to salvage a weekend and begin to change the destructive way they recover from conflict.

EXPRESS YOUR FEELINGS

Perhaps the most common communication advice from popular psychology is to "express your feelings." Pop psychology tells us not only that this is a good thing to do, but also that if we don't express our feelings, particularly our negative feelings, something bad may happen to us. This advice is based on a "balloon model" of negative feelings: if we push them down in one spot, they will pop up in another. Unexpressed, our feelings may "build up" inside and then "come out" physically as ulcers, headaches, and the like or "come out" psychologically in impulsive reactions such as emotional outbursts or rash decisions. Even if the feelings don't emerge in other ways, they may create stress that promotes illness and damages well-being. There seems to be nothing good about holding in our negative feelings.

Not surprisingly, the scientific evidence for these notions suggests much more complexity than the balloon model would indicate. The impact of expressing feelings depends on what the feelings are, how they are expressed, and to whom they are expressed. Sometimes the expression of feelings can prolong or amplify those feelings. Yet, despite these caveats, emotional expression has clear positive effects on our relationship. Appro-priate expression of feelings can lead to greater intimacy and influence. Confiding feelings—especially hidden emotions—to our partners is one of the best ways to feel emotionally closer to them. And by listening to us, they may feel emotionally closer to us. In addition, as they learn about our feel-ings, they may take our feelings into account when they deal with us. They may alter their behavior out of consideration for our feelings.

Despite all the potential good that can come from communicating our feelings to our partners, many problems arise when we try to express our negative feelings to them, especially when those feelings concern them.

Certainly, it will not be pleasant for them to hear the negative reactions we have to them. They may have trouble listening; they may interject their own negative feelings about us. But apart from their reactivity to what we say, it may be difficult for us to express our feelings honestly.

First, we may simply not know exactly what we feel. Take fear as an example. Psychologists measure fear in three different ways: by looking at behavior (people display fear by avoiding or escaping from a feared object), by assessing physiological arousal (people have faster heart rates, higher blood pressure, and sweat more when they are afraid), and by asking about subjective feelings (people report feeling afraid). Psychologists have found that these three measures of fear are consistently high when fear is great. If a husband took out a knife to threaten his wife, she might run away from him, her heart would be pounding, and she would certainly report terror. However, if fear is low—if a husband raised his voice with his wife, who was intimidated by anger—she might not show such consistency. She might turn away from him, her heart rate might rise slightly, but she might report no feelings of fear. She genuinely wouldn't label her internal state as fear because she simply wasn't aware of it. If we had clear evidence of her history of intimidation by anger, we might say she was not aware of her feelings of fear in this instance.

This example of fear is simple in that only one emotion was aroused. When more than one emotion is aroused but all at a low level, being "aware of your feelings" becomes more complicated. For example, assume that a husband and wife are out to dinner with friends. His contributions to the conversation aren't particularly interesting or amusing, but hers are. Encouraged by the attention and interest she commands, she interrupts him a couple of times. She does nothing rude or dramatic, but she slights his contributions and assumes control of the discussion. If we could inspect his feelings with a magnifying glass, we might see that he feels competitive with his wife, that he is envious of her ability to entertain others, and that he is annoyed at the interruptions. Yet because the things that she did were subtle and because his feelings of competition, jealousy, and annoyance are at such a low intensity, he may not be able to articulate them. He may only experience some vague sense of dissatisfaction. On the way home from their dinner, she may express her pleasure with the fun evening they had, while he seems in a bad mood.

Another reason we have difficulty expressing our feelings honestly is that we may not be comfortable with certain feelings and may not want to experience them. The husband above not only has trouble detecting his true feelings because they are at a low intensity; he does not *want* to identify these true feelings within himself. Either he is not comfortable feeling competitive with or envious of his wife, or he believes these feelings are not justified in this instance and is therefore embarrassed by them.

When we can't or won't express our feelings honestly, we often resort to acting on them instead of voicing them. When we walk out of the room and refuse to discuss a matter with our partner, we are acting on our feelings of anger, not voicing them. When we withdraw and sulk, we are acting on our hurt rather than verbalizing it. Even when we talk to our partner, we may be acting on our feelings rather than voicing them. As we explained in Chapter 9, our words may be stimulated by our hidden emotions, but those words may make no mention of those emotions. When we call our partner a jerk or yell "Don't you ever do that to me again," we may think our feelings are perfectly clear, but we're really adopting the diversionary tactic of focusing on the other person's faults instead of our hidden emotions.

When I ask partners in couple therapy to express how they feel about an issue of concern to them, I am asking questions about one person, but I often get a reply about the other. Here's a typical response from a husband asked about his feelings about their marital communication: "She doesn't know how to communicate very well. She either blurts out her feelings no matter what—whether the situation is appropriate or not—or just clams up. She just cannot have a simple, straightforward discussion about any disagreement without it getting all tense. I think she is afraid that she will lose out if she tries to deal with a problem rationally." Notice that the husband never mentioned anything about his feelings or even about himself.

Don't be surprised if you catch yourself "expressing your feelings" in this way. You may end up feeling hurt and frustrated that your partner has not heard your feelings. But you may never have voiced them.

USE "I" STATEMENTS

A common piece of communication advice designed to help couples express feelings rather than judgments like those above prescribes messages that begin with "I feel" rather than "You." A statement that begins this way is more likely to be about one's own feelings and less likely to be a judgment, an accusation, or a blameful comment. In contrast, a "you" statement is about the other and will often be accusatory. The comment "You blew it again" could easily communicate judgment and blame and invites argument. In contrast, "I feel angry when you do that" focuses on the speaker's feelings and is less subject to debate. It's a lot tougher to argue about whether someone has had a certain emotional reaction than about whether certain behavior was appropriate, so therapists and other advice givers advocate the "I" statement to filter out blame and judgment from communication.

If you hope to promote change and intimacy in your relationship with the help of this advice, however, beware of the ease with which this advice can be sabotaged. Partners in conflict often preface unadulterated judgments with an "I feel," as in "I feel you are shirking your responsibility" or "I feel you are being selfish." In fact, partners may try to sanitize their most accusatory or demeaning statements by putting them under the guise of expression of feelings: "I feel you are a jerk." "I feel you don't have the capacity to love." "I feel you are worthless as a spouse."

More specific advice about using I statements suggests that the "I feel" be followed by an emotion word. Messages such as "I feel angry" or "I feel disappointed" or "I feel hurt" clearly communicate feelings rather than judgments. But, of course, there's a way around this for the person bent on blaming and name calling: "I feel angry that you are being so selfish." "I feel disappointed when you are so cruel." "I feel hurt that you are being such a jerk about this." The listener is likely to hear the accusation—selfish, cruel, jerk—more than any expression of feelings.

There's an answer to this twist too: exclude all references to the other person. Instead of "I feel angry *that you* are being so selfish" or "I feel disappointed *when you* are so cruel," try "I feel angry about this whole incident" or "I feel very disappointed."

Yes, of course, there's another loophole. Depending on the context, voice tone, and facial expression, a statement like "I feel angry about this whole incident" can communicate "You know exactly why I am angry, you did the dastardly thing that made me angry, and you are going to pay for it." When anger is intense, it may be impossible not to communicate some sense of judgment and blame, no matter what the word choice. The expression of anger may then lead to defensiveness and counterattack in a partner, a situation that the focus on the speaker's feelings was designed to avoid.

If you are to approach change in the context of acceptance, you need to be aware of these misuses of "I" statements. Nevertheless, a pure statement of feelings, without any reference to the partner, is often a good place to start a discussion. And it is particularly a good place to start a discussion if that expression of feelings includes your hidden, soft feelings. Recall from Chapter 4 the distinction between surface and hidden emotions. We may feel angry but also feel hurt. We may feel resentful but also disappointed. We may feel irritated but also neglected. Those softer, less obvious, hidden emotions may capture our partner's interest, attention, and empathy.

Although comments such as "I am really angry," "I am really disappointed," and "I feel neglected and ignored" are a good place to start a discussion, clearly more needs to be said. Unless the trigger for these feelings is obvious, your partner may wonder or ask directly: "What are you angry

about?" or "What made you disappointed?" That brings us to the next section: how we can talk about our partners without attacking them.

TALK ABOUT YOUR PARTNER'S SPECIFIC BEHAVIOR RATHER THAN HIS OR HER PERSONALITY CHARACTERISTICS

To avoid the accusation inherent in a statement such as "I feel angry that
you are so selfish" and to avoid the lack of reference in a statement such
as "I feel angry," one common piece of advice is to express your feelings in
reaction to your partner's specific behavior: "I feel angry when you come
home late and don't call" or "I am disappointed that you forgot I had a
doctor's appointment today." With this kind of message, we express our
feelings and we indicate what we are reacting to, yet we don't attack our
partners' character or call into question their personality and put them on
the defensive. Contrast "I feel angry that you are so selfish" with "I felt
ignored when you didn't ask me about my day." Although a partner may not
like to hear either comment, the first invites defensiveness and argument
("I'm not selfish. You're the one who's selfish.") while the second invites
understanding.

Just like "I" statements, specific comments can be sabotaged, however.
Adrianna could get specific about Malcolm's behavior of paying attention
to other women by saying "I get angry when you leer at other women"
or "when you gawk at other women." While these statements contain no
personality descriptions, each one contains some negative evaluation that
could lead to defensiveness and argument: "I was not leering."

A more constructive approach would be for Adrianna to avoid loaded
words such as "gawk" or "leer" and instead describe his behavior more neutrally. For example, she might say "I didn't like it when you glanced at
Susan's cleavage" or "I got angry when you did a top-to-bottom checkout
of Esther." With messages like these, she will communicate in clear and
detailed language her exact feelings and exactly what behavior of his led to
those feelings.

Will this approach be easy for Adrianna to take? Maybe not. She might
find it phony to use such toothless language that does not accurately express
her experience. Or if Malcolm's behavior was subtle, she might not be sure
exactly what caused her feelings, the same way the husband who ended
up feeling competitive with and envious of his wife following a party was
unable to pinpoint the source of his bad mood. Or she might be wrong
about what caused her feelings. Adrianna may attribute her unhappiness to
her dislike of Susan or Esther and their provocative clothing, for she is only
dimly aware that it was Malcolm's actions more than their manner of dress

that upset her. Finally, focusing on the specific behavior may be ill-advised for Adrianna because it could obscure a larger issue of concern, such as Malcolm's commitment to their relationship. Without addressing this, he could forswear ever looking at women's cleavage again, but the commitment problem would remain.

Despite these difficulties, a focus on specific behavior will be more constructive than a focus on broad personality traits. When we know the difficulties of such a focus, we may accept some struggle and confusion and persist until we discover the things that really bother each other.

Tip 1: When discussing problems with your partner, first find a time and place where both of you feel comfortable, reasonably calm, and receptive to the other. Then talk about your own emotional reactions to your partner's specific behavior. Keep the focus on what you feel rather than on what your partner feels. If you can, try to describe your softer, hidden emotions as well as your surface emotions. Describe the behavior of your partner's that bothered you as specifically and neutrally as possible.

Guidance for Listening to Your Partner

While we typically think of communication as meaning "how we talk" or "how our partners talk," there is another important part of communication to consider: how we and our partners listen. Here again, when taken with a mindful grain of salt, some general advice can be helpful.

LISTEN TO WHAT YOUR PARTNER IS SAYING

Listening is one of the first casualties of couples' conflicts. As disagreements between partners escalate, they each make their points and produce their evidence, which fall on deaf ears. Active interruption by each makes it impossible to maintain even a pretense of listening. If partners do allow each other an uninterrupted turn at speaking, they use their silence to plan for their turn rather than to hear what the other says.

Therapists and other advice givers have gone beyond simple exhortations to listen and devised a way to ensure that partners not only attend to what the other is saying but also truly understand it. The strategy is called "active listening," and it requires that partners alternate between speaker and listener roles. The listener must paraphrase or summarize what the speaker has said, to the speaker's satisfaction, before the listener gets a chance to say his or her piece. The listener does not have to agree with the speaker's position but must demonstrate his or her understanding of that position. Here is an example in which Tony tries to listen to a concern of his wife, Rose.

> *Rose:* I am bothered by all our arguments over the kids. I think they are unnecessary—we shouldn't have to have them—and they upset the kids.
>
> *Tony:* So you don't like the arguments and you don't think the kids do either.
>
> *Rose:* Yes, but it is more than that. I think we should be able to discuss our differences without arguments. And I think the arguments may be harmful to the kids.
>
> *Tony:* You think the arguments are harmful to the kids' mental health?
>
> *Rose:* Yes. I think it makes them feel insecure. Maybe they wonder if we are going to stay together.
>
> *Tony:* So you think we ought to be able to discuss our differences without getting upset, and if we did, you think that would be better for the kids. They would feel more secure.
>
> *Rose:* Yes, that's right.

In this example, Rose got her message across to Tony. Whether he agrees or not, he genuinely understood what she had to say. Communication took place. Rose would feel heard, understood, and validated by Tony. She would likely be more open to his point of view should he want to voice it. Even if Tony did not agree with Rose, he would have understood something important about her. The connection they made about this concern of hers could easily enhance the closeness she felt to him and they felt to each other.

There was nothing particularly complicated about Rose's message, but it would be easy for even this simple communication to go awry. If she stated the message accusatorily, Tony would have a hard time hearing it. Rose could have said: "I don't know why you always argue with me about the kids. It really hurts them." In this message she puts the blame on Tony (it is "you argue," not "we argue"), and she uses the inflammatory word "always." So Rose communicates that Tony is culpable and that he always does this blameworthy behavior. Tony would probably react strongly to such a message. Even if he didn't defend himself and counterattack, he might turn off to Rose and distance himself from her. Most likely he would not be receptive to hearing anything further from her.

Even if Rose did not openly attack Tony and conveyed the messages as in the example, Tony could still feel defensive and respond in ways that distorted the message and derailed the discussion.

> *Rose:* I am bothered by all our arguments over the kids. I think they are unnecessary—we shouldn't have to have them—and they upset the kids.
>
> *Tony:* (*defensively*) So you can't take the simple arguments we have.

Here Tony subtly twists Rose's statement, interpreting her revelation that "I am bothered by all our arguments" as a weakness in her: "you can't take" the arguments. Calling the conflicts "simple arguments" implies that she cannot take what any other ordinary person could take. See where this might lead.

> *Rose:* I didn't say I couldn't take it; I said I was bothered by it.
>
> *Tony:* Well, you seem to be so bothered that I think you can't take it.
>
> *Rose:* It is not an issue of whether I can take it; I have taken it for far too long. It is an issue of whether it is good or appropriate for the kids.

Now they are off on an argument about their arguments over the kids. A listener can make an even more subtle perversion of the speaker's message by restating the speaker's words precisely but adding a *seemingly* innocent word or two.

> *Rose:* I am bothered by all our arguments over the kids. I think they are unnecessary—we shouldn't have to have them—and they upset the kids.
>
> *Tony:* So you want to feel bothered by all our arguments over the kids.

By throwing in the "you want to feel," Tony accuses Rose of intentionally getting upset. He implies that her distress is her own fault. Let's see where this could go:

> *Rose:* I didn't say I want to get bothered. I said I *was* bothered.
>
> *Tony:* But you have some control over your emotions, don't you? You are not a victim of your emotions, are you?

> *Rose:* Of course I am not a victim of my emotions.
>
> *Tony:* So if you feel bad, you must want to feel bad.

So now the two are off on an argument that may seem to plumb philosophical and psychological issues about control of emotional reactions, but it is really an argument over who is to blame for the conflict. Tony feels blamed for the arguments over the children and thus tries to blame Rose for being upset about those arguments.

Attempts to summarize the speaker's words can include much more obvious distortions than those in the preceding examples. The listener can editorialize about the speaker's message or ridicule that message in his or her supposed summaries of the speaker's message.

> *Rose:* I am bothered by all our arguments over the kids. I think they are unnecessary—we shouldn't have to have them—and they upset the kids.
>
> *Tony:* You think we have too many arguments about the kids. More than the ideal couple who never have conflict and are always sweet and agreeable.

Here Tony editorializes about what might be going on in Rose's mind—namely, that she is comparing their arguments to some ideal. However, Tony's message really serves to invalidate Rose's statement. In so many words, he is saying: Your feelings are not justified because you are comparing our normal arguments to your unrealistic ideal.

Let's look at a final example in which the listener, under the auspices of summarizing the speaker's message, ridicules that message.

> *Rose:* I think we should be able to discuss our differences without arguments. And I think the arguments may be harmful to the kids.
>
> *Tony:* So you think our little tiffs are going to make the kids go crazy!

Here Tony minimizes the arguments ("little tiffs") and exaggerates the possible impact ("make the kids go crazy") in a message that is far from capturing Rose's concerns, but rather invalidates those concerns by ridiculing them.

So far we have focused only on the verbal content of the listener's message. The way the listener communicates nonverbally—the posture, the voice tone, and the facial expression—can overshadow that message. For example, Tony might make a verbally accurate comment such as "You are really worried that our arguments are going to make the kids feel insecure" but say it with a tone of voice and manner that communicate understanding and sympathy. Or he could say it in a voice tone and manner that communicate "That's the craziest idea I've ever heard."

Why is it that listeners have such a difficult time with the simple request to summarize what the partner is saying? The difficulties usually arise when the listener feels blamed or challenged by the speaker's message. The listener then makes a statement that may attempt to capture the speaker's concerns but at the same time invalidates those concerns.

The complication for couples is that any conversation over a common problem is likely to include some implication of blame. When the focus is on something that one is upset about in the relationship, it is impossible to communicate that without also communicating some accusation. For one last time, let's consider the speaker's initial message:

> *Rose:* I am bothered by all our arguments over the kids. I think they are unnecessary—we shouldn't have to have them—and they upset the kids.

Even if Rose matched these nonblaming words with a nonaccusatory style of speech, there is a clear message of culpability. She is suggesting that Tony should not be doing what he is doing to contribute to the arguments. Certainly, she is not shifting all the blame onto him. But Tony, knowing Rose far better than we do, might accurately see that the nice message is a cover for the real underlying message that "you are the cause of our arguments that upset me and the kids." Or Tony may be so defensive that he responds to even an implication of shared blame with defensiveness.

The challenges of listening to your partner when he or she is describing a difficulty in which we have some role are great, as the illustrations above indicate. However, the payoff is immense. When we are able to voice our deepest concerns and issues and have the person we love the most listen to them and validate them as reasonable, even if our partner doesn't agree with them or see them in the same way, it is a powerful boost to emotional intimacy. We no longer feel alone with our concerns. Even if these concerns are not or cannot be readily addressed by problem solving or appropriate changes in behavior, the mere fact that they are heard and understood can be soothing.

Because of the challenges of listening to our partners describe problems in their relationship with us, we will inevitably stumble at times, as they will in trying to listen to us. Acceptance of those stumbles and persistence in the face of those stumbles can mean that we provide our partners,

and they provide us, with that special experience of being heard and validated while we express something of great importance—a concern about
our relationship with the person we love the most.

> **Tip 2:** Try showing your partner that you understand by summarizing his
> or her message before adding your own. Don't editorialize or impose your
> own spin. Try to see the validity in what your partner is saying and com-
> municate that validation. Remember that understanding does not mean
> agreement and that there are many ways of viewing any situation. Commu-
> nicating to your partner that he or she has a valid point of view will increase
> the chances that your partner will hear your valid point of view.

Guidance for Negotiating Reasonable Compromises

Better bend than break.
—SCOTTISH PROVERB

A compromise is a settlement by which each side
gets what neither side wanted.
—EVAN ESAR, *20,000 Quips and Quotes* (1968)

The man who says he is willing to meet you
halfway is usually a poor judge of distance.
—EVAN ESAR, *20,000 Quips and Quotes* (1968)

The idea that marriage involves compromise is probably as old as marriage
itself. What is more recent is the emphasis on the process of problem solving, in which partners negotiate and compromise as a means of dealing
with their differences. Business and law, in which people hammer out
detailed agreements with others, have been influential on marriage. Many
have noted that getting married and raising a family is in part a business
and is governed in part by law. The sheer frequency of divorce has alerted
most of us to the possibility that our marriage may not last forever and has
encouraged a pragmatic view of self-protection in the face of that possibility. Young love has been forced into an uncomfortable relationship with
prenuptial agreements and estate planning.

Some approaches to couple therapy and many self-help books have
advocated rational problem solving in marriage. Partners should sit down,
in a businesslike manner, and discuss their differences, negotiate and bar-

gain to fashion compromises, write down their agreements, and let these guide their behavior almost as if they were legal contracts. Sometimes couples are encouraged to engage in this process early in their relationships so that expectations can be clarified and problems averted. Let's look at some of the specific advice commonly offered to couples.

SET THE STAGE FOR PROBLEM SOLVING

Often couples try to solve problems when they are most upset by them. At those points the problems seem dramatic, and they have the energy to focus on them. But they may also be too angry to compromise or too upset to evaluate possible solutions. They may also not have discussed the problem enough to fully understand it. So similar to the advice above about communicating about relationship difficulties, couples are advised to engage in problem solving only when they are calm and unhurried and in a place that is comfortable for them both. The only problem with this advice is that couples often don't want to focus on controversial issues when they are relaxed and feeling good about each other. So this advice could lead couples to avoid the issues of concern altogether. Nevertheless, a problem is more likely to be solved when both are in a comfortable and positive frame of mind.

FOCUS ON ONLY ONE SPECIFIC PROBLEM AT A TIME

Discussions of problems often escalate in intensity and expand in content, both horizontally and vertically. Horizontally, the content includes more and more specific topics; vertically, content may expand from specific topics to broad categories. Rose and Tony may start out with a discussion of their arguments in front of the children but end with a discussion of their abilities as parents and how much each really loves the children. The advice to focus on one specific topic at a time is meant to counter this tendency.

However, it may be important for couples to explore broader themes as well as specific problems. For example, Rose may have a more important point to make to Tony than just that they shouldn't argue in front of the kids. She may be concerned that they as a couple and Tony as a father do not attend to the impact of their actions and words on the kids. Not observing the impact of their arguments on the children may be just one example. She may also be concerned that he doesn't seem to notice the impact of his moods on the children. The challenge for Rose and Tony is to be able to discuss this broad theme, and maybe even Tony's related theme about Rose overprotecting the children, without the discussion's escalating into a confusing and distressing confrontation that brings in "the kitchen sink."

Thus, our challenge is to narrow our focus on a particular problem but without limiting a full and broad exploration of that problem.

SEPARATE PROBLEM DEFINITION FROM PROBLEM SOLUTION

Often one or both members of a couple may generate solutions before the problem has been clearly defined and agreed on. As we saw in Chapter 8, this tendency leads to oversimplified solutions that are toxic. So it makes sense to first take a systematic, logical approach to defining the problem. And common advice to couples suggests that they carefully define the problem before attempting to solve it.

But human thought and emotion rarely follow the lock-step sequence that logic might dictate. Sometimes consideration of possible solutions helps define the true problem. Let's assume that Rose raised the problem of arguments in front of the kids and that Tony, ignoring our advice, proposed that he would be willing to move their arguments into a private setting away from the kids if she would simply request it at the time. Although this solution would solve the problem as Rose initially defined it, she was not satisfied with the solution. In her consideration of this solution and her discussion with Tony about it, she came to realize two important facets of the problem: (1) In addition to whatever direct impact they had on the kids, the arguments upset her and made her less able to deal with the kids. Merely keeping the kids away from their arguments would therefore deal with only the direct impact of their arguments on the kids. It would not deal with the indirect impact: how the arguments upset her and made her less capable as a mother. (2) She was in part concerned that Tony was not tuned in to the kids. She wanted him to notice the impact of arguments as well as the impact of his own behavior on the kids. If she had to notify him when the kids were affected, it would not resolve her concern.

GENERATE SOLUTIONS AND NEGOTIATE AN AGREEMENT

Once a problem has been defined so that both members agree on exactly what it is, they can move to the solution stage, where they generate, evaluate, and negotiate ideas to resolve the problem. A common piece of advice is to "brainstorm" solutions, that is, to generate as many ideas as possible without evaluating their quality. To focus on evaluating solutions may thwart creativity in generating them. Often an enthusiastic partner proposes a possible solution only to be deflated by the reaction of the partner who says in so many words "That will never work."

After all possible solutions have been generated, couples are advised to go through their list and systematically evaluate them, identifying the pros and cons of each. This evaluation process becomes a negotiation over possible solutions, in which couples give and take until they reach a compromise on a solution or set of solutions to implement. At this point couples are encouraged to write down the solution; the mere act of putting it on paper will make it more concrete to them. They are then advised to implement the solution and see if it is helpful. They can later sit down and discuss how the solution worked and perhaps modify it accordingly.

In Tony and Rose's evaluation of possible solutions, Rose might push for delaying their arguments until later. Tony would be reluctant to accept that plan because he knows Rose would push "later" back later and later. He might agree to a delay in their disagreement if they agreed to set a specific time period to resume the discussion that is sooner rather than later. Even if they could work out some agreement on this solution, Rose would be concerned, based on her experience with Tony, that he might push for the last word before they delayed their discussion. It would be hard for her to return her attention to the children if she were still fuming over Tony's ending remark. Thus, even apparently simple, concrete solutions, such as agreeing to delay discussion of a conflict, require discussion and negotiation before agreement is possible.

Problem solving can be a difficult and tedious process, but if it results in new behavior that solves an old problem it is well worth the effort. Problem solving is most likely to be successful when it addresses actions in which emotions play little or no role. Couples can use rational problem-solving strategies to handle conflicts over household chores, work schedules, and child care more easily than they can use these strategies to solve conflicts about how they argue or how they express anger. Tony and Rose can negotiate about who does the laundry more easily than they can negotiate about their arguments in front of the kids. Especially difficult are negotiations about behaviors that normally require positive emotions. Being "in the mood" is largely irrelevant for complying with an agreement to vacuum the house or pick up the kids on Tuesday. However, it is hardly irrelevant for an agreement about being more affectionate or sexual or attentive. You can easily follow through with the former, even if you don't feel like it. Not so with the latter.

Even when the strategy of rational problem solving works—when partners address a problem that lends itself to the strategy, when partners are able to follow a logical sequence, and when partners can agree on a workable solution—the outcome is often surprising. Partners may come to an agreeable solution but never implement it! Rose and Tony struggled with the issue of their arguments in front of the children. After considerable effort they worked out a plan in which they would delay their discussions until later; they would agree on a particular time for the later discussion; Tony would not level a zinger at Rose before the delay; and Rose would stop what she was doing and talk at the agreed-upon time. In the weeks that followed the agreement on this plan, Rose called for a delay only once. Tony agreed, but both forgot to return to the topic later. On a number of occasions neither Tony nor Rose initiated the solution when they got into a disagreement about the kids in front of the kids. This failure to implement the agreement was due in part to the fact that their disagreements in front of the children were not as intense as they were before. In reflecting on the problem, it was clear to Rose that she just wanted her concerns to be heard and taken seriously by Tony. The process of problem solving accomplished that. Afterward they both were more careful about how they dealt with disagreement in front of the kids. So their "solution" became irrelevant almost as soon as it was created. Yet their problem solving had been successful.

Tip 3: Try to problem-solve when both of you are relatively calm and not upset about the issue. Try to define the problem as carefully as possible before considering possible solutions. Consider as many solutions as either of you can think of and evaluate them for their possible effects before choosing any of them. Negotiate the most appropriate solution and try it out, revising it as needed based on how it works. However, be flexible in your problem solving because, as our examples illustrated, sometimes it can be helpful to bend these guidelines. When in doubt, let your in-the-moment and hindsight awareness of your relationship tailor general guidelines—they're not written in stone.

RECAP

In this chapter, we reviewed some of the most common rules of communication. We dismissed the "apple pie" advice that simply exhorts people to maintain a particular attitude or emotional state without any information about how to achieve that state. Then we focused on three broad categories of advice that give behavioral prescriptions about what to do, leading us to suggest three tips for communication.

1. When discussing problems with your partner, first find a time and place where both of you feel comfortable, reasonably calm, and

receptive to the other. Then talk about your own emotional reactions to your partner's specific behavior, including your softer, hidden emotions as well as your surface emotions and describing your partner's behavior as specifically and neutrally as possible.

2. When listening to your partner, summarize his or her message without any editorial comments or spin and try to capture the validity in that message. Remember that understanding does not mean agreement.

3. Problem-solve when both of you are relatively calm and have carefully defined the problem. Then consider all possible solutions, evaluate their pros and cons, negotiate a possible solution, and try it out, revising it later as needed.

Like most advice, these tips can be useful if you understand and accept their limitations, are flexible in their use, adapt them mindfully based on your understanding of you and your partner, and are prepared for occasional failure.

Exercise: Communicating Better with Your Partner

Although some of the rules discussed in this chapter are useful for everyday conversation, they are applicable primarily for discussions about relationship problems. It is these discussions that are most likely to deteriorate into accusation, defensiveness, counterattack, and withdrawal. Therefore, it is these discussions that need the structure that rules can provide.

Applying these guidelines to your core relationship conflict, answer the questions below.

• What is normally a good time and place where both of you are comfortable and receptive and might be able to discuss this issue constructively?

_____

• How could you tell your partner about your emotional reaction to a particular behavior of his or hers related to the core conflict? Write down a message that you might give.

_____

_____

_____

- You probably have some idea of the message that your partner wants to get across to you related to the core conflict. What is something you could say that would summarize that message in a validating way?

_____

_____

_____

- If you and your partner get to a point of problem-solving this issue, what are some concrete solutions that might be helpful (list at least one thing that you could do differently and one thing that your partner could do differently)?

_____

_____

_____

If both you and your partner have read this book up through this chapter, you could try using these communication guidelines to share with each other the DEEP analyses that you have done about a central problem in the relationship. For example, in describing the DEEP analysis that you have done, you could describe the emotional sensitivities that get touched in you when your partner engages in certain behaviors. You could also use the skills of listening and summarizing your partner's message when your partner describes his or her DEEP analysis. Even if your partner is not reading this book, you could at an appropriate time use these guidelines to share with him or her your DEEP analysis of a central problem and get your partner's reactions. Once you have gotten to understand each other's views better, you might even try to see if you can problem-solve to make some behavioral changes using the advice above.

Next Steps

As we have illustrated amply in this chapter, there will be times when mood and emotion prevent either you or your partner from using these rules appropriately. Sometimes these good rules will be bad advice for your relationship. However, they often can be helpful in communicating with your partner about your core conflictual issues. Using these rules while being mindful of the traps that you and your partner often get stuck in will enable you to use the rules more effectively.

Despite our best efforts, sometimes our attempts at communicating with our partners will go awry. Even these significant stumbles in our efforts to talk about the things that matter to us most emotionally can also provide opportunities to us. We may learn how to prevent a bad situation from getting worse. We may learn how to turn a bad situation into something beneficial for our relationship. In our next and final chapter on change, we consider change under the most difficult of circumstances— when things go bad between us.

CHAPTER 14

The Silver Bullet of Deliberate Change

TAKING CHARGE OF CHANGE EVEN WHEN THINGS GO BAD

Be the change that you wish to see . . .
—MAHATMA GANDHI

I wanted to change the world. But I have found that the only thing one can be sure of changing is oneself.
—ALDOUS HUXLEY, *Point Counter Point* (1928)

The sweetest pleasure arises from difficulties overcome.
—PUBLILIUS SYRUS, *The Moral Sayings of Publilius Syrus: A Roman Slave* (1855)

At least occasional defeat is inevitable for those seeking change—as the last three chapters have demonstrated. Efforts to seek sudden and dramatic change usually fail and often make the problem worse. New approaches to each other are often unmasked as simply more of the same old behavior because it's so hard for us to recognize how our relationship story comes into play in every encounter between us. Good advice is bad for us because it doesn't consider the emotional context of our conflicts. Rational rules become nonsensical because they fall into the trap captured by W. C. Fields, whose advice for conquering insomnia was "Get plenty of sleep." Even when we do everything right, our partners may have good reasons for not responding well to our efforts to change them.

Now for the good news: Being prepared to accept lack of change and being aware of how your current pattern of interaction doesn't solve the problem and often makes it worse opens up a wealth of opportunities for transforming your relationship into the peaceful, intimate union you've wanted all along. When you accept the failure of your efforts, you head off arguments about the change you believe should have occurred. Your partner may even respond to your acceptance in ways that lessen the need for change. Finally, you may end up less discouraged and frustrated than if you had been intractable, which may open you up to pursuing other, more successful avenues of change.

In this chapter we shift our attention to situations in which things between you and your partner go bad. Disappointment in the outcome is inevitable in efforts to create change, but you can take positive steps to minimize the instances of failure or to profit from them when they do occur. Instead of better rules for communicating and behaving, we will offer flexible guidelines that incorporate acceptance of whatever may come and that bend to accommodate your unique circumstances.

With this forgiving, adaptable, accepting, and mindful approach, you can succeed in bringing about improvement in your relationship whether any particular effort to make change succeeds or fails. You can win even when you lose.

To Change Your Relationship, First Change Yourself

As you've now seen many times, most efforts to improve relationships are directed at changing our partners. A fundamental shift occurs when we focus on changes *we* can make rather than on changes *they* can make. Rather than implying that we are culpable for whatever problems exist, this shift acknowledges that we have direct control over and responsibility for our own behavior alone. Likewise, only our partners have direct control over and responsibility for their behavior. It is empowering to know that we can make a change, rather than waiting in frustration for our partners to make a change. This notion of changing yourself first as a means of changing your relationship is the "silver bullet" of deliberate change.

Gerda appreciated Nat for his many fine qualities. He was a good man: honest, generous, hardworking, and committed to the family. She knew he loved her and would never be unfaithful to her. Yet some of his difficulties in communication were frustrating to her. He often didn't listen to her, he was easily distracted when she talked to him, and he would interrupt her in midsentence.

She first tried to talk to him about the problem. At times he would acknowledge the problem; at other times he would defend himself. But nothing seemed to change, so Gerda bought him a book on communication. With some persistent prodding on her part, Gerda got him to read a few chapters. He acknowledged some valuable points in the book, but again his behavior did not seem to change. Finally, Gerda proposed they go to a communication training class that was offered through the local college extension program. But Nat put his foot down at that point. The class was not held on a good night for him. Furthermore, he was tired of her constant complaints about his "inability to communicate." She should just accept him for what and how he was.

That confrontation precipitated a minor depression for Gerda. She didn't want to break up the marriage over some seemingly simple problems in communication. Yet these problems were a daily frustration to her that dimmed the value of Nat's more positive qualities and eroded her positive feelings for him. In her despair over the problem, she withdrew from Nat. This prompted more attention and concern on his part; he really wanted her to be happy. Gerda responded to his attention, became more engaged with him, but knew their problems wouldn't go away.

At this point, a fundamental shift occurred for Gerda. In her frustration over the possibility of never effecting a change in Nat, she decided that she could stop one annoying event from happening: his habit of continuing to watch television or trying to read the newspaper while he listened to her. In the past when she had complained about this diversion of his attention, he would argue that he could listen to her and still keep one ear turned to the television or one eye on the newspaper. So the television stayed on and the newspaper remained in his lap.

Mustering her courage, one evening Gerda told Nat she wanted to talk to him but wanted the television off and the newspaper off his lap before she did. He was annoyed by the request and launched into his argument that he could easily do two things at once. He recalled a previous occasion where she had accused him of not listening but where he had proven to her that he could recall everything that she had just said even though he had been glancing at the television. Because Gerda had carefully considered her approach to him and had already anticipated his reaction, she was prepared for this argument. She accepted his point but made her request anyway: "You may be able to listen to me and watch television or read the newspaper, but it is uncomfortable and distracting for me. I can't concentrate on what I'm saying when I'm wondering whether you're actually listening, so I would prefer to have your undivided attention when I have something important to say."

She had added the word *important* to justify her position, which she felt might be too extreme. However, that word served to stimulate Nat's curiosity. He argued with her a bit, but when he became convinced that she would not be swayed, he turned the television off with annoyance and said, "All right, what is it?" Gerda persisted that he needed to put the newspaper aside also. Frustrated, he threw the newspaper on the table, but he was all attention. Intimidated by his anger, she told him of an event that had happened at work that day, trying to make it as interesting as possible. At the end of her story, he commented sarcastically, "Well, that was certainly worth turning off the television and putting aside the newspaper for." He went back to his television. Gerda went upstairs and cried.

Because this first incident had gone so badly, Gerda almost gave up her struggle with Nat over the television and the newspaper. However, she knew that getting Nat to change his habits would not be easy, and she told herself that she was worth his full attention. She persisted with her plan; she would only greet him and exchange minimal information while he was involved with his television and newspaper. She would request time to talk to him without either. Sometimes he refused or delayed any conversation. There were also frustrating times when he would turn off the television and put away the newspaper with resentment or argue with her about her position. But gradually they established a new pattern in which he listened to her without the distractions of the television or newspaper.

Even during these diversion-free conversation times there were problems. Sometimes Nat's attention would wander, particularly if Gerda went on and on. At times she was so needy for conversation time with Nat that, given his undivided attention, she would luxuriate in it, without thought to what he was experiencing. Also, he would often interrupt her and talk over her. In an attempt to deal with these problems, Gerda tried to curb her tendency toward monologue. She also decided to confront Nat's interruptions directly.

Gerda was so accustomed to Nat's interruptions and so used to yielding to them that she often was not aware of them at the time. Only later in the conversation, as her frustration with being unable to voice her ideas increased, did she realize that he had been interrupting her. Then sometimes she would criticize him for his interruptions, he would defend himself, and an argument would ensue. Only as she became aware of his interruptions at the moment of their occurrence was she able to intervene in ways that allowed her to prevent the interruption but without creating an argument. She would say, "Wait. I'm not finished yet," or "Excuse me. You interrupted me. I am not done." These comments would often allow her to continue her communication to Nat.

Needless to say, Nat was not particularly pleased with these comments.

They were interrupting his interruptions. Even though they did not necessarily create an argument, he was frustrated by her efforts. He would let her continue with what she had to say, but he was often irritated by her comments. Although Gerda wavered at times in her efforts, wondering if she had a right to be so insistent, questioning whether it was worth dealing with Nat's negative reactions, feeling guilty for upsetting the status quo between them, she persisted. She counseled herself: Of course he is going to react negatively; I am upsetting his usual style. But I have a right to be fully heard by him.

A turning point came, paradoxically, when she was so frustrated with the tension her efforts created that she was ready to give up. She burst out to Nat: "I really don't want to create tension between us, but I am in such a bind. I can let you interrupt me and keep peace, but then I feel bad about myself, that my ideas are not worth your attention. Or I can stop your interruptions and complete my thoughts, but then I create tension between us. Neither way seems to work."

Because her emotions and words rang so true, Nat heard her message. He was sympathetic to her position. Surprisingly, he encouraged her in her efforts, and he tried to interrupt her less often.

Dealing with his interruptions in public created different challenges for Gerda than dealing with them in private. She feared creating a scene; she didn't want their friends to detect tension between them. But after achieving some success in stopping his interruptions in private, she went public with her efforts. At first she intervened cautiously, almost apologetically, when he interrupted her in public. The tension that her action created was painful for her. What she had not anticipated and what was even more difficult for her was seeing the hurt look on his face when she stopped him.

Over time, Gerda's efforts paid off. Nat would not only attend to her without television and a newspaper as distractions; he would also interrupt her less. Occasionally he surprised her by stopping himself in mid-interruption and letting her finish her comments. Although he would never be inducted into the "Listeners' Hall of Fame," he did listen to her more attentively. He changed in some very clear and concrete ways—but only because Gerda had changed first.

Although Gerda was not blameless—she had a tendency to ramble in her conversation—most of this problem was clearly in Nat's corner. It would have been easy for Gerda to persist in trying to get him to change his inconsiderate ways. In changing her own behavior, Gerda not only had to get over her self-righteousness; she had to face her own doubts, fears, and frustrations; she had to deal with Nat's negative reactions; and finally she had to deal with the repeated failure of her efforts. At first it seemed unfair that the burden of change fell on her, the one who was in the right, but toward the end, as she started to see Nat changing gradually, the experience was empowering for her. She did not have to wait—impatiently—until he changed. She could take matters into her own hands.

Perhaps more important than the specific changes Nat made, though, were the changes that occurred in their relationship. Because a frequent source of her resentment diminished, Gerda felt more positive about Nat, she was able to be lighter with him, and he responded in kind. Also, because Nat was now more attentive to Gerda—she had insisted that he be so—he adapted more to her feelings and opinions. Thus Gerda felt more important to Nat and he in turn became more important to her. The "little" changes that Gerda had made created "little" changes in Nat, but in combination they had large ripple effects on their relationship, enhancing their intimacy with each other.

Do Less of the Same—and More of the Different

There is always the danger that change, even a change in ourselves, will turn out to be more of the same—that what seems new is really but a variation of the old. Awareness of what is happening in the relationship—awareness of the "story" you composed and have been using since Chapter 8—can prevent this kind of false change. With awareness of what is going on, you can make a genuine effort to do something different.

In the previous section, we urged you to change yourself first. In this section, we urge you to change yourself by doing something truly different. In the sections that follow, we target specific areas where you can do something different.

RATHER THAN COMPLAIN AND CRITICIZE, TAKE CONSTRUCTIVE ACTION

A common trap in relationships is to get caught in the pattern of complaining to or criticizing your partner about a problem but doing nothing else about it, even though constructive action could change it. To paraphrase a line from Eleanor Roosevelt, some would curse the darkness rather than light a candle.

In trying to create change in communication, it was easy for Gerda to complain *after* Nat had tuned her out and turned on the television or to complain *after* he had interrupted her. But her complaints only created arguments without ensuring the changes she wanted. What was harder for

Gerda—and would be for most of us—to do was to intervene at the moment rather than complain afterward. She had to push herself to ask Nat to turn the television off and to put the newspaper aside before she talked to him. She had to achieve an in-the-moment awareness of Nat's interruptions as they occurred so she could intervene at the time of an interruption and thus prevent it.

Let's consider another example of constructive action rather than complaints. Zack is upset over how controlling Samantha is. Everything has to go her way or, in Zack's words, she "throws a fit." She is adept at managing the situation so that the only reasonable alternative seems to be the action she desires. It is easy for Zack to grumble about Samantha, to say sarcastically, "I guess we should do what you want to do—because you never get your way," or to whine, "Let's do it your way again." In a calm moment, not near the scene of any relevant incident, he can even bring up the problem of her control as an issue to be discussed. Samantha usually ignores his sarcasm and whining. When he brings the problem up for discussion, she usually tries to justify her position.

It is hard for Zack to state his desires constructively and to push for them assertively in the moment of decision making. Samantha usually has a blueprint for their activities before Zack has thought of an alternative. Because everyday decisions are so much more important to Samantha than to Zack, she can trump his casual predilection with her decided preference.

Although any particular decision is usually not that important to Zack, his cumulative lack of influence *is* important to him. To alter this pattern, Zack will have to decide when to push his own preference and when to go along with Samantha's. On the one hand, he doesn't want to precipitate a struggle over an issue that matters little to him. On the other hand, if he just defers to Samantha because the decisions are not important to him, he feels bad about her, because she is so controlling, and bad about himself, because he lets himself be controlled. Once he decides to push for his preferences, he has to confront her questioning and resistance. "Do you really want to do that? It's so boring." He also may have to confront realistic limitations on what he can do, limitations that are sometimes exacerbated by Samantha's careful planning. For example, one Saturday morning they were driving to visit friends a couple of hours away when Zack saw a scenic area he wanted to stop and visit briefly. Samantha explained that she had told their friends they would arrive by noon for lunch so there was no time for this detour. To take the detour he wants, Zack would have to call the friends and make a potentially disruptive, last-minute alteration of the plans Samantha had made without his input. Of course, she makes plans without him because he often shows little interest in them at the time.

Zack decided to speak up in this instance and said, "I am going to call them and see if it is a problem if we are a little late." Samantha protested, arguing that it would be a problem but their friends would not say so, and suggested that his desires were selfish and trivial: "I can't believe you want to delay our friends just to see some stupid little piece of scenery." Zack resisted an impulse to attack back and just said tensely, "I believe my desires are as important as yours and theirs." Samantha responded tartly, "So you are creating a stupid little power struggle?" Rather than getting drawn into an argument, Zack ignored her comment and simply called their friends who, as he had predicted, were fine with their being a little late. Zack resisted the temptation to deliver an "I told you so." He and Samantha drove in tense silence to look briefly at the scene, which didn't quite live up to its advertisement. Zack was surprised that Samantha didn't point out its inadequacies but just rode in silence. Once they got to their friends' house, they relaxed with each other and had a good time. Because he felt better about himself for his assertiveness, he was more affectionate with Samantha for the rest of the day. To his pleasant surprise, she did not resist.

One positive incident like this did not change the dynamics between Zack and Samantha. Zack will need increased in-the-moment awareness of his own desires and increased involvement in Samantha's planning so that he can see to it that he gets more of what he wants rather than complain, after the fact, about not getting his needs met. He will have to sort out what is important for him and what is not because he will never be as concerned about planning as Samantha is and most details don't matter to him the way they do to her. It won't be easy, but it will probably be worth the trouble. When Zack feels powerless in the relationship, he feels bad about himself and angry with Samantha. He withdraws from her, which exacerbates her own feeling that she has to go it alone in the relationship, and deprives them both of the intimacy they desire. Any movement that Zack makes toward developing greater awareness, either in-the-moment or even hindsight awareness, and asserting his own desires, as he did in the example above, would be a step toward altering their dilemma.

DO SOMETHING POSITIVE FOR YOUR PARTNER—WITH NO STRINGS ATTACHED

When partners are in conflict, much of the daily positive attention they normally give each other may cease. Therefore many advice givers urge us to make a point of extending to our partners the little courtesies and considerations, the tokens of appreciation and affection, that we have been denying each other out of anger and resentment. Unfortunately, this advice falls into the W. C. Fields category: If we could follow the advice, we wouldn't have the problem; if we have the problem, we can't follow the advice. As we saw in Chapter 13, our hurt and anger over our partners' offenses may make following such advice all but impossible. Either we can't give these gifts freely or we can't face the way they might be received. For this reason, positive gestures toward your partner should probably not be offered unless you can make them without requiring your partner to respond in kind—without, in fact, predicating your action on any kind of response at all. The most powerful positive act is offered in the context of acceptance—an acceptance of your partner's negative feelings, which may lead him or her to reject your positive action. When your positive gestures are made independent of your partner's reaction, they remain positive no matter what the response.

After a particularly unpleasant confrontation, Samantha says to Zack, "I know that I can be controlling and hard to deal with at times. I just want to say that I love you a lot and I am willing to work on this or any other problem." This statement acknowledges her role in their problems, assures him of her love, and indicates her willingness to work on the problem. We could hardly imagine a more positive gesture. However, Zack may be too upset to respond in kind. He may be suspicious of her positive response and test it. He might reply angrily: "Well, you have finally acknowledged some responsibility. Now what are you going to do about it?"

If Samantha reacts to his negative reaction, they are back into another argument. If she can accept his negative reaction, perhaps because she has some compassion for his struggle with her, she may say: "I know you are angry now. Maybe we should talk later, but I want you to know that I do understand your feelings." Granted, these positive words would require considerable strength on Samantha's part. But when she offers them to Zack, she is giving the only genuine gift—one that comes without strings. If Zack takes a moment to review this interchange later, he may very well be touched by his wife's generosity and courage. In fact, it would be difficult for him not to be affected by a positive action that withstood even his own attempts to test it. Her simple unencumbered gesture toward him could in time lead to a powerful reconciliation between them. Beyond the resolution of their immediate conflict, her message communicates to Zack that she hears his. She gets it. As a result, he may have less need for protective distance from her.

DO WHAT YOUR PARTNER HAS BEEN ASKING YOU TO DO

One clue about what we can do that is really different, that is not more of the same, lies in our partners' complaints. What they accuse us of not doing, what they request or demand that we do more of, may include pre-scriptions for constructive action on our part. As long as the request is not something that triggers our vulnerable, soft emotions or would require us to compromise our core identity and values, we may be able to comply with our partners' requests at least some of the time. For example, if our partners want us to visit their parents with them more often, join them in attending a sports event or concert or movie, or simply help them with a project, their desires provide guidance for constructive action on our part. Even if we are not enthusiastic about these events, they all involve contact with our part-ner. We can participate in them occasionally without committing to doing so as often as our partners might ideally like. We might be able to use our creativity to make the experience, even though not our first or even second choice, something pleasurable for us both.

Doing something for our partners rather than with our partners can be more complicated, but it is sometimes a more powerful gift. As an example, let's consider a conflict between Enrique and Rosa about child care and housework. She complains, with considerable justification, that he does not take his share of the responsibility for child care and housework. He com-plains that she insists child care and housework be done to her exacting standards and that she does not acknowledge his contributions. A simple, positive action that he could take would be to do what she has been asking him to do: get more involved in child care and housework. Because of his flair for the dramatic and surprising, he decides to offer Rosa a complete Saturday off. He will take care of the children, and she can have the day to herself.

This seemingly simple, positive action could, however, be complicated for Enrique to implement. First, he has to deal with his own feelings that making such a positive gesture to her will indicate weakness, that he has given in to her, and that his position has no validity. A second challenge for him is to make his offer of a Saturday off without a grudge on the one hand or martyrdom or heroism on the other. If he comes in with an attitude that smacks of "You've been complaining so much, I guess I'll finally do some-thing to shut you up," he won't get a good reception for his offer, and his offer, contaminated by his resentment, will just lead to another argument.

Third, Enrique may also need to be prepared for skepticism and suspi-cion. Rosa may not know what to make of his offer and therefore may not respond to his first effort with wild appreciation. Fourth, he may face some practical obstacles. Maybe the Saturday that he wants to "give her" doesn't work for her. Finally, Rosa may have difficulty "letting go" for a whole day, perhaps because she feels guilty about being away from the kids or feels guilty that Enrique is taking the entire burden this Saturday. Just because she genuinely wants him to take more responsibility doesn't mean that she can easily give up that responsibility herself.

Even if Enrique and Rosa meet all of these challenges, some unexpected comment by one or the other could rock their precarious boat of genuine change. Let's say he makes the offer of a free Saturday to Rosa, she takes him up on it, and he carries it off well. On her return home, he shares his experience with her. Perhaps he had some difficulty with the kids and now has a greater realization of how challenging it can be to spend a whole day with them. He recounts his difficulties and his frustration and says, "Now I know more what you mean about how hard it is to take care of them for hours on end and keep your sanity at the same time."

Rosa may feel guilty about being gone all day. She may anticipate that he will use this day against her—that he will hold it up as evidence of what he does for the kids, that this one day will invalidate all her charges of noninvolvement. As a result, she may jump on his expression of frustration. "Well, now you know how difficult it can be. Maybe from now on you will be a little more sympathetic with me and offer to help more than once in a blue moon."

If Enrique were strong, he might hold on to the positive change and not be drawn into an argument: "I know it is difficult. And I plan to get more involved. Today was just a start, but it was a genuine start." However, after a day with the kids, this might be too much to ask. He responds to her provocative comment with an angry retort: "I can't believe it. Here I spend the whole day with the kids and all you can do is jump on me."

She responds: "Well, you think one day is all you need to do. So your work with the kids is done for the year, right?" And an argument is off and running.

However, this argument need not signal the white flag of defeat; it need not destroy the positive effort to change. A couple can salvage an argument and recover the thrust of change. After this unpleasant argument, Rosa mulls over her day alone and the fight they have just had. She achieves some hindsight awareness of what has just happened. She realizes that her husband did make a genuine effort and that she, out of her own anxieties, used his expression of frustration against him. Although she still has her fears about what one day of action on his part will mean, she apologizes to him. She expresses appreciation for what he has done.

Enrique's actions show Rosa not only that he has heard her message but also that he is willing to take constructive action about her message. Her apology shows him that she is willing to admit error and to acknowledge his efforts. Those actions could do more than start them on the difficult road to changing responsibility for child care. They are the kinds of actions, even when born out of argument, that can foster appreciation and closeness with each other.

TAKE BETTER CARE OF YOURSELF

A handful of guilt is better than a truckload of
resentment.
—PROVERB

Our genuine desire to protect our partners' feelings may make us conceal our own feelings and curb the behavior of ours that hurts their feelings. Although these loving acts of protection may ensure peace in the short term, if extensive, they may create resentment in us that, ironically, generates more distress than had we not been so protective. If we took better care of ourselves, we might have to deal with conflict in the short run, but we might increase our satisfaction over the long run.

In our sexual relationship, for example, we may forfeit potential pleasure rather than risk injury or embarrassment to our partners. To mention that something feels uncomfortable or that we need a slower pace might upset our partners or create tension in our relationship. To ask for some action that might arouse us could embarrass our partners and ourselves. Our sexual relationship could be disrupted. Our effort to improve our sex life could backfire and make things worse. So we endure discomfort or forgo pleasure to preserve what we have. We pass up opportunities to improve our own, and ultimately our partners', level of sexual satisfaction.

Although our sexual relationship is often a particularly sensitive area in which we may protect our partners' feelings, we can do so in almost any area. For example, you may be watching a television show that interests you, but your partner interrupts you to tell you something. Not wanting to hurt your partner's feelings, you do not say honestly, "I really want to watch this show. Can you tell me later?" Instead, you give your partner half your attention, leave the other half focused on the television, and feel vaguely resentful. Meanwhile, your partner may feel irritated at the less-than-full attention you provide.

These examples are not meant to oversimplify. Voicing your wishes may create hurt feelings, generate tension, or precipitate an argument. The distress may not be worth the freedom of expression. Because your partner's feelings do matter to you, it may be better to suppress your reactions and let the situation pass under certain circumstances. A useful guideline, like taking better care of yourself, can never substitute for good judgment.

When a problem comes up repeatedly, however, confrontation may be better than protection. Cara would like to spend more time away from

Diane. She enjoys a few hours shopping by herself and would like to go out with her friends without Diane more often than she does. In contrast, Diane prefers doing things with Cara and will adjust her schedule to go with her on almost every occasion, from social events to errands. Cara usually does not have the heart to tell Diane that she wants to do her shopping alone or that she would prefer to go on her errand by herself. So Diane tags along, and Cara finds herself mildly irritated by her partner's presence. Her only solution so far is to be slightly devious: she times her errands for when Diane is away or seems too busy to join her, or she makes up excuses for not taking Diane along when she gets together with a friend. She feels slightly guilty about these deceptions, and then she gets angry at Diane for putting her in this defensive position. But to take better care of herself and assert her right to independent activity would mean doing things that would hurt Diane's feelings, which in turn would mean more guilt for Cara. It might also precipitate an argument or spur Diane to withdraw in resentment.

There is no easy way for Cara to resolve her need for independence. But by taking the more devious avenue—carefully timing her errands or her shopping, offering half-truths about what she and her friends are going to do—she forces herself to repeat these measures every time she wants some time without Diane. Confronting Diane more directly about her needs would require her to handle Diane's emotional responses and her own, but in time genuine change might take place. A new pattern of greater independence for her in their relationship could emerge.

Cara might start by discussing her concerns with Diane. It would be important for her to focus on her desire for time apart from Diane rather than on any presumed deficiency in Diane, such as her insecurity. If the conversation emphasizes Diane's inadequacies rather than her own desire for independence, it will almost surely fail. However Cara approaches the subject, Diane will certainly be hurt by it. At some level, she will see Cara's desire for more independence as a rejection. Diane may well try to reframe her desire for independence as lack of love, or she may withdraw and sulk in a guilt-inducing way. It will be a challenge for Cara to maintain both that she does love Diane *and* that she needs more independence. It may help for Cara to share her own vulnerable, soft emotions with her partner: her guilt about hurting Diane, the appeal her constant presence had for her early in their relationship, her fear that Diane's constant presence may dampen her love for her. It is possible for them to be allies rather than adversaries in this effort.

Whether Cara starts with a heart-to-heart discussion or not, the real challenge for her will come in the everyday decisions about how to spend her time. She will need to tell Diane in so many words "I want to go shopping by myself today" or "I want to spend some time alone with Candace." Undoubtedly, she will have to deal with some negative reactions on Diane's part. At times she may decide not to push the issue; at times she may need to reassure Diane that greater independence is not her only goal. At other times, despite their best efforts, her actions may precipitate an argument.

If Cara persists in this struggle, she will achieve her immediate goal of more time apart from Diane. However, she may achieve much more. Once she has more independence and feels less guilt about achieving it, she may find that she values her time with Diane even more. Rather than tolerating Diane's presence with mild irritation, she may enjoy her company. Although Diane may find the initial rejection from Cara painful, she may end up with a more loving and appreciative partner. She may decide that a smaller portion of a genuine Cara is worth a greater portion of a half-hearted Cara. Furthermore, her insistence on greater independence may force Diane to reevaluate her own dependence on her and her connection with other friends and family.

Genuine change threatens conflict, but it offers the potential for greater personal growth and increased intimacy.

> **Tip 1:** The most powerful way to create change in your partner and in your relationship is to change yourself first. Rather than complain about your partner, take some constructive action yourself. Try doing considerate, positive things with and for your partner, without expecting anything in return. If you can, do some of what your partner has been asking you to do. Finally, always care for yourself as well as your partner. Don't forget your own needs or allow your concerns about your partner's reactions to prevent you from pursuing your own reasonable and valued goals.

Minimize Damage

Love puts us in harm's way. Although physicians try to follow the adage "First do no harm," lovers cannot. Because we care so much about our partners, who are different from us in what they want and think and feel, they will inevitably do things that disappoint, sadden, hurt, and anger us. They will, of course, also do things that excite, please, relax, and gladden us. But pain will always be part of love.

One important feature of good relationships is "pain management" and "damage control." Partners in any long-term relationship inevitably will experience tension and distress. The challenge is to contain these experiences, to prevent them from escalating out of control. An argument, a disappointment, a misunderstanding can create hurt and angry feelings that escalate into damaging statements ("I never really loved you") or intimidating threats ("I am going to leave you and this relationship"). These are the kinds of damaging words and actions we want to prevent. The following guidelines are designed to control damage.

IF YOU CAN'T GET YOUR MESSAGE ACROSS, CHANGE THE MEDIUM

It may be impossible to talk constructively about some issues with your partner. A controversial topic may have such a history of conflict that neither of you can bring it up without tension. The mere mention of the topic can initiate a chain of emotional arousal that leads to an impasse. However, the topic is important enough that it cannot be ignored.

You can change the circumstances of your discussion. You may bring up the topic when both of you are calm. You may talk about the topic when you both are at a restaurant, where neither of you would want to make a scene. You may talk on the phone since the extra distance that comes with a phone call may prevent the escalation of your emotions. All of these strategies are reasonable attempts to create a setting where constructive discussion may take place. However, if they are unsuccessful, a more dramatic change may be necessary.

You can change the medium of your message. Rather than talking in person or on the phone, you can write a note, send a text or e-mail, leave a voice-mail message, or make a video. This change in the medium may catch your partner's attention, particularly if you don't normally communicate this way. Your partner may be intrigued by getting a note, an e-mail, or a video from you. Changing the medium also allows you to say your piece without feedback or interruption. You will not be deterred by your partner's looks of annoyance, thrown off by his or her attempts to "correct" your version of events, or riled up by the rolling of her or his eyes. You can also deliver a more considered, thoughtful, and deliberate statement of your position. You can prepare what you're going to say, deleting a phrase that doesn't seem right or cutting a section of video that may be inflammatory. If you use the written word, there will be no angry voice tones or tense facial cues to distract from your message. Finally, if your partner chooses to respond in kind, he or she will enjoy some of the same benefits: freedom of expression without feedback or interruption and the opportunity to prepare a more thoughtful response. As a result, the process of communication may be less accusatory and less defensive. The change in medium may change the message.

WHEN DISCUSSION DETERIORATES INTO ARGUMENT, FOCUS ON EMOTIONS RATHER THAN CONTENT

Listen for the melody, not the words.

Tara and Ned are discussing their planned summer vacation in California. Although she is not fully aware of it, Tara is feeling increasingly irritated that Ned is taking over the discussion and the planning of the trip. He mentions that they can easily drive in one day from Los Angeles to San Francisco. She objects strenuously.

Tara: No, we can't drive from LA to San Francisco in a day.

Ned: Of course we can. People do it all the time in less than a day.

Tara: No they don't. Unless they're race car drivers.

Ned: Look. You're no judge of distance and time. We can take the 5 freeway; it's only a few hundred miles!

Tara: Bullshit! It's more like 500 miles. And is that your idea of a vacation—driving on a freeway?

Ned: My idea of a vacation is to get where you want to go as quickly as possible.

Tara: Well, I may want to take the scenic coastal route.

Ned: Great, then we can spend all our vacation in the car.

In this example Tara and Ned focus on details—the distance between LA and San Francisco and whether to take the inland or the coastal route—but ignore the growing tension between them that will prevent them from ever coming to a decision. Like the story of the family who has an elephant in their living room but never discusses it, they ignore the powerful emotional interplay going on between them and focus only on the superficial details of their discussion.

In *The Talk Book*, Jerry Goodman, a former colleague at UCLA, offers the following advice: "When in trouble, self-disclose on the double." Statements such as "I am beginning to feel tense" or "I dread where this conversation seems to be going" or "I think we are getting stuck" can shift a conversation away from its often superficial content to its more important emotional tone. A self-disclosure can put the emphasis on the melody in a conversation rather than the words. With this attention to emotion, it is possible to calm the discussion rather than inflame it further. Or at least postpone the discussion until a later time when emotions are calmer. Let's see how this might happen.

> *Tara:* I'm not sure why, but I'm getting really irritated by this conversation.
>
> *Ned:* I can tell.
>
> *Tara:* Well, you're not exactly Mister Calm.
>
> *Ned:* That's true. I'm frustrated too. I have this incredible urge to go online and prove to you that LA and San Francisco are less than 500 miles apart.
>
> *Tara: (smiling)* Please don't. Even if you were right, you'd win the battle but lose the war. Because I might refuse to go to California with you at all.

By talking about her emotional state, Tara was able to stop the escalation of emotion and inject some welcome lightness into their discussion.

Like all interpersonal advice, this advice comes with no guarantees. It is hardly a surefire solution to tension-filled talk. One danger is that we will comment on our partners' emotions or behavior rather than disclose about ourselves. Statements such as "You're overreacting to this whole thing" and "Why are you getting so angry?" change the focus from the content of the discussion to the emotional tone of the discussion. However, rather than disclosing how we're feeling, they make a judgmental evaluation of how our partners are feeling. Furthermore, even if we make a genuine disclosure about our own emotional state, we may imply that our partners are to blame for causing those emotions. For example, the comment "I'm getting really frustrated" can be made as simply a statement of one's emotions or with an overtone of "and you are such a jerk for making me frustrated." Even when we do it right—we are getting tense in a conversation so we change the focus from the content of our discussion to the emotions we are feeling—our partners may be so distressed themselves that they ignore what we have said and barge forward with their own points.

WHEN ALL ELSE FAILS, TAKE A TIME-OUT

There comes a point in arguments when nothing good will happen. Emotions are too high. Your partner is not listening, and neither are you. The looks and words that pass between you are only angry condemnations. It's time for a "time-out," a break in the communication where you can get out of each other's presence. You may mentally rehash the argument and get more inflamed, but at least the destructive comments have stopped. And eventually you will calm down. The retreat offered by a time-out can be a victory for the relationship.

Time-out is widely advocated because it has the compelling logic of a cease-fire. The first constructive act is to stop the fighting. And implementation seems simple: Just part company. Leave the immediate scene. Don't talk to each other until you're both calmer.

Of course, nothing is that simple between lovers, and time-out is no exception. It may be overused by those who want to avoid conflict and resisted by those who prefer to push ahead at all costs. And whether time-out is effective depends to a great extent on how it's initiated. The initiation itself can contain a heavy accusation, as in "You're getting hysterical, so I'm going to take a time-out" or "I can't talk to someone who is unreasonable, so I'm going to leave until you calm down." Or time-out can be the punctuation following a telling point or a dramatic summary of our position, which is precisely the wrong timing for our partners. It leaves us with the last word and our partners recoiling from our final shot. Not surprisingly, they may not cooperate with our proposal.

We can initiate a time-out with hints that it may be more than temporary or with the overt statement or covert implication that we will refuse to talk about this topic ever again. Or we can simply leave the scene, insulting and confusing our partners with our sudden departure.

Perhaps the best way to think about time-out is as a self-protective strategy for use in cases of failed discussions. If you view time-out as a way of taking care of yourself and the relationship when you're too upset to be reasonable or constructive, you're less likely to invoke it accusatorily or to use it to get in the last word. Even if your partner is the one who is hysterical, while you are still able to be reasonable, you can use time-out as a self-protective strategy. Sometimes when your partner is very upset, you can act in ways that soothe and comfort, but when the hysteria is directed at you, engaging with your partner will only upset you too. So calling a time-out still delivers the same message: I cannot act constructively in this current situation. I want a time-out as a way of protecting myself and our relationship.

The best way to call a time-out is to do it simply and briefly, requesting it for yourself and indicating your willingness to continue the discussion at a later time. For example, "I am getting frustrated and want to take a time-out. I am willing to continue the discussion later." Or "I don't think we are getting anywhere. I need a time-out—but will be able to talk about it later."

When you view time-out as a way to protect yourself and the relationship, you may become more respectful of your partner's needs for self-protection and thus more accommodating when your partner calls a time-out. Rather than preventing your partner from leaving the room or following your partner, you will allow him or her privacy and freedom of movement. You will accept your partner's calls for time-out even if you wanted to continue the discussion.

When you use time-out appropriately, you acknowledge a mutual failure: neither of you was successful at making the conversation constructive. This acceptance of failure, however, can prevent further damaging escalation in the argument. Moreover, it allows you to recover more quickly from the argument and renew your efforts to relate to each other. Your acceptance of failure can plant the seeds of later success.

Conflict is a window on both the best and worst of human relationships. During conflict, otherwise loving partners can relentlessly attack a vulnerable other or withdraw from a needy other, emotionally wounding the other even as they themselves are wounded. Conflict is often the tortuous road to separation and divorce. However, conflict can also spark powerful reconciliations, inspire intimacy and commitment, and invigorate relationships. It is often the occasion when partners voice, albeit in exaggerated form, what they have not been able to voice before. It can lay bare vulnerabilities and incompatibilities but in so doing stimulate efforts to address them rather than avoid them. These positive features of conflict can occur only if damage during the conflict is kept to a minimum. Thus time-out, by limiting damage, can pave the way for a more fulfilling, intimate relationship.

> **Tip 2:** Try to minimize the damage that conflict can cause. If a certain topic usually triggers unproductive conflict, try using a different setting or different medium to communicate about the topic. Intervene early if tension begins to overtake discussion. Focus on your emotional reactions rather than persisting with a focus on the topic of conflict. If your efforts to prevent or alter a conflictual discussion fail, take a time-out to prevent further escalation.

RECAP

Making positive, deliberate changes in our relationships is not easy, but it can be done. Although our tendency is to focus on what our partners should change, we will be more successful if we focus on what *we* can change. If we do less of what we normally do and more of what we typically don't do, we may achieve positive change. In particular, we can take constructive action instead of complaining and criticizing. We can do something positive for our partners even though there is negativity between us. We can do what our partners have asked us to do. None of these seemingly simple acts will be simple to implement. We may run up against our own resentment or a less-than-enthusiastic response from our partners.

Sometimes we can make a genuine change in our relationships by taking better care of ourselves. If we do not protect our partners so much, we may find ourselves less resentful. But we must deal with our own inhibitions and guilt about upsetting them by doing what we want to do.

At times, our disagreements with our partners may veer out of control. Our feelings and their feelings are so strong that constructive discussion becomes impossible. A positive change may simply be to minimize damage. If certain topics seem impossible to discuss constructively, we can change the circumstances or medium of those discussions. At the first signs of emotional distress, we may be able to salvage a discussion by focusing on the emotional interplay between us rather than by persisting with the particular topic that led us astray. When a discussion is not salvageable, we may need to call a time-out to cease the discussion between us and allow for a cooling-down period. A time-out represents an overt acknowledgment of the failure of our discussion, but, by preventing damaging escalation, it can facilitate reconciliation after the conflict and a quicker recovery to "normal." We get less painful conflict and sometimes, with a compassionate reconciliation, greater intimacy.

The discussion in this chapter led to two specific tips:

1. Rather than complain about your partner, take some constructive action yourself. Try doing positive things with and for your partner, without expecting anything in return, including some of the specific things your partner has asked you to do. But always care for yourself as well as your partner.

2. If a certain topic usually triggers unproductive conflict, try using a different setting or different medium to communicate about the topic. Intervene early if tension begins to overtake discussion. Focus on your emotional reactions rather than persisting with a focus on the topic of conflict. If your efforts to prevent or alter a conflictual discussion fail, take a time-out to prevent further escalation.

Exercise: Taking Charge of Change

The most fundamental and far-reaching change you can make in your relationship is to focus more on what you can do differently and less on what your partner can do differently.

- Consider some of the things you complain about. What kinds of constructive action could you take to improve those situations?

  _____

  _____

  _____

  _____

- What are some simple positive actions you could take for your partner or with your partner (think of what he or she has been asking that you do or complaining that you don't do)?

  _____

  _____

  _____

  _____

- Do you protect your partner's feelings unnecessarily, at the expense of your own resentment? What are some ways that you could care for yourself better, while still being kind to your partner?

  _____

  _____

  _____

  _____

One important way to improve your relationship is to minimize damaging interactions.

- If you are completely unable to communicate about a particular topic constructively, try changing the circumstances or medium in which you communicate. What is a different setting or different medium that might lead to more constructive communication?

  _____

_____

_____

- If a particular discussion begins to deteriorate, focus on the emotions, not the content. What emotions are typically raised in you and your partner that interfere with productive discussion (think back over your DEEP analysis, particularly the emotional sensitivities)?

_____

_____

_____

_____

- Try using time-out as a way to protect yourself and the relationship when an argument is no longer salvageable as a constructive discussion. Is there a recent argument when it might have been better to use time-out? Write out the best way for you to implement time-out with your partner without further exacerbating a conflictual situation (e.g., by explaining that you are upset rather than accusing your partner of being too upset, by leaving without a parting shot, and by suggesting your willingness to talk about the topic in the near future).

_____

_____

_____

_____

Where Are We Now, and Where Are We Going?

At this point, we hope that reading this book and doing the exercises have helped you achieve several broad goals. First, from Part I, you should have a greater understanding of the complexity of intimate conflict and how entrenched it can become when your efforts to resolve it begin with fault finding and blame laying. In Part II you should have gained an understanding of how your Differences (D), Emotional sensitivities or vulnerabilities (E), and External stressors (E) lead to initial problems between you and your partner and how your efforts to cope with these problems, your Pattern of communication (P), can lead to more serious reactive problems. Second, from Part III, you should have taken this general knowledge of conflict and applied it to your own particular struggles with your partner and created a "story of your relationship problems." Based on this story and your reading in Part III, you should have more understanding and compassion for your partner's position in the conflict and should have been able to communicate that compassion. You should be able, at times, to see your struggle with some healing distance, as more of an "it" and less of a "you." All of this can make you more accepting of the struggles in which you find yourself. Finally, from Part IV, you should have a greater understanding of the difficulty of making genuine, deliberate change and an awareness of how often efforts at change create more of the same.

Hopefully, you also are empowered with the notion that genuine change, though difficult, is possible if you start with the only person you have control over: yourself. Furthermore, genuine change is worth the struggle because it not only reduces conflict but also leads to greater intimacy. Ideally, the total impact of this book will lead to a softening of your position vis-à-vis your partner and to an appreciation of your partner's human limitations and vulnerabilities as well as your own, even as you struggle to create a better, more fulfilling relationship. Perhaps you have now begun to move away from adversarial incompatibilities to reconcilable differences.

At this point, you might find it helpful to evaluate your progress. To get an objective indication of your progress, you could take the relationship satisfaction questionnaires in Chapter 1 again and see if there has been improvement. If you have not achieved some of the objectives described above or if your level of improvement in satisfaction is not what you wanted, it might be wise to reread a chapter or section or to redo some of the recommended exercises (or do them now if you skipped over them). It is also possible that some special problem—an affront by your partner, such as an affair, violence, or verbal abuse, or a serious disorder in your partner, such as depression or alcoholism—prevents the kinds of positive change we have envisioned. It is also possible that your difficulties, whether or not they are exacerbated by special problems, require more than either of you can do. You may need professional assistance for your difficulties. In Part V we address each of these special problems.

PART V

When Acceptance
Is Not Enough

CHAPTER 15

"Don't Do That to Me!"

VIOLENCE, VERBAL ABUSE, AND INFIDELITY

Throughout this book we have promoted several important ideas: There are at least two sides to every conflict. No one partner is responsible for an interpersonal problem; both members contribute to it, usually unintentionally. Interpersonal pain comes in part from the action perpetrated and in part from a vulnerability to that action. Crimes of the heart are usually misdemeanors, but our vulnerabilities make them feel like felonies.

Yet sometimes true felonies are committed in relationships. Sometimes one partner does something that is really, objectively wrong. The problem is not that we are sensitive, although we may be. The problem is that our partners have done something that no one should have to accept or even tolerate.

This chapter discusses three all-too-common categories of action in relationships that should not be accepted because they raise moral as well as interpersonal issues: (1) violence, destruction, and physical coercion; (2) psychological, emotional, and verbal abuse; and (3) infidelity. These three kinds of behavior are very different and have different consequences. We don't want to equate their degree of seriousness. Clearly, violence is the only one that can literally be deadly. Also, specific acts within each category range dramatically in their severity: being pushed is very different from being beaten. Yet each of these three types of action is destructive in relationships. In each case, there are victims. The victim of all three types of action can convincingly say, "Whatever I did that was problematic in our relationship, I didn't deserve this."

Violence, Destruction, and Physical Coercion

It seems obvious that violence, destruction, and physical coercion should not be accepted in any relationship. Yet they are so widespread that they bear discussing in the context of acceptance and change. We envision home as a safe haven, a place where we are protected from the struggles of the world. Unfortunately, instead of being a sanctuary of safety and support, homes are all too often dangerous sites of violence and destruction.

In 1985 Murray Straus and Richard Gelles conducted a national telephone survey of more than 3,500 couples who were married or living together and representative of the U.S. population at large. Among other questions, the researchers asked about specific violent acts that might have occurred in the last year between husband and wife. Their results showed that violent acts, such as pushing, shoving, slapping, hitting, kicking, and beating up, occurred in 16% of couples. Severe violence, which they defined as kicking, biting, hitting with a fist, hitting with an object, beating up, threatening with a knife or gun, or using a knife or gun, occurred in 6% of couples. Because these reports were made to a stranger over the phone, they probably underestimate the true prevalence of violence in couples. More recent surveys have found even higher levels of abuse. For example, Breiding, Black, and Ryan (2008) estimated that 29.4% of women and 15.9% of men experience at least one lifetime occurrence of physical or sexual violence in an intimate relationship.

Not surprisingly, rates of physical aggression are higher in distressed couples seeking counseling than in the general population. Studies suggest that 50% or more of all couples who seek therapy engage in at least some physical aggression. For example, in our clinical trial of couple therapy, 273 couples showed interest in the program and completed initial measures. Of these, we classified only 21% as no-violence couples. The remaining couples were approximately equally divided between low-level-violence couples, who had engaged in behaviors such as pushing and shoving, and moderate-to-severe-violence couples, who experienced punching, injury, etc. Even after excluding couples with potentially dangerous levels of violence from our study, a full 45% of couples reported one or more incidents of low-level violence in the year preceding therapy. Thus violence, particularly low-level violence such as pushing, grabbing, and shoving, is unfortunately quite common among couples, particularly those in distress.

Both men and women are violent, and most studies find that men and women are about equally likely to perpetrate low- and moderate-level violence. Similar rates occur in same-sex as well as cross-sex relationships, data that counter stereotypes that men could not be victims of violence by their male partners or that women would not be violent with their female partners. However, in heterosexual relationships, the physical and psychological effects of violence on women tend to be more damaging than those effects are on men. Because men are generally bigger and stronger than women, they are more likely to prevail in any violent episode. In fact, women are twice as likely as men to experience physical injury from violence. Furthermore, women are more likely than men to suffer psychological consequences, such as lowered self-esteem, depression, and stress as a result of the violence. In their landmark study of battering, Neil Jacobson and John Gottman reported that men virtually never experienced or reported fear during altercations, whereas women were typically terrified before, during, and after. Male violence is also more likely than female violence to escalate in intensity.

Another important difference between the violence men and women perpetrate is that men are more likely to commit severe violence, often referred to as "battering." Battering seems to have a different purpose for men and women. Men are more likely to use violence as a method of control, intimidation, and subjugation, whereas women are more likely to be violent as an act of self-defense or as an ineffectual expression of anger.

In contrast to the information on violence, there is little information on the frequency of destruction and physical coercion in the population. *Destruction* occurs when one partner deliberately damages a possession of the other. *Physical coercion* occurs when one partner physically forces the other to do something, such as have sex, or physically prevents the other from doing something, such as going out with a friend. Although there is not much information on these kinds of acts, they go hand in hand with violence.

CAN COUPLE THERAPY OR THE TECHNIQUES ADVOCATED IN THIS BOOK HELP STOP VIOLENCE IN A RELATIONSHIP?

To answer this question, we need to distinguish between battering on the one hand and the more common, low-to-moderate physical aggression on the other. In battering situations, almost always perpetrated by men, partners are afraid of the batterer because of current or past injuries they have experienced at the hands of the batterer. Battering includes acts such as hitting with a closed fist, kicking, hitting with an object, throwing the other down or against a wall, biting, and beating up. Even if there are no such acts of violence, there may be intimidation. Partners may be afraid for their physical safety or too scared to speak their minds, lest the batterer retaliate.

We do not do couple therapy, nor do we recommend it, for couples in which there is battering; therapy could be dangerous in these situations. Because therapy engages both partners in discussions of conflict-laden topics, the therapy could precipitate violent episodes. For example, as therapists we could encourage a wife to explain her point of view, her husband might become furious at her for what she then says in front of us, and he could retaliate at home by beating her up. As therapists, we would have then unwittingly precipitated violence.

Furthermore, if we agree to do couple therapy where there is battering, we are treating the batterer's problem as if it were a *couple* problem. This comes in handy for the batterer, who typically blames the partner for the violence, but it is destructive for the partner. It places the therapist in the untenable position of implicitly blaming the victim. In fact, stopping battering is solely the batterer's responsibility. Furthermore, by treating the pair as a couple, we imply that this is a relationship worth saving. We are endorsing the couple's staying together rather than separating. But that is seldom the right course for a couple where there is battering.

Finally, there is little evidence to suggest that any treatment will stop battering, including couple therapy. The evidence in favor of rehabilitation of any kind is meager and suggests that batterers will be batterers as long as they are physically able. The best solution to battering is for victims to leave, which they usually do once they have an adequate safety plan. But the short-term risk can be to place battered victims in even greater jeopardy if they try to leave. Although many battered victims escape abusive relationships eventually, the escape is all too often followed by more serious beatings, stalking, harassment, and even murder. *We advise battered victims interested in escaping safely to call the National Domestic Violence Hotline: 1-800-799-7233.* This hotline refers battered victims to local low-cost help from trained advocates, who can assist them in their safety needs. This may be the most important phone call that battered victims ever make. We also suggest going to National Domestic Violence Hotline website: *www.thehotline.org.*

Reading this book is not going to help battered victims any more than couple therapy would. If you are in such a violent relationship, you are reading the wrong book. In the Resources section, we recommend several books that can be helpful in dealing with violence in relationships.

What about physical aggression where there is no battering? What can be done about those angry exchanges that lead to low-level violence, such as pushing, grabbing, or shoving, but where there has not been injury or intimidation?

TAKE VIOLENCE, EVEN A PUSH OR A SHOVE, SERIOUSLY

One of the troubling things about violence in couples is that neither partner may take it seriously. In our study of 147 couples who were recruited as part of our clinical trial, both partners were asked to "Please list the main factors that led you personally to seek marital therapy." Only one couple reported physical or sexual abuse as the reason for seeking therapy, yet 52% of the couples had experienced an incident of minor physical aggression in the previous year, such as grabbing and pushing, and 24% had experienced an incident of severe aggression, such as punching or slamming into the wall, during the previous year. Our findings are consistent with others in the field. Clearly most couples with violence don't report it as a major problem.

The tendency to ignore violence is especially likely when the level of violence is low. Why make a big deal out of an occasional push or shove? Actually, there is a very good reason. *Mild violence should always be taken seriously because it can easily escalate into more serious violence.* The shove can be reciprocated; then the shoving match can turn into kicking or hitting. What was once seemingly innocent can become dangerous. Mild violence can also cause accidental injuries—for example, a person who is shoved can trip and fall. If you have children, you have another good reason to take mild violence seriously. Any display of violence between parents is harmful to children, not only because it sets a terrible example for them and increases the chances of their being physically aggressive in conflict situations but also because it triggers anxiety in the children toward their parents. They may feel scared and protective of the parent who gets shoved or pushed. It may complicate their feelings toward the two people most important in their lives. Additionally, violence between parents that occurs in front of the child could reasonably endanger that child (from thrown objects or other unintended actions), and such violence is considered potential child abuse in many states.

What does it mean to take violence seriously? You need to acknowledge it openly as a problem. You need to talk about it with your partner and establish a goal of nonviolence in your relationship. You need to insist on a standard of "zero tolerance" for violence. The remaining sections will discuss steps to achieve this goal.

ESTABLISH RESPONSIBILITY FOR VIOLENCE

A primary assumption in this book is that both partners contribute to problems between them. Unfortunately, those who have been violent, destructive, or physically coercive often use this rationale to justify their own behavior: I would not have pushed you if you had not been so insulting. I would not have torn up our wedding picture if you had not been so rejecting. I would not have kept you trapped in the kitchen had you been willing to talk to me.

There is, of course, a certain logic to these arguments. Without the insult, there might not have been the pushing incident. Without the rejection, the wedding picture may have remained intact. And with a willing-ness to talk, there would have been no necessity for coercion. This does not mean, however, that insults, rejection, or uncommunicativeness directly causes violence or that violent acts are of a kind with insulting words or rejecting words or refusal to talk. Freedom of speech, even insulting speech, is guaranteed for all, as is freedom of movement. Violence, destruction, and physical coercion are illegal acts, except in cases of self-defense. Therefore, the one who was violent, destructive, or physically coercive owns full and sole responsibility for these actions. Both partners are responsible for con-flict and arguments, but only the perpetrator is responsible for violence, destruction, and physical coercion.

REMEMBER THAT PERPETRATORS CAN CONTROL VIOLENCE

Violent partners may argue that they get so upset that they can't control their violence. Conflict provokes their anger so that they can't help grabbing or shoving, breaking things, or hindering the other's free movement. In fact, mildly violent partners can control themselves and are already control-ling their violence. They have not crossed certain lines. Despite their anger, they have not engaged in wanton destruction or actually battered their part-ners. They have demonstrated repeatedly that they can and do control their impulses, proving that the insults or whatever made them angry are not controlling their violent reaction.

The task in these cases is to move back the line of what is acceptable, to shift that control so that any violence, any destruction, or any physical coercion is off-limits. You can verbally insist on this standard of "zero toler-ance." More important, you can refuse to engage in violence, destruction, or physical coercion yourself, even in retaliation. You can discourage the initiation of violence by vowing never to respond to violence with violence. Unless it is critical to your self-defense, any retaliatory act of violence may signal your partner that you find mildly violent behavior as acceptable as he or she does.

END ARGUMENTS BEFORE VIOLENCE

The low levels of violence that are the focus of this section usually develop out of an argument. There is a buildup of conflict, an increase in intensity, until you are not listening to your partner and your partner is not listening to you. No constructive discussion is taking place. And then the shoving or grabbing or pushing begins.

This buildup may be rapid. Like a souped-up car in a drag race, you may go from a zero of calm conversation to the 100 miles per hour of intense anger and frustration in less than a minute. But it is possible to be aware of that transformation, no matter how rapidly it occurs. And it is possible to take control, to apply the brakes, before violence breaks out.

Chapter 14 discussed time-outs, stopping an argument in midstream. You and your partner can use this strategy to end arguments and postpone discussions and thus avert violence. You must become aware of the buildup, be tuned in to the shift from constructive engagement to futile argument. And then it is possible to stop the discussion before violence happens.

Even if you are not violent yourself, you can assist in this process. If your partner requests a time-out, you can honor it. You can even assist in the detection of a futile argument. You can say, even if your partner doesn't, "This argument is getting out of control. Let's take a break." It is not your responsibility to prevent your partner from being violent, only to prevent yourself from being violent. However, if you can stop an unproductive discussion, you will help your relationship. And if your partner is the violent party, you may make it easier for your partner to control his or her violence.

SEEK PROFESSIONAL ASSISTANCE

If you are unable to end violence on your own, seek professional assistance. Even though we do *not* recommend couple therapy for battering, our research demonstrates that it *is* useful for low- to moderate-level violence that erupts from arguments. Specifically, couple therapy is effective in improving overall relationship satisfaction when couples report mild to moderate levels of aggression and does not usually pose a risk for escalating violence. If one partner has a problem managing anger without resorting to low-level violence, destruction, or coercion, individual therapy may also be helpful. The next chapter discusses professional assistance in more detail.

Verbal, Psychological, and Emotional Abuse

> Sticks and stones may break our bones, but words
> will break our hearts.
> —ROBERT FULGHUM, *All I Really Need to Know I
> Learned in Kindergarten* (1988)

Words can hurt. The carefully aimed criticism, the dismissive comment, the blunt rejection, and the taunting joke can create psychological suffering that makes physical pain seem mild in comparison. Even the absence of words can create comparable emotional anguish. Physical withdrawal in response to affection, a bored look that greets excitement, or preoccupation that shuts down emotional expression can all break our hearts.

Although most of us know that love brings its share of pain, some words are more hurtful than should be allowed. But where does "unkind" or "unfair" or "mean-spirited" end and "abusive" begin?

DEFINING ABUSE

The term *verbal abuse* focuses on the actions of the abuser, the unacceptable words that the abuser uses. We often use this term to describe epithets and insults that anyone would consider unacceptably cruel. A pattern of cursing, swearing, or name calling can certainly be abusive. No one should have to tolerate personally degrading expressions like "You ugly bitch!" or "You worthless loser!" or "You miserable cunt!"

Certainly, threats of physical violence, *even if they are not carried out,* are another form of blatant verbal abuse. You should never have to hear threats such as "You say that again and I'll smash your face in" or "You do that again and I will hit you so fast you won't know what happened to you." Even if violence is not specifically threatened but only implied, it is abusive: "You won't do that if you know what's good for you" or "You do that again and you're going to regret it."

Other kinds of extreme threats, involving illegal or unacceptable actions, are also abusive, whether they are carried out or not. You should not have to hear threats involving the deprivation of your freedom ("I won't let you leave the house") or threats about contact with your children ("You do that again and I will take the kids, and you will never see them again") or threats about access to your friends and family ("I won't let you go see them") or threats that deny you normal adult autonomy ("I won't let you have any money, and then see what you can do") or threats about the destruction of your property ("Next time I will burn your stupid little diary"). All these actions are abusive; the threat of them, whether carried out or not, is verbal abuse.

Apart from these obvious examples of verbal abuse, it is difficult to specify which actions and words are verbal abuse and which are merely undesirable. Defined too broadly, the term loses its meaning and the impetus to stop the behavior. In a study by Julian Barling and associates of 398 New York couples 6 months after marriage, none of whom was seeking marital therapy, 89% checked off the item "insulted/swore at him/her," 82% checked "did/said something to spite him/her," 84% checked "stomped out of the room/house/yard," and 97% checked "sulked/refused to talk about an issue." Not surprisingly, rates are higher for couples in treatment: 90%

or more admit to each of these behaviors. These behaviors are probably not abuse but the result of the common relationship difficulties we've laid out in Parts I through IV of this book.

Instead, the term *abuse* refers to some action that is morally wrong, that is unacceptable human behavior, that should be condemned by all. We may be tempted to use the word to describe something that is merely negative or unpleasant for us, because it adds weight to our protest, invoking moral sanctions against our partners. Even if we use it in the desperate hope of deterring the unpleasant behavior, however, the charge of "abuse" may be another form of accusation that inflames an argument. Furthermore, it can backfire. For example, one husband's description of his wife's criticisms of him as "abusive" did not change her behavior. Instead, it gave her the opportunity to discount his objection altogether: that he would see her criticism as abusive just showed how ridiculously sensitive he was to her "constructive criticism."

How, then, do we distinguish the verbally abusive from the nonabusive? Perhaps we can find a clearer definition of abuse if we shift our focus from the abusive actions of the perpetrator to the emotional reactions of the victim. Some actions are termed *psychological abuse* or *emotional abuse* because the effect on the victim is abusive. What does it mean to feel emotionally or psychologically abused? It is much more than simply feeling hurt or upset by something, even if that hurt or upset is extensive. We can be very hurt that our partners forgot our birthday or flirted with someone else or made a critical comment about our appearance, but their behavior, in and of itself, is not abusive.

Feelings of emotional abuse involve fear, intimidation, and degradation. You are emotionally abused when you feel subjugated and controlled by your partner. When you are emotionally abused, you are frightened, you feel bad about yourself, even dehumanized, and you may blame yourself solely for the problems in the relationship.

Of course, it is possible to have feelings of fear, inadequacy, intimidation, degradation, and self-blame even when your partner is not being particularly abusive. These feelings can come more from yourself than from your contact with your partner. Furthermore, even if your partner is clearly abusive—yelling, swearing, and threatening you—you may not experience these bad feelings about yourself. You may fight back by yelling and swearing and threatening in return. Although the communication is clearly destructive, no one is feeling abused, just angry.

Therefore, to get a clear understanding of emotional and psychological abuse, we must consider both people in the relationship. If a woman feels intimidated and her husband is trying to dominate her; if she is feeling unworthy, and he looks at her contemptuously and tries to put her down; if she is feeling self-blame, and her partner is heaping on the accusations; or if she is feeling weak and inadequate, and her partner is trying to control her, then emotional and psychological abuse is occurring. Abuse happens only in a context of power inequities. When one is on top and trying to take advantage of it and the other is on the bottom and feeling scared, the situation is abusive.

Thus, words that are abusive in one relationship may not be abusive in another relationship. What is merely unpleasant for one couple may be poison to another. A wife could deride her husband with comments such as "You really blew it. You messed up royally. Can't you get it right for once?" If he found her comments annoying and simply fought back verbally ("Oh, get off my case"), this would be an argument, not abuse. However, if he said the same things to her, and his attack occurred within the context of a history of violence and intimidation, the same message would be abusive.

Battering is almost always accompanied by psychological abuse. When men batter their wives and girlfriends (or their husbands and boyfriends if they are in gay relationships), their threatening words carry the memories of or potential for real violence. Their words are often used in conjunction with their fists to subjugate and control. We noted above that this book is not helpful for couples in a battering relationship. Nor is it helpful in dealing with the psychological abuse that accompanies battering.

How often does psychological abuse or emotional abuse occur in the absence of battering? It is certainly possible for someone in a relationship to be intimidated, subjugated, and controlled even without the threat or actual occurrence of violence. A powerful man might use money, along with his abusive words, to control his wife, without ever beating her or threatening to beat her. We simply don't know how often this occurs. However, many of the concepts in this book—especially regarding acceptance—are not appropriate for those cases of control any more than they are appropriate for cases of battering. We would recommend that someone in this kind of relationship begin with the resources we described above for battering.

DISCOURAGING CRUEL AND UNACCEPTABLE LANGUAGE

The suggestions that follow do *not* apply to cases of battering or abusive control and subjugation. Following these suggestions could easily precipitate violence in a battering relationship or additional abuse in a psychologically or emotionally abusive relationship. These suggestions apply only to cases of cruel and unacceptable language such as cursing, name calling, and nonviolent threats. We will not use the term *abusive* for this kind of language, reserving that term for situations in which there is subjugation and control. We also encourage you not to use the term *abusive,* as that can be counterproductive in attempts to change the language that your partner uses. You may get into fruitless arguments about whether the "F word" is abusive or not or whether it is wrong to call the other an "ass" and miss the major point, which is that certain language may be painful for you to hear. And if certain language is painful or cruel or unacceptable for you, then it deserves your partner's attention. Your emotional or psychological reaction is the key to determining whether a behavior warrants action. Some partners can occasionally tell the other to "go to hell" or call the other a "jerk" or an "ass" or threaten separation or divorce without causing serious harm. Although these are hardly laudable acts, they may be just part of the way one or both express anger. If these acts are extremely painful, a serious affront to your dignity, then you should take action.

Talk to Your Partner

It's important to talk to your partner about a comment that is a painful affront to you, but only in a calm situation, not during the heat of the argument. Tell your partner the specific words or comments that offend you and focus on the impact of these words on you. Railing vaguely against "the way you talk to me" may leave your partner unsure of exactly what you find offensive and may invite defensiveness and arguments about your own sensitivity.

Consider how April tells Kerry of her feelings and resists being drawn into defending them.

> *April:* I need to talk to you. I really don't like it when you call me a "bitch" during an argument. I find that term degrading and offensive.
>
> *Kerry:* Oh, I just say it when I'm angry. I don't really mean it.
>
> *April:* You may not mean it, but I find it offensive, and I would appreciate it if you wouldn't say it anymore.
>
> *Kerry:* I think you're making a mountain out of a molehill. It's just a word.
>
> *April:* It is just a word, but for me it's an offensive word. And I would appreciate, out of consideration for me, that you not use that word.

Take Action in the Moment

An effective way to deal with language that is unacceptable to you is to take action that shows you will not tolerate it when it occurs. By "action" we don't mean a discussion such as just described but instead quick action to end the language right now. If your partner is cursing you or calling you an unacceptable name, you can simply announce, "I won't listen to you talk to me like that," and leave. Or you can leave without comment. You don't have to tolerate threats or name calling or insults. Take a time-out from the situation and leave your partner without an audience.

Ending a conversation when your partner makes an objectionable comment communicates a powerful message about that comment, but it's not an easy action to take. You may be so stung by your partner's attack that you want to attack back. You don't want to leave the situation; your impulse is to stay and fight. Often this leads to more objectionable language, perhaps on both sides. Similarly, if you are invested in the conversation or if there is some urgency to the conversation, you may not feel like ending it and waiting for a better time.

Don't Use Objectionable Language to Your Partner

If you want your partner to talk to you without name calling, yelling, cursing, or threatening, give your partner the same respect. Objectionable language is often the end product of an escalating argument. Stop the escalation by avoiding such language on your own part and you may decrease the chances that your partner will escalate into such language. You may need to invoke time-out to stop the escalation.

Infidelity

Most serious, committed romantic relationships endorse monogamy. In fact, the agreement to be monogamous is fundamental to most relationships. That is why having sexual relations with someone else is considered infidelity—literally, "not faithful": more than being simply an act of intimacy with a third person, it means betrayal of a fundamental trust—and often a great deal of deception as well.

Infidelity can occur even in relationships that allow sexual contact with others. Those relationships often have agreed-upon rules about that sexual contact. For example, some gay relationships allow sexual contact with others as long as those others aren't mutual friends or as long as it is a one-time occurrence with that other individual. Having sexual contact that broke these rules would be infidelity.

Infidelity can even occur apart from sexual contact with others. For months Clayton met secretly with his coworker, Alicia. Although he told his wife that work demands were keeping him late at the office, it was really Alicia. He poured out his soul to her, revealing all his marital problems, including difficulties in their sex life. She became his primary confidant. Behind his closed office door, Clayton and Alicia not only talked to each other; they kissed and fondled each other. They deliberately avoided intercourse, however, because Clayton felt that intercourse would clearly be a violation of his marriage vows. Furthermore, Alicia wanted to save sex for the day when Clayton left his wife.

Although Clayton took moral reassurance from the fact that he had not actually had intercourse with Alicia, it would have provided little solace for his wife. She would have been outraged by his secrecy, lies, and misleading comments. She would have been furious that he had shared their marital secrets with another woman. She would have felt foolish for comforting him after he came home late after a long workday. The fact that his physical contact with Alicia had never crossed the line into intercourse would not have consoled her. Even if Clayton had never kissed and fondled Alicia, his wife would have viewed his relationship with Alicia as an affair of the heart that violated their marriage.

In a national survey of human sexual behavior, about 20% of women and 25% of men indicated that they had been sexually unfaithful in their marriages. A British survey with an expanded definition of infidelity that included "adulteries of the heart" found, however, that 40% of their participants were unfaithful. And one report suggests that 60% of couples seeking therapy had been affected by extramarital relationships that were either completely sexual or were affairs of the heart. It seems clear that, although most couples manage to stay faithful to each other, there are many who do not.

THE IMPACT OF AFFAIRS

The discovery of an affair may be a pivotal point, like the death of a family member, which burns itself into your memory and changes your life forever. If you have no inkling of the affair and then get an anonymous letter or catch your partner with someone else, you may feel shocked and stunned. If you are strongly attached to your partner, you may experience the event as a trauma, more severe in its emotional impact than a car accident or a robbery at gunpoint. You may experience trauma's incumbent symptoms: constant and intrusive thoughts about the affair, inability to experience the emotions you normally experience, or hyperarousal and supervigilance, such as scrutinizing your partner for further evidence of affairs.

Even when the discovery is not traumatic, it can be destructive in other ways. If you suspected your partner's infidelity, finding out the truth may give you a strange sense of relief because it shows you that your suspicions were not crazy, as your partner may have implied. Still, confirmation of your suspicions can cast a dark shadow of distrust or erect a wall of anger that affects all your contact with your partner.

Is an affair a terminal condition for a relationship? Infidelity certainly presents a crisis, and it may signal the end of the relationship. Sometimes infidelity brings an already severely deteriorated relationship to a sudden, crisis-ridden end because neither partner has the desire to put the relationship back together. But even if a relationship is capable of recovery, the experience of moral and emotional violation may be so vast that the betrayed partner is unwilling or unable to give the relationship another try. There is much good in the relationship, but the infidelity crossed a line that could not be uncrossed.

Although infidelity can and often does end relationships, it clearly doesn't have to. In our clinical trial, we showed that couples in which there was infidelity could improve substantially during couple therapy and stay together, as long as they revealed the infidelity in couple therapy. Those whose infidelity was discovered after treatment termination almost all ended in divorce. However, even if both partners want to recover from the infidelity and mend the relationship, it can be difficult. Their efforts at recovery may create such powerful additional problems that they eventually break up. This is a special case of the reactive problem ending up causing more trouble—the end of the relationship—than the initial problem, the affair. It is such a common trap for couples that the rest of this section is devoted to helping you steer through the difficulties of getting past infidelity.

FIND OUT INFORMATION ABOUT THE INFIDELITY

You may have a strong need to know what happened. Your partner's affair may feel like community property, as much your business as your partner's. You certainly have a right to know about any risk to your physical safety. Did your partner practice safe sex? Is there a risk of sexually transmitted disease or of pregnancy? Should your partner be tested? Should you be tested?

Once questions about physical safety have been settled, you may desperately want to know details about the infidelity so you can understand what has been violated and gauge its impact. How long did the relationship last? How serious was it? Did they ever discuss marriage? Did they go to the same special, romantic places that you as a couple frequent? Did they ever have sex in your bed?

Often a struggle will develop over revelations about the affair. Because your partner doesn't want to anger you further or stoke his or her own guilt, your partner may conceal details of the affair. He or she may minimize the time spent or the gifts purchased or the intensity of feelings. As you sense his or her unwillingness to disclose what really happened, you may fear the affair was a bigger deal than it actually was. You may push for details, while your partner resists. You may wonder if you will ever get the whole story. Because your thirst for information never seems satisfied, you might find yourself slipping in questions at the oddest moments. Passing a hotel in town, you may ask, "Did you ever go there with him/her?" Your partner will surely get frustrated by what seems like a never-ending stream of questions: "Can't you ever give this up?"

In couple therapy we often set up a limited period for full disclosure. We find out whether the perpetrator of the affair is willing to answer any and all questions during a limited number of therapy sessions, say two or three. During these sessions we ask the unfaithful partner not to minimize involvement in the affair. In fact, we may ask him or her to "round up" rather than "round down." For example, if a husband saw his affair partner once or twice a week, he should say twice a week rather than once a week. In this way his wife may get a clear, unminimized picture of the affair and his involvement in it.

We ask the partner who has been violated to agree to ask questions only during these specially designated sessions. We encourage this violated partner to think of all possible questions and even to write them down before the session. We also ask the violated partner not to just ask the questions but to reveal their concerns in asking the questions as well. For example, a husband may want to know the intimate, physical details of the wife's affair to discover whether she was more adventuresome with her lover than she has been with him. If he felt she was resistant to sexual exploration with him, he may want to know if she was more open with her lover. Such revelations can lead to a useful though perhaps painful exploration of the couple's own sexual relationship. The payoff in these discussions for the violated partner is complete disclosure as long as the violated partner is willing to keep the questions within these specially designed therapy sessions. The payoff for the unfaithful partner is that the questions will cease if full disclosure is made as agreed.

If you are struggling with the aftermath of your partner's affair and have a strong need to know what happened, you may want to set up something similar. A few sessions of full disclosure may enable you to get the information you want without either of you enduring a constant struggle over what happened.

CLOSE THE DOOR ON THE OTHER RELATIONSHIP

To move your relationship forward, the affair must stop. Your partner will probably understand this. He or she may have considered a termination or even attempted it before you discovered the affair. But it is a decision that affects three people, and it is important to keep that in mind. The third party is often a victim too, perhaps having been deceived by your partner in some of the same ways that you were. For example, Clayton misled Alicia about his intentions to divorce, one time telling her he had consulted an attorney when he had not. Even if your partner has not misled the "third party," he or she may have legitimate concerns about that person's feelings. Your partner may need to consider how best to end the relationship.

You may want your partner to terminate not just sexual relations but any relationship with his or her lover. Because of the strong feelings that were generated in this other relationship, your partner may want to maintain close ties, even if no sexual relationship. He or she may still wish to have intimate conversations. He or she may want to keep that other relationship open just in case the relationship with you fails to heal.

You will have a hard time ever trusting your partner again, but it may be impossible if your partner doesn't cut off the other relationship completely. It would be perfectly natural to worry that if a so-called platonic relationship continues, a casual conversation will turn into an intimate conversation or an intimate conversation will turn into sexual intimacy. The progress of your relationship will be hampered if your partner maintains even a warm connection with the person who once had a more intimate and intense connection with your partner than you did. Nevertheless, your partner may be unwilling or unable to cut off all ties. The other person could be a coworker, and your partner may be unwilling to make a career sacrifice. You may walk a tightrope: Do you press your partner to make a sacrifice for your relationship or try to accept your partner's limited relationship with the other person?

Reviving trust may be easier if you can participate in the termination of this other relationship or at least be privy to its termination. Perhaps you and your partner can compose a letter that tells the other that the affair is over and that the two of you are going to put your relationship back together. Or perhaps you can listen in as your partner talks on the phone and tells the other that he or she wants to end the affair and work on your relationship.

What is important in this process is to shift the balance of intimacy and secrecy. During the affair, their relationship was secret from you. They talked about your relationship and its problems. You knew nothing of their relationship. Now you, the victim, have an understandable desire to know about their relationship, now past, and an equally understandable need to deny the third party any further information about your relationship as it now stands. You quite naturally want to shut the door to the person who had an affair with your partner so you can open it to your relationship.

This approach will feel right to you, who have been violated by another relationship, but it may not feel right to your partner, who still has feelings for the other man or woman. Your partner may claim, rightly, to be unable to turn off his or her feelings for this other person. But you are not asking your partner to turn off feelings, only to turn off the behavior toward this other person, behavior that your partner can control. Your partner may feel bad about hurting the other person by terminating all contact. And if the other person did care about your partner, the termination will hurt her or him. But the problem of a lover's triangle can never be solved without pain. Usually it is pain for all three. And one person must be eliminated from the triangle.

ESTABLISH RESPONSIBILITY FOR THE AFFAIR

Your partner may blame problems in your relationship for the affair. The fact that the relationship wasn't close or that the sex wasn't great drove your partner into someone else's arms. Or your partner might take it one step further and blame you directly. Because you did not listen to your partner's concerns, or because you were so selfish, or because you were not sexually responsive, your partner sought comfort elsewhere. Thus, the affair is as much your fault as your partner's—maybe more so.

In your own thinking about the affair and in your discussions with your partner, you need to clarify and separate two points. First, there may well have been problems in your relationship or problems in your responsiveness to your partner's needs. Affairs always happen in context; they don't happen when both partners are completely satisfied with their current relationship. But the second point is even more important: affairs are not designed to solve relationship problems, and they usually make those problems worse, not better. There are many other constructive ways of responding to relationship problems that don't involve secrecy and betrayal. Although you and your partner are jointly responsible for problems in the relationship, your partner is solely responsible for choosing an affair as a bad solution to those problems.

LET GO OF THE AFFAIR

Three weeks after he had confessed his affair, Joe felt there was no letup in Mary Louise's anger. It seemed that every conversation eventually turned to the affair. Her looks cast a thousand knives at him. Couldn't she realize that it had been a mistake on his part? He was hardly the first human being to make such a mistake. And he had been honest enough to admit the affair and strong enough to end it. Couldn't she focus on that?

For her part, Mary Louise found Joe's stance incredible. He seemed to want compliments for the fact that he had confessed the affair and ended it rather than criticism for the fact that he had had the affair to begin with. Why couldn't he focus on her pain and distress rather than justify his own position? Why couldn't he give her a genuine, heartfelt apology? She didn't need him to cry her a river, but she did need him to make amends.

Joe found it difficult to apologize to Mary Louise because of her intense anger. He read in her anger, "You have committed a horrible crime" or "You are less than human for doing what you did to me." An apology would feel to him like admitting to being inhuman or confessing to an unforgivable sin. Instead of offering an apology or displaying remorse, he tried to convince her that the affair was not serious and that the other woman meant little to him. But to Mary Louise, Joe's attempts to explain the affair came across as efforts to invalidate her feelings. She heard in his comments the message "You shouldn't be so upset; I didn't do anything very bad." So his efforts to explain himself made her angrier. And her anger made it more difficult for him to see her pain and respond to it.

A struggle, like that between Joe and Mary Louise, often develops over letting go of the affair. Naturally, your partner wants you to move on, to stop focusing on it. Your partner may encourage or even insist that you not dwell on the past, that you look to the future. Your partner may question why you bring it up when it only creates upset. But the affair may have so shaken your confidence or been so emotionally traumatic that you have difficulty letting go. You cannot avoid thinking about it. You are frequently reminded of the affair. You bring it up.

Even if your partner verbally acknowledges responsibility for the affair, you may not feel much relief or satisfaction. Your partner may come to that acknowledgment only reluctantly, after you pushed him or her on the point. Your partner may put more energy into justifying the affair by pointing out the inadequacy in you or in the relationship than in acknowledging his or her own personal responsibility.

If you saw that your partner understood your pain and was truly sorry for what he or she did to you, you could let go of the affair more easily. But instead you see defensiveness about the affair. Your partner's apologies may seem too cheap and easy. In response, your anger is heightened and your focus on the affair more intense.

Your partner may find it difficult to express genuine remorse. In the face of your angry accusation, he or she may resist making even a nominal apology. Your partner cannot see the suffering behind your accusations.

To break this kind of struggle requires one of three possible actions. Your partner can put aside his or her own feelings, realize that your anger masks your suffering, and respond to your suffering with genuine remorse and apology. Conversely, you can let go of some of your accusation, allow your pain and vulnerability—your hidden emotions—to be more obvious, and create a context in which your partner can experience empathy for you. Either one of these actions, if taken unilaterally, is difficult and for many people impossible. A movement by both you and your partner is a more likely avenue for letting go of the struggle and ultimately of the affair. If your partner makes an effort to understand the depth of your feelings and you show the hidden, softer side of those feelings, then your partner may move toward genuine remorse and you toward genuine forgiveness.

THE ONGOING ISSUE OF TRUST

You may wonder if you will ever trust your partner again. He or she betrayed you once; it could happen again. Going down a strange path is easier the second time around. How can you recapture your trust in your partner once it has been broken?

You may try to restore trust by seeking evidence of your partner's faithfulness or unfaithfulness. You may question your partner about his or her activities while not in your presence. You may carefully note the times your partner leaves home and returns from work. You may interrogate your partner if his or her behavior deviates from the usual—he comes home a little late, she is not at the office when you call, he has "errands to do" on Saturday morning.

In response, your partner may get irritated at your distrust. You also may wonder if you can ever trust again. From your seemingly innocent questions about his whereabouts to your interrogation of her over anything suspicious, your partner may fear that he or she will never be free again. Your partner will be boxed in by your mistrust.

Battles over trust can sometimes create as many as or more problems than the infidelity itself. You get angry at your partner because he or she won't tolerate your distrust. Here you had to tolerate infidelity, but your partner is annoyed that you won't suddenly trust again. Your partner gets angry at you because of your suspicions, your questions, and your vigilance. Your partner may feel tortured by your distrust.

When your partner has been unfaithful, you may look for evidence that will be as convincing. However, the problem with evidence is that it is only convincing in the negative, that is, when it points to an affair. Positive evidence is always suspect. If you find no evidence of suspicious calls on the phone bill, it may mean only that your partner used a disposable cell phone or work phones to make calls. If you find no suspicious credit card receipts, your partner may have simply paid in cash. Even in the extreme case of hiring a private investigator, an absence of evidence could simply mean that your partner's lover was out of town or otherwise unavailable during the period of surveillance.

For building trust, what is more important than evidence about what your partner does when he or she is not with you is the experience you have with your partner when he or she is with you. You can have experiences together with your partner that build trust apart from any evidence about what your partner does when you are not present. Some of these experiences occur as part of the process of discovery of the infidelity. For example, if your partner felt so guilty about the affair that he or she stopped it and revealed it to you, even when you had little or no suspicion, you may find in that revelation a basis for trust. Your partner could not persist in the infidelity; the commitment to you and personal integrity made your partner stop. Certainly, this kind of experience, no matter how upsetting, sets more of a basis for future trust than a case in which you yourself discover the infidelity in full bloom.

Even if you discovered the infidelity, there are experiences around it that can promote trust. If you see your partner's genuine guilt and remorse, you can be reassured that your partner has strong feelings for you and an intact sense of integrity. If you experience empathy from your partner for the pain you endured, you have a reason to believe your partner won't hurt you again.

Your partner's sensitivity to your feelings can also bolster trust. He may make extra efforts to call you when he is away on business trips, so you can feel the security of contact with him. She tolerates your insecurity and your questions. He can pass up a party at which his former lover may be present.

Greater openness is a direct antidote to distrust. Secrecy and deception are a necessary part of infidelity. If your partner makes efforts to be more open, so there is less that is unknown between the two of you, your partner will promote your trust. He may offer more information about what goes on with him. She may include you in her social circles at work so you know her colleagues and friends.

What ultimately will build your trust are your partner's efforts within your own relationship. If your partner addresses the problems in your relationship, you know your relationship is important to him or her. You know your partner wants to be with you.

What complicates all of these trust-building experiences is that they cannot be mounted by your partner alone. Your accusatory fury can dispel your partner's empathy. Your demands can quash his sensitivity. Your interrogation can prevent much openness. To have trust-enhancing experiences with your partner, you must give as well as receive. You may want and need your partner to make the first moves, but the process of rebuilding trust will require you both.

SEEK PROFESSIONAL ASSISTANCE

If you are not able to deal successfully with an affair on your own, by reading either this book or special books in the Resources that focus specifically on infidelity, you may need professional assistance. Couple therapy could help you get past the infidelity and resolve some of your relationship problems. In the next chapter, we discuss couple therapy.

RECAP

Three common ways in which we can be mistreated in relationships are (1) through violence, destructiveness, or physical coercion; (2) through verbal, emotional, or psychological abuse; and (3) through the infidelity of our partners. These kinds of actions are very different from each other, particularly in their danger to us, but are all similar in that they are objectively wrong. For most of this book, we have tried to get you away from moral judgments, to get you to see your problems instead as differences and emotional sensitivities exacerbated by external stressors and patterns of communication. However, some actions, even if they are common, are simply wrong. You should not have to endure violence, abuse, or betrayal from someone who loves you.

The actions encompassed by these three categories are not equally wrong. Being pushed is very different from being beaten up. Being called "an ass" is very different from having your life threatened. We made an important distinction between battering on the one hand and low-level physical aggression on the other. Battery involves injury and intimidation and is almost always committed by men. If you are in a battering relationship, this book is not for you. It is important that you seek help elsewhere, such as by calling the National Domestic Violence Hotline at 1-800-799-7233 or visiting its website at *www.thehotline.org*. Our comments on violence, destruction, and physical coercion concerned only low levels of these acts.

Like battering, psychological and emotional abuse involves fear and intimidation. They often go hand in hand with battering, and people in these kinds of relationships should consult the resources we provided for battering. Our comments focused more narrowly on objectionable language, such as name calling and cursing.

Finally, we discussed infidelity, the betrayal of relationship vows. Unless a partner reveals his or her actions immediately, infidelity also involves deception. Infidelity almost always creates a crisis for a relationship, challenging a core assumption that partners have made about the relationship and raising an enduring question about whether the restoration of trust is possible.

Although coping with each of these threats to the relationship has its own special requirements, there was one similarity across these issues. Our partners may believe that we contributed to their infidelity or their psychological abuse or their violence by what we did in the relationship. Even though they were the perpetrators, our actions led them to do what they did. We too may believe that we bear responsibility for our mistreatment at their hands. Maybe we deserved it.

It is important that we and our partners establish responsibility for the infidelity, the psychological abuse, and the violence, destructiveness, and coercion. Yes, we bear our share of the responsibility—along with our partners—for problems in the relationship. But our partners bear the *full responsibility* for reacting to those problems by being unfaithful, verbally abusive, violent, destructive, or physically coercive. No relationship problems force individuals to resort to these kinds of actions. No one deserves to be treated with lies or with abuse. These actions do not mean our partners are monsters or inhuman, but they do mean they were wrong. Recovery from infidelity, cruel or unacceptable language, and low levels of violence, destructiveness, and physical coercion is possible, particularly when appropriate responsibility for these acts is first established.

CHAPTER 16

Calling In the Professionals

COUPLE AND INDIVIDUAL THERAPY

If you've been quite unhappy in your relationship for several months or more, and your constructive efforts to talk to your partner, to implement the suggestions in this book, and to make positive changes in yourself have failed to improve your relationship substantially, you may want to try other alternatives. Of course, there are many other self-help books that focus on relationships, some that generally focus on relationship problems such as the current book and others that focus on particular problems, like infidelity. In the Resources, we list several other self-help books that are based on sound principles of relationship functioning and principles that have some support in the scientific literature.

Another entirely different and growing area of self-help is through online relationship programs. Two of the authors (B. D. and A. C.) have developed an online program (*www.OurRelationship.com*) based on the principles in this book. *OurRelationship.com* has two programs: one for couples to complete together and another for individuals to complete on their own if the partner is unwilling to participate. If your partner has not been reading this book with you or talking with you about what you have learned but might find an online program more appealing, completing the online program together might be a good way to get your partner involved in improving your relationship.

The online program, which is interactive and tailored to fit the specific needs of the participants, consists of three sections, an "observe" section where participants complete brief questionnaires about their relationship and get individualized feedback, an "understand" section where participants are taken through a DEEP analysis of their particular relationship problem, and a "respond" section that helps participants decide on specific changes to address the problem and improve their relationship. In the program for couples, these three sections each culminate in a conversation: first to clarify the problem or problems the participants want to work on (observe section), second to share what each thinks causes the problem (understand section), and finally to share what each would like to do to solve that problem (respond section). In the program for individuals, participants go through the three sections alone with the option of involving the partner only at the conversation stage. However, since you've gotten this far in *Reconcilable Differences*, doing the online program on your own probably would not be the best use of your time, especially if the ideas from *Reconcilable Differences* are fresh in your mind.

Self-help, whether through a book like this one or through an online program such as *OurRelationship.com*, has its limitations. If these programs do not work for you or you desire more professional attention, you may want to seek couple therapy. If you do, you will not be alone: relationship problems are one of the most common issues that send people to mental health professionals. The first half of this chapter explains who might benefit from couple therapy, what kinds of help are available, and how to find the best person to assist you.

Self-help is particularly likely to fall short when either you or your partner has serious individual problems that are affecting the relationship. Throughout this book we have tried to steer you away from laying blame for intimate conflict on your partner. But sometimes one of you does have a behavioral or emotional problem, and this problem clearly does play an important role in your struggles and in recovery from them. Research has indicated that the quality of intimate relationships is associated with the presence of anxiety, depression, substance abuse and dependence, and sexual dysfunction—the behavioral and emotional problems for which people most commonly seek help. A poor relationship can contribute to your partner's depression or anxiety or substance abuse or sexual difficulties, but these problems can also contribute to a poor relationship, in a kind of vicious cycle.

If your partner has an individual problem, you may have an important role to play not only in getting your partner to seek professional help but also in assisting your partner with his or her individual problem. The second half of this chapter will explain how.

"We Need Help!"

It's not hard to understand why so many people seek couple therapy. Almost half of all first marriages end in divorce, and the prospects are even dimmer for second marriages. Even many of those who stay married are not happy in the relationship—many couples stay together only because financial or religious barriers prevent them from separating or because they believe staying together will be best for their children. If your relationship has ceased to be a positive factor in your life, a pleasure or a support for you, and is instead an emotional burden, couple counseling may help. Even if you are extremely dissatisfied with the relationship—either because of a preponderance of negative emotions like anger, resentment, guilt, and disappointment or because there is little emotion of any kind, positive or negative—you are a good candidate for couple therapy if you are still committed to the relationship.

WHAT IS COUPLE THERAPY LIKE?

Asking what couple therapy is like is a little like asking what treatment for cancer is like. Just as the treatment that one patient receives for cancer will depend on the type of cancer, the variety of treatment options available, the philosophy of the doctor, and the receptiveness of the patient, your experience in couple therapy will vary depending on your specific problem, the treatment approach chosen, the type of therapist you consult, and what the two of you are willing to do.

Couple therapy is usually done conjointly. Although the therapist may want to see each of you alone at times, both of you will be present during most of the sessions. It is possible to undergo couple therapy without your partner, but the willingness of both partners to come to treatment will certainly increase its effectiveness.

You should also be aware that therapists normally take a neutral position about the conflicts that divide couples. Many couples come to therapy seeking specific advice on how to solve a particular conflict, but therapists usually will not simply hand over a point-by-point plan for how conflict ought to be resolved or how they would solve the same problem in their own relationship. Although they may make suggestions, therapists serve primarily as mediators who assist couples in understanding their problems and, based on this understanding, assist couples in coming up with their own solutions.

People who seek couple therapy sometimes want not advice but affirmation of their own righteousness. Many clients mentally rehearse the "evidence" against their partners before the first session. Others come fearing that the therapist will find fault with how they have behaved in the relationship. Because there is usually an excess of fault finding in couples who seek therapy, the therapist will work toward helping partners communicate better and find common ground rather than at directing blame.

This does not mean, however, that the therapist is passive. Those who have not experienced therapy before often hold in mind a stereotypical image of a patient lying on a couch, complaining about his or her problems, while the therapist sits nearby, quietly taking notes. This image is truer of psychoanalysis than of psychotherapy. Most individual therapy today would not proceed this way, and certainly couple therapy would not. Typically, partners in a couple sit so that they can speak directly to the therapist as well as to each other. Furthermore, the therapist is an active participant in the communication, rather than a note-taking observer. Because a couple in therapy can easily get into arguments, the therapist often serves as an active mediator in their conflicts.

WHAT TYPES OF COUPLE THERAPY ARE AVAILABLE?

In a very real sense, there are as many types of therapy as there are couples in therapy. Each therapist develops his or her own way of working with couples and adapts that strategy to each individual couple. However, there are several broad approaches to working with couples that have influenced therapists.

One broad distinction is between those approaches that focus on the past and those that focus on the present. A substantial portion of therapists, who call themselves psychodynamically oriented or psychoanalytically oriented, look to the past for answers to the puzzles of the present. They believe, for example, that spouses' marital difficulties stem from their past relationships with their mothers and fathers or other important figures from their past. Therefore, these therapists will be interested in the childhood histories of the spouses and will be on the lookout for connections between the present relationship and patterns in the past. For example, maybe the husband had a critical mother and learned to deal with her by withdrawing inward and avoiding direct communication with her. Now, when his wife is critical of him, he feels like he did with his mother and copes in the same way, by withdrawing. Or a wife may have gotten generous praise and admiration from her father when she was a girl. If her father was not forthcoming with adoration, she may have pouted and sulked. Perhaps she behaves similarly with her husband, seeking his praise but pouting if she doesn't get what she feels is an appropriate response from him. Therapists who focus on the past believe that when people achieve insight into the childhood origins of their own behavior and their partners' behavior, they will learn new and more constructive strategies for dealing with each other.

Therapists who focus on the present don't deny that the past is influential. But they don't believe it is necessary to attend to the past to solve the problems of the present. Furthermore, they wonder about the accuracy of people's recall of their childhood histories. In any event, they examine couples' present behavior, emotional reactions, and thought processes to help them approach their problems more constructively.

One major approach, called *behavioral couple therapy*, focuses couples on positive actions each could take to solve their problems and promote a better relationship. These therapists have partners generate lists of actions they could take that would make the other more satisfied, they encourage partners to engage in behaviors from these lists, and they debrief any actions that are taken to be sure that partners are acknowledging each other's efforts. This strategy of focusing on positive changes is also a mainstay of clinicians who call themselves *solution-focused therapists*.

In addition to this focus on positive actions, behavioral therapists teach partners communication and problem-solving skills, such as those discussed in Chapter 13. Similar to how coaches teach athletic skills, therapists may have couples practice the skills in session, give them feedback about their performance, and then assign them exercises to do at home to enhance their communication skills.

A group of clinicians who call themselves *cognitive-behavioral therapists* may use all the strategies just described, but they add an emphasis on the interpretation of behavior. Will interprets Claire's lack of interest in physical affection one evening as her punishing him by withdrawing affection. In fact, her intention may not at all be to punish him; she is simply not interested in being affectionate. In this case, a cognitive-behavioral therapist would analyze Will's interpretations of Claire's behavior in an effort to help him understand her better and respond to her more appropriately.

Other therapists focus on the present but attend more to emotions than to cognitive interpretations. A group of clinicians who call themselves *emotionally focused couple therapists* look at the primary emotions that partners arouse in each other. For example, partners may get so distressed with each other because they feel hurt by the other or fear abandonment by the other. These therapists help partners express these primary emotions of fear and hurt rather than engaging in verbal attacks of the other or withdrawal from the other. The expression of these primary emotions will often generate a positive, sympathetic response in the other that can lead to closeness and intimacy.

Researchers have studied the effectiveness of each of these approaches in couple therapy. More research has been conducted on behavioral couple therapy than on any other approach. In fact, studies conducted in the United States, Canada, Europe, Australia, and South America have consistently shown that this form of therapy helps a majority of heterosexual and gay/lesbian couples, at least in the short run. However, research has shown that many couples relapse 1 to 4 years following treatment. Although less research has been done on the other approaches to couple therapy, evidence from several studies shows that cognitive-behavioral therapy and emotion-focused therapy also help couples.

We have developed an approach called *integrative behavioral couple therapy* (IBCT) that utilizes strategies similar to a number of the therapies already discussed, as well as new strategies, but focuses on emotional acceptance in relationships. This book is a description of that approach but written for couples themselves. Research that we have done, as well as studies that others have conducted, suggest that IBCT is an effective treatment, perhaps more effective than behavioral couple therapy, the most studied therapy to date. Because of our research, the National Institute of Mental Health funded us (A. C. and N. J.) to conduct a large clinical trial comparing *IBCT* to *traditional behavioral couple therapy*. One hundred and thirty-four chronically and seriously distressed couples in Los Angeles and Seattle each received up to 26 weekly sessions of couple therapy. The data from this study indicated that IBCT led to superior outcomes that persisted over 2 years of follow-up. A full 69% of couples showed clinically significant improvement even 2 years after treatment termination. Over the next 3 years of follow-up gains tended to diminish and differences between the two treatments dissipated. We concluded that *IBCT led to superior outcomes* but that *for seriously and chronically distressed couples additional treatment in the form of booster sessions may be needed to maintain gains.* The Resources section lists links to websites where you can find therapists who practice this and other treatment approaches.

WHO DOES COUPLE COUNSELING?

There is no such thing as a couple counseling profession. Several different professions with different kinds of state licenses or certification engage in couple counseling. State licensing laws mandate what kind of professional practice a person holding the license can engage in. State certification laws mandate who can use a specific professional title.

Psychiatrists

Psychiatrists are first of all medical doctors. Just like their colleagues who will later become surgeons or radiologists or specialists in some other area of medicine, they go through 4 years of medical school, complete an internship or residency, and must pass a state licensing exam to practice medicine.

Specialty training in psychiatry comes primarily during a residency in psychiatry, which happens after receiving an MD and lasts for 3 or more years. Typically, this residency focuses on medical treatments, such as the use of drugs and hospitalization, to treat serious mental disorders such as depression and schizophrenia. Psychiatrists also learn how to consult with other physicians about patients with physical disorders that may be complicated by psychological factors. Couple therapy is usually not an important focus of their training.

Clinical Psychologists

Clinical psychologists have a PhD or PsyD (doctor of psychology) rather than an MD (doctor of medicine) degree. They go through 5 or more years of graduate school in psychology, where they study the assessment and treatment of psychological disorders. Their training also includes a year's internship, often in a hospital or mental health clinic, before they receive their doctorate. Prior to licensing or certification as psychologists, they must complete an additional year or more of postdoctoral training in assessment and treatment. Some exposure to couple therapy is usually a part of training, although only a small number of psychologists, such as the authors, specialize in it.

Social Workers

Social workers attend a 2-year graduate program before obtaining a master's degree in social work, an MSW degree. Before becoming licensed or certified as a clinical social worker, they need 2 additional years of supervised training. Those social workers who specialize in psychiatric social work will learn about mental disorders and individual, group, couple, and family therapies.

Counselors

Most states have licensing or certification laws for other kinds of counselors or therapists, such as mental health counselors. Of most relevance to the current discussion are those trained as marital and family therapists (MFTs, sometimes called marriage, family, and child counselors). They usually complete 2 years of graduate school leading to a master's degree. Prior to certification or licensing, they usually complete 2 years of postgraduate supervision. The content of these graduate programs varies considerably, but MFTs are specifically trained in couple counseling.

CHOOSING A COUPLE THERAPIST

Which of these mental health professionals is best at couple counseling? If we assume that those who have the most overall training are best, we would choose psychiatrists. Generally, they have spent a longer time getting their education and training than any of the other professions. Furthermore, if we assume that cost and quality are related, we would also choose psychiatrists, since they are generally the most expensive. However, much of the training of psychiatrists is completely irrelevant to couple therapy, particularly if the couple's problems are not tied to physical or mental health problems. In fact, most psychiatrists have had little or no formal training in couple counseling. One could pay out a lot for very little.

If we exclude medical training and look for the professional with the largest amount of psychological training, then we will naturally choose doctorate-level psychologists. During their training, they may spend more time and effort studying human behavior than the other mental health professions. However, unless they specialized in couple or family therapy, they may not have had much experience working with couples.

If we assume that it is not the overall amount of training that matters but rather the amount of specific training in couple counseling, we might choose a marital and family therapist. Although less educated overall than the doctoral mental health professions, these counselors have had special training in marital and family therapy. Furthermore, they will be less expensive than the doctoral-level providers. However, the programs that train master's-level clinicians show great differences in quality. Admissions standards tend to be lower than for doctorate-level programs. Therefore, the therapist who has a counselor license or certification may not be a better couple counselor than one with another professional identification.

Furthermore, the qualities that make a good couple therapist may have less to do with professional training and experience than with the therapist's own personal qualities. There is considerable evidence for this point in individual therapy. A number of years ago we reviewed the large research literature on training and experience in individual psychotherapy and found that it has little to do with client success. Thus clients are as likely to have a successful result of psychotherapy with a less experienced and less trained therapist than with a more experienced and more trained therapist. However, it may be that specific training in an approach with empirical support—such as those trained in IBCT or emotionally focused therapy—may achieve better outcomes for their clients.

We believe that couple therapy is more challenging than individual therapy simply because there are two people in the room rather than one and these two people are often adversaries. Being a good listener can take one a long way in individual therapy. Much more is required in couple therapy. Therefore, training and experience in couple therapy may make much more of a difference than training and experience in individual therapy. Nevertheless, no good research exists at this time on how training and experience in couple therapy affects the success of that therapy. The research literature on individual therapy should give us pause and make us look at factors other than simple training and experience when we choose a couple therapist.

The best couple therapist is one who has been successful with other couples. Therefore, a good place to get a referral is from friends who have been helped by couple counseling. Another good place to get a referral is from professionals, such as therapists, physicians, and ministers, who have referred people for couple therapy and gotten reports of their success. Getting in touch with professionals who can provide such referrals might mean calling a university psychology clinic or a community mental health center or the intake counselor at your health care organization. But be sure to ask whether the referring person knows couples who have been satisfied with the therapist being suggested to you. Reports of satisfied clients are probably still the best way to find satisfactory therapy yourself. Also inquire if the therapist is practicing any of the empirically supported approaches discussed above. That information will also increase the chances of a successful experience.

In choosing a therapist, remember that costs can vary widely and are not necessarily an indication of quality. Psychiatrists may charge $200 or more a session, clinical psychologists $150 or more a session, and master's-level therapists $100 or more a session. If asked, these therapists will sometimes take clients for less than their normal fee. Furthermore, your health insurance may provide some coverage of your couple therapy, particularly if you use a therapist who is employed by or who has a contract with your health care company.

The website *http://ibct.psych.ucla.edu*, devoted to IBCT, lists hundreds of therapists throughout the country who have been trained in this approach. Most of these therapists were trained through the U.S. Department of Veterans Affairs training program in mental health. These licensed therapists spent several days at a training workshop where they learned about IBCT from the first author (A. C.). Then for approximately 6 months, they saw couples using this approach while they were supervised each week by IBCT consultants. These consultants listened to audiotapes of the actual therapy sessions of these therapists so they could see how they were performing and give them accurate feedback on their performance. Only those therapists who saw a sufficient number of couples, participated in a sufficient number of supervision sessions, and demonstrated on the audio tapes sufficient competence in IBCT were approved by the VA and are listed on this website. These therapists include primarily psychologists and master's-level mental health professionals such as social workers. Many of them see couples only through the VA facility in which they are affiliated, but many also see private couples. If there is a therapist on this website who is near you and available, we would recommend calling that person first.

EVALUATING YOUR COUPLE THERAPIST

Just because you have carefully chosen a therapist who has been successful with other couples does not mean that this therapist will be successful with you. Even if the therapist has had 100% success before, if he or she cannot help you, you have not found the right therapist. The process of being a discriminating consumer does not end with the selection of a therapist. You should evaluate how your therapist affects you and your partner.

First, both of you should feel comfortable with your therapist. Being in therapy means disclosing your personal feelings, some of which may be uncomfortable or embarrassing. You certainly don't want to feel that your therapist is judging you for your feelings and positions. But more than that, you want to feel that it is easy to talk in front of your therapist, that he or she encourages open communication.

Second, both of you should feel that your therapist is an understanding ally. He or she should be neutral about your particular issues, not taking sides with you or your partner. But neutrality does not preclude understanding. Both of you should feel that your therapist understands your point of view, that he or she can see why you feel the way you do.

Third, discussions about your problems should be more constructive in therapy sessions than they have been elsewhere. You came to therapy because you avoided talking about your problems or got into destructive arguments. Unless your therapist can keep you from arguing with each other or refocus the discussion so it is more productive, you are not gaining anything from therapy.

The ultimate measure of success, however, is not what happens in the therapy session but what happens at home. No matter what wonderful things happen in session, if tension between the two of you does not decrease at home and satisfaction between the two of you does not increase outside of session, then therapy is a failure. Furthermore, these positive effects of therapy should not take forever. Couple therapy is not psychoanalysis. It does not take years. Most of the research on couple therapy shows that couples can improve with as few as a dozen or so sessions (about 3 months). In our research, which is more extensive than any research published to date, we achieved large and lasting gains in relationship satisfaction with couples who were chronically and seriously distressed in 26 sessions or less (about 6 months).

Improvement in your relationship, like improvement in any other important endeavor in life, is not a straight line upward. There are setbacks. Sometimes couples experience an initial "honeymoon effect" of therapy followed by some setback, as they see the problems are deeper or more complex than they first thought. However, despite some ups and downs, by 10 to 15 sessions of therapy you should experience some genuine progress. The two of you are confronting issues directly. You are able to talk about them more constructively. Even if you have a way to go, you should have a sense of progress.

If therapy isn't helping, discuss your concerns with your therapist. Perhaps the three of you can chart a more productive path. If therapy still isn't helpful, try another therapist. Couple therapy is hardly a panacea, but in the right hands it can definitely alter relationships for the better.

"_You_ Need Help!"

When does a personal problem become an interpersonal problem? Almost invariably, when one partner in a relationship has a serious personal problem, that problem intrudes on the relationship, causing conflict and sometimes preventing effective resolution of conflict.

When Justin started complaining about chest pains, he attributed them to indigestion, dismissing Selena's concerns that they might be something more serious. When he started perspiring and getting nauseous, he continued to insist that it must be something he ate, but Selena insisted that he go to the emergency room. "If you won't do it for yourself," she said, "at least do it for me."

At the hospital, their deepest fears were confirmed: Justin was having a heart attack. However, because Selena had insisted he go to the emergency room, the doctors were able to intervene early and minimize the damage to his heart. He later told her, "You may have saved my life."

Selena's efforts did not end with this dramatic event. When Justin returned from the hospital, both he and Selena decided to make some dramatic lifestyle changes. He quit smoking and cut back on his drinking. They both tried to eat less saturated fat and more fruits and vegetables. They started an exercise program. At first, Selena's enthusiasm and support for these changes was a welcome aid for Justin. She cheered him on and was sympathetic to his suffering, particularly when he gave up cigarettes. She was even tolerant of his bad moods.

But gradually Selena took on a supervisory, parental role with Justin. She monitored his diet and looked on disapprovingly when he indulged in a steak or treated himself to ice cream or cookies. She served him vegetables even when he didn't want to eat them. She reminded him when he didn't do his exercises. Concerned about his stress level, she urged him not to stay up so late.

Justin's contact with Selena created its own stresses for him. He resisted her efforts to control him, no matter how well-intentioned they were. He found himself sneaking cookies when she wasn't looking. He looked forward to eating without her because it was more relaxing for him. Occasionally he lied to her about going to the gym. He felt diminished by the whole process: somehow he had gone from a competent, respected husband to an errant child.

For her part, Selena felt increasingly frustrated at Justin's lame efforts on his own behalf. Didn't he realize how close to death he had come? Did he want to bring more stress on himself and the family? Why couldn't he do what everyone agreed was healthy for him? In a moment of insight, Selena realized that she cared more about Justin's problem than he did. She had gone from helping him with his problem to taking it on as her own.

In this example, Justin is clearly the one with the health problem. It is his heart that suffered the damage. It is he who must take medication and change his lifestyle. In a marriage, however, one can rarely have a problem in isolation. His heart attack affected Selena in dramatic ways—she was faced with the possible loss of her mate or with the potential of caring for an invalid. It was almost as if their marriage had suffered a heart attack as well.

As any loving partner would, Selena tried to help Justin with his problem. But over time her help turned into pressure and control. Maybe Justin needed some of that pressure, but it created its own stress for him. And Justin's difficulties making lifestyle changes created stress for Selena. A health problem became an interpersonal problem.

With a physical health problem, it is relatively easy to sort out who has the problem, what should be done about it, and how a mate can help out with the problem. When someone in a relationship has a psychological problem, it is more difficult to make these simple distinctions. Psychological problems all exist on a continuum, and unless the problem is extreme, partners may not even agree on whether a problem exists. A husband who suggests that his wife has a problem with depression may be met with the response that any depression on her part is only the result of his bad treatment of her. Even if both partners agree that one has a psychological problem, they may differ about what should be done about it. The wife may suggest marital therapy while the husband proposes antidepressant medication. Furthermore, they may differ on the role the "well" partner should take. Our depressed wife may want active emotional support from her husband as she struggles with depression, while he may point to all the ways he has taken on extra responsibilities in an effort to relieve some of the stress on her. In each of these situations, whatever personal problem exists can rapidly become an interpersonal problem. Furthermore, the personal problem may have had its genesis, in part, in the relationship.

If your partner has a serious personal problem, how can you avoid rejecting your partner for having the problem and abandoning your partner to deal with it on his or her own without taking on the problem as your own? If you can navigate these difficult waters, you will not only help your partner with his or her problem, but you may increase the intimacy in your relationship. A joint struggle against an important problem can bring about greater closeness. If you are the one with the individual problem, your openness and willingness to examine yourself will help not only you but also your relationship. It also may enable your partner to assist you more actively.

It is beyond the scope of this book to deal specifically with all the possible psychological problems that you or your partner can have, or even to deal specifically with the most common of these psychological problems, such as anxiety, depression, alcohol and drug problems, and sexual dysfunction. Each of these problems is complicated on its own and can impose specific challenges on an intimate relationship. What we can do here is offer some general guidelines, based on the principles of this book, for dealing with a partner who has a psychological disorder. In the Resources we have provided information to help you or your partner locate appropriate books or treatment if either of you is experiencing individual problems.

THINK OF YOUR PARTNER'S DIFFICULTIES AS A PSYCHOLOGICAL DIFFICULTY OR DISORDER, NOT AS A CHARACTER FLAW

It is relatively easy to handle a partner's physical problems. If your husband is injured in an accident or has a bona fide illness, you feel genuine concern and sympathy for him. If your wife needs surgery, you gladly visit her in the hospital. You don't begrudge your partner time away from responsibilities but instead take on some of your partner's share of the load while he or she cannot handle it.

Emotional and behavioral difficulties are harder to handle. You may believe your partner brought an emotional problem on himself and thus is responsible. You may suspect your partner of malingering out of laziness. You may view emotional difficulties, such as anxiety or depression, as a personal weakness, an inadequacy in handling life's stresses. You may fear your partner is manipulating you emotionally.

Behavioral difficulties, even more than emotional difficulties, may suggest character flaws. People may not be responsible for their emotions, but they certainly are responsible for their behavior. An alcohol abuser makes a decision to drink; he or she is not forced to do so. Because behavioral problems such as alcohol and drug abuse involve such clearly voluntary behavior, it may seem inappropriate to dignify them by calling them psychological disorders. Doesn't that allow your partner to escape responsibility for his or her behavior?

Not at all. Viewing your partner as having a psychological disorder does not absolve your partner of responsibility or rob her of the choice to take care of or not to take care of this disorder. Just as cancer victims make the choice to seek treatment even when the treatment is painful and scary, people with alcohol or gambling problems can seek and cooperate in difficult treatment.

There are many good reasons for us to think of emotional and behavioral problems as psychological difficulties or disorders rather than as character flaws. First, an abundance of evidence suggests a genetic vulnerability to almost all of the psychological disorders. Anxiety, depression, sexual dysfunction, and alcoholism are not flaws in something as nebulous as character; they are complicated products of biological and environmental factors over which we may have little control.

Second, if emotional and behavioral problems are accepted as psychological problems, some of the shame and blame associated with them can be dispelled. Rather than propelling them toward change, the shame and guilt that many people feel over depression or alcohol abuse may sink them more deeply into their problems. When self-blame is echoed by blame from family and friends, a downward spiral can easily occur.

Third, people can admit that they have a difficulty or disorder more easily than they can admit that they are bad, inadequate, or failures as people. Coming to the realization that they have a drinking or gambling problem or a problem with depression is often the first major step for people with a psychological disorder. This step, no matter how difficult, is usually easier if the admission doesn't destroy their dignity.

Finally, viewing emotional and behavioral problems as disorders makes it easier to seek help for them. There are specific treatments for psychological disorders. Concrete steps can be taken to seek those treatments: making an appointment, participating in an evaluation, going to a meeting. It is unclear how to treat character flaws, a failure of will, an inadequate personality, or failure as a person.

You may find it easier to think of your partner's problem as a psychological disorder if you learn more about the disorder. The appendix lists resources for several common psychological disorders that may be a starting point in your search for more information about a particular disorder. However, disorders always occur in unique human beings. If you want to know more about your partner's problems, you will need to talk and listen to him or her.

TALK ABOUT THE PROBLEM

Sometimes psychological problems are the elephant in the room that no one discusses. A husband rarely discusses his wife's difficulty in leaving the house because of her anxiety; nor does she. A wife notices but doesn't mention the quantity of alcohol her husband consumes each day; neither does he. The spouse with the problem may deny the seriousness of the condition; the partner may be afraid to bring it up.

Other couples may discuss the problems of one partner frequently but unproductively. A husband complains of his wife's drug problems, but she dismisses or ignores his complaints. A wife complains about her husband's complete disinterest in sex, but he passively tunes out her concerns.

If you have a partner with a serious psychological disorder, you may suggest that your partner seek treatment; you may even apply pressure in that direction. Yet your recommendations, especially if they are based on some readings about the problem, may come across as domineering advice from self-designated "experts." Or your recommendations may carry an accusatory subtext: "You are so bad you need a psychiatrist." Your advice may come out of your own frustration and carry the message "You are impossible for me to deal with; maybe the professionals can deal with you." These recommendations reflect your own needs and not your partner's needs: "I don't want to have to deal with this anymore. Go to a professional." These recommendations are often personally rejecting: "Take your problems elsewhere."

It is hardly surprising when a partner reacts negatively to recommendations that contain these messages. Your partner may argue with you, reject your calls for treatment, or criticize you in return. He may resist your suggestions, simply because you made them. Your recommendations for treatment can then prevent your partner from seeking it or at least delay it.

It is best to talk to your partner about her problem when you are not frustrated by it. When you are not upset, you can approach your partner with concern for his or her well-being; your message is less likely to have overtones of accusation. Also, it is usually better to talk about your partner's problem when she is not angry with you. For then she is less likely to anticipate accusation and more likely to hear your concern. Finally, it is usually best not to mention treatment right away. Your partner will need to admit to his problem before he will be willing to seek treatment for it. If he is defensive about his problems, it may take considerable constructive talk before he can face the possibility of treatment.

YOU CANNOT CONTROL YOUR PARTNER'S EMOTIONS OR BEHAVIOR

A special kind of pain comes when we see those we love do damaging things to themselves. We watch an alcoholic partner take the first drink, knowing what will follow. We watch a depressed partner berate himself relentlessly. Usually these actions not only bring us vicarious pain but affect us directly as well. We are embarrassed by our partners' drinking binges and clean up after them. We fear that the downward spiral of depression may lead to a job loss. We want to stop this self-destructive emotion and behavior, for their sake as well as our own. We cannot sit by helplessly and watch. So we try to control their destructive behavior. We may pressure a depressed partner to get out of bed and try to enjoy the day. We may remind an alcoholic partner not to drink at a party. We may try to distract an anxious partner.

If the problem is serious, it is unlikely that these prompts and reminders will have much impact. We may become more of a nagging partner than a helpful one. As we see the failure of our efforts to control our partners, we can get angry. We complain about their destructive behavior. We criticize them for their problem.

In our foiled efforts to help our partners by controlling their behavior, we may inadvertently contribute to their difficulties. There is considerable research on how family members respond to a spouse or child with a serious emotional disorder. Criticism, hostility, and even overinvolvement in the patient's life and problems have consistently been shown to have negative effects on the patient. For example, Jill Hooley, a psychologist at Harvard University, examined relapse in depressed patients. She and her colleagues followed depressed patients after they were released from the hospital and looked at what predicts whether their depression would return. Those patients whose spouses had critical and hostile attitudes toward them were most likely to relapse. In fact, in one study, the response of depressed patients to the question "How critical is your spouse of you?" was the best predictor of relapse—better than the overall marital satisfaction of the couple and better than another variable previously shown to predict depression, and even better than these two variables combined!

It may be difficult to accept that you cannot control your partner's destructive emotions and behavior. However, you have some power to influence your partner in several positive ways.

VALIDATE YOUR PARTNER'S EMOTIONS, NOT NECESSARILY YOUR PARTNER'S BEHAVIOR

Those with psychological problems often feel distressed as part of the problem or as a result of the problem. A depressed person by definition is unhappy but may also be depressed that he is depressed. Similarly an anxious person is distressed by definition but may also be distressed that she is anxious. Finally, someone with an alcohol or drug problem or a sexual dysfunction may be embarrassed by his or her problems. This distress is real, and you can help by showing some sympathy for that distress.

Sometimes partners are hesitant to sympathize with emotions that seem excessive, in the fear that their sympathy may exacerbate or reinforce the emotions. Although that can happen if the emotional expression is the only way for the person to get attention, a more common occurrence is that the "well partner" resists or minimizes the emotions of the "sick partner" so that the "sick partner" exaggerates his or her emotions in a vain attempt to prove to the other that the pain is real. Or the "sick partner" feels even worse due to feeling alone in the pain. In both of these situations, the response of the "well partner" actually exacerbates the distress of the "sick partner."

Your partner's pain is real. You can validate that pain in ways that show your partner you believe and understand his or her distress. This validation will likely ease your partner's pain and facilitate taking constructive action to address his or her difficulties, especially if you follow the additional advice below.

NUDGE BUT DON'T NAG YOUR PARTNER TO TAKE CONSTRUCTIVE ACTION

If your partner feels you are an ally and not an adversary, he or she will likely be open to your gentle suggestions. For example, encouraging your anxious partner to make a phone call he is anxious about making can facilitate his making the call. Your suggestion that your depressed partner get out of bed and go shopping with you may alter her behavior and her mood. Your request that you and your partner leave a party early before he drinks more than his limit may prevent a drunken episode.

There is a fine line between nudging and nagging, however. If your partner starts to resist you, it is better to back off. It is still your partner's life and his or her right to decide how to behave. You cannot be your partner's ally if you take on the role of parent or judge.

REINFORCE CONSTRUCTIVE BEHAVIOR

Virtually everyone with a psychological difficulty attempts to take constructive actions at times to deal with it. Your partner will also, and you can be there to support those efforts. If your depressed partner makes an effort to engage in constructive activity, despite feeling down, you can support that action by reinforcing it appropriately, showing your partner that you appreciate the effort she is showing to get moving despite feeling depressed. If your anxious partner makes an effort to face one of his fears, you can be there to cheer him on. And if your partner requests that you remove the liquor from the home so it won't be a constant temptation, you can support that healthy request.

Sometimes partners are stingy about their support. They don't want to reinforce anything but a dramatic change in behavior. However, evidence shows that we usually change not in dramatic leaps and bounds but by making small changes in behavior. Reinforcing those little changes that your partner makes can have a cumulative effect over time.

Dealing with a partner with a serious problem is emotionally difficult and, at times, dangerous. Such problems can affect you dramatically. It is important to give up some of your fruitless efforts to try to control your partner and to help your partner as described above. However, you will be able to do that optimally only if you also take good care of yourself.

PROTECT AND CARE FOR YOURSELF

Some emotional and behavioral problems in your partner can present threats to your own safety and security as well as to your partner's. A focus on taking care of yourself, even if you can't take care of your partner, is essential. You may not be able to prevent your partner from driving under the influence of alcohol or drugs, but you can refuse to ride along. You may not be able to prevent your partner from gambling, but you can take steps to protect your money and perhaps the family money.

Even in less dramatic circumstances, you may need to take better care of yourself. Dealing with a partner who has an anxiety disorder or depression can be demanding. Your life can become focused on his needs to the exclusion of your own. You take over his responsibilities because he has such difficulty with them. Your antennas are precisely tuned to his emotional state, so you detect his mood changes even before he does. As your life becomes restricted by his demands, you naturally feel resentful toward him and criticize him for depressed and anxious behavior. This criticism may then exacerbate your partner's own difficulties with anxiety or depression and create tension between the two of you. Furthermore, you may feel guilt along with your resentment, because you see your partner's struggle. This is another example of the effort to cope with an initial problem creating an additional, reactive problem.

By not losing yourself in your efforts to help your partner, by taking care of your own needs as well as hers, you may have to face some disappointment, possibly even anger, from your partner. However, you may limit your own resentment and guilt and be able to be more energetic and supportive toward your partner. By taking care of yourself, you may also be better able to take care of your partner.

SEEK PROFESSIONAL HELP

Psychological disorders usually require professional assistance. Once your partner has admitted to a serious psychological problem, you may be able to assist with obtaining treatment. In fact, it may be helpful if you participate in treatment. Sex therapy is best done with both partners. Some treatments for substance problems, such as alcoholism, involve both partners. Couple therapy is a useful treatment for depression, especially when relationship problems were one of the original causes of the depression or serve to maintain the depression. Even if you don't participate in the treatment itself, you can support your partner's efforts in treatment.

Some of the suggestions we made about finding couple therapy are applicable to individual therapy. Contact friends and professionals to find a mental health professional who specializes in the disorder and who has successfully treated the disorder. Your partner needs to feel comfortable with the therapist and confident in him or her. The therapist should practice a treatment that has scientific evidence to support it. For example, of the psychological treatments, behavior therapy and cognitive-behavioral therapy have proven effective with both anxiety and depressive disorders. Interpersonal psychotherapy has also been proven effective for depression. There are also medications that are effective for depression and anxiety, particularly for depression. Don't be afraid to ask your therapist about the scientific evidence in support of the treatment he or she is to provide or to ask for readings about the treatment.

RECAP

Despite your best efforts, you may be faced with relationship problems that you are unable to resolve through reading this book alone. Online relationship programs may also be of benefit, such as *OurRelationship.com*, which is based on the principles in this book. However, your problems may be such that you need professional help—couple counseling or couple therapy—to improve your relationship. Dozens of studies done throughout the world have shown that therapy can help couples improve their satisfaction with each other. Couple therapy is certainly no panacea for relationship problems: some couples are not helped, and others relapse after treatment. But therapy can help a majority of couples resolve their problems and improve their relationship. Consult the Resources section about sources for obtaining therapists.

Your or your partner's psychological difficulties, such as anxiety, depression, sexual dysfunction, or alcoholism, present problems for both of you. In the worst of all cases, the relationship problems contribute to the individual psychological disorder and the disorder contributes to the relationship problems. In the best of all cases, the relationship can support and even heal the individual problems of your partner, contributing to a greater intimacy between you. If you both are able to discuss the problem constructively, if you accept your limitations in influencing your partner's behavior, and if you can protect and care for yourself while helping your partner by validating his or her emotional distress, nudging your partner toward constructive action, and reinforcing those constructive actions, you can join forces to face the problem together rather than letting it alienate you. You can seek professional help and use that help effectively.

Resources

Authors' Websites

Andrew Christensen, PhD
www.psych.ucla.edu/faculty/faculty_page?id=24&area=2
www.DrAndrewChristensen.com

Brian D. Doss, PhD
www.psy.miami.edu/faculty/bdoss

Integrative Behavioral Couple Therapy

Integrative behavioral couple therapy (IBCT) was developed by Andrew Christensen and Neil S. Jacobson and is the therapeutic approach behind this book. For information on that approach, including the research that supports it as well as referrals to therapists trained in it, see the following website:

http://ibct.psych.ucla.edu

To participate in the online program of IBCT described in Chapter 16, go to

www.OurRelationship.com

Intimate Partner Violence and Abuse

HOTLINES

1-800-799-SAFE (7233)
1-800-787-3224 (TTY)

WEBSITES

www.thehotline.org
www.ncadv.org

SELF-HELP BOOKS

General Relationship Problems

Gottman, J. M., & DeClaire, J. (2002). *The relationship cure: A step guide to strengthening your marriage, family, and friendships.* New York: Three Rivers Press.
Johnson, S. (2008). *Hold me tight: Seven conversations for a lifetime of love.* New York: Little Brown.
Markman, H. J., Stanley, S. M., & Blumberg, S. L. (2001). *Fighting for your marriage: Positive steps for preventing divorce and preserving a lasting love.* New York: John Wiley.
Notarius, C., & Markman, H. C. (1994). *We can work it out: How to solve conflicts, save your marriage, and strengthen your love for each other.* New York: Berkley Books.
Wile, D. B. (2008). *After the honeymoon: How conflict can improve your relationship.* Oakland, CA: Collaborative Couple Therapy Books.

Violence in Relationships

Bancroft, L. (2003). *Why does he do that?: Inside the minds of angry and controlling men.* New York: Berkley Books.
Dececco, J., Letellier, P., & Islan, D. (1991). *Men who beat the men who love them: Battered gay men and domestic violence.* New York: Routledge.
Evans, P. (2010). *The verbally abusive relationship: How to recognize it and how to respond.* Holbrook, MA: Bob Adams.
Lobel, K. (1986). *Naming the violence: Speaking out about lesbian battering.* Berkeley, CA: Seal Press.
NiCarthy, G. (2004). *Getting free: You can end abuse and take back your life.* Seattle: Seal Press.

Infidelity

Glass, S. P., & Staeheli, J. C. (2004). *Not "just friends": Rebuilding trust and recovering your sanity after infidelity.* New York: Atria.
Snyder, D. K., Baucom, D. H., & Gordon, K. C. (2007). *Getting past the affair: A program to help you cope, heal and move on—Together or apart.* New York: Guilford Press.
Spring, J. (2012). *After the affair: Healing the pain and rebuilding trust when a partner has been unfaithful.* New York: William Morrow.

Professional Organizations

The websites of the major professional organizations that deal with mental health issues provide information on the particular profession, provide assistance with getting a therapist, and provide information on mental health problems.

American Association for Marriage and Family Therapy
www.aamft.org

Association for Behavioral and Cognitive Therapies
www.abct.org

American Psychological Association
www.apa.org

American Psychiatric Association
www.psych.org

National Association of Social Workers
www.socialworkers.org

Registry of Marriage and Family Therapists in Canada, Inc.
www.marriageandfamily.ca/?ww_pageID=953C55F2-1372-5A65-3BD54999BE76B41F

International Association of Marriage and Family Counselors
www.iamfconline.org

Family Therapy Association of Ireland
www.familytherapyireland.com

Resources for Mental Disorders

We have listed several sites where information on some of the most common mental disorders, which were mentioned briefly in Chapter 16, can be found.

National Institute of Mental Health
www.nimh.nih.gov

National Institute on Alcoholism Abuse and Alcoholism
www.niaaa.nih.gov

National Institute on Drug Abuse
www.nida.nih.gov

Anxiety and Depression Association of America
www.adaa.org

Australian Psychological Society
www.psychology.org.au

Canadian Mental Health Association
www.cmha.ca

Mind
www.mind.org.uk

Mental Health Foundation
www.mentalhealth.org.uk

Mental Health Association Australia
www.mentalhealth.org.au

Australian and New Zealand Mental Health Association
www.anzmh.asn.au

Bibliography

Chapter 1

Christensen, A., Atkins, D. C., Baucom, B., & Yi, J. (2010). Marital status and satisfaction five years following a randomized clinical trial comparing traditional versus integrative behavioral couple therapy. *Journal of Consulting and Clinical Psychology, 78,* 225–235.

Christensen, A., Atkins, D. C., Berns, S., Wheeler, J., Baucom, D. H. & Simpson, L. E. (2004). Traditional versus integrative behavioral couple therapy for significantly and chronically distressed married couples. *Journal of Consulting and Clinical Psychology, 72,* 176–191.

Christensen, A., Atkins, D. C., Yi, J., Baucom, D. H., & George, W. H. (2006). Couple and individual adjustment for two years following a randomized clinical trial comparing traditional versus integrative behavioral couple therapy. *Journal of Consulting and Clinical Psychology, 74,* 1180–1191.

Fincham, F. D., & Rogge, R. (2010). Understanding relationship quality: Theoretical challenges and new tools for assessment. *Journal of Family Theory and Review, 2*(4), 227–242.

Funk, J. L., & Rogge, R. D. (2007). Testing the ruler with item response theory: Increasing precision of measurement for relationship satisfaction with the Couples Satisfaction Index. *Journal of Family Psychology, 21,* 572–583.

Jacobson, N. S., Christensen, A., Prince, S. E., Cordova, J., & Eldridge, K. (2000). Integrative behavioral couple therapy: An acceptance-based, promising new treatment for couple discord. *Journal of Consulting and Clinical Psychology, 68,* 351–355.

Chapter 2

Karney, B. R., & Bradbury, T. N. (1995). The longitudinal course of marital quality and stability: A review of theory, methods, and research. *Psychological Bulletin, 118,* 3–34.

Peterson, D. R. (1979). Assessing interpersonal relationships by means of interaction records. *Behavioral Assessment, 1,* 221–236.

Chapter 3

Bagby, R. M., Parker, J. D. A., & Taylor, G. J. (1994). The twenty-item Toronto Alexithymia Scale: I. Item selection and cross-validation of the factor structure. *Journal of Psychosomatic Research, 38,* 23–32.

Christensen, A., Eldridge, K., Catta-Preta, A. B., Lim, V. R., & Santagata, R. (2006). Cross-cultural consistency of the demand/withdraw interaction in couples. *Journal of Marriage and the Family, 68,* 1029–1044.

Gosling, S. D., Rentfrow, P. J., & Swann, W. B. (2003). A very brief measure of the big-five personality domains. *Journal of Research in Personality, 37,* 504–528.

Huston, T. L., & Houts, R. M. (1998). The psychological infrastructure of courtship and marriage: The role of personality and compatibility in romantic relationships. In T. N. Bradbury (Ed.), *The developmental course of marital dysfunction* (pp. 114–151). New York: Cambridge University Press.

McCrae, R. R., & Costa, P. T. (1997). Personality trait structure as a human universal. *American Psychologist, 52,* 509–516.

McGue, M., & Lykken, D. T. (1992). Genetic influence on risk of divorce. *Psychological Science, 3,* 368–373.

Pope, H., & Mueller, C. W. (1976). The intergenerational transmission of marital instability: Comparisons by race and sex. *Journal of Social Issues, 32,* 49–66.

Widom, C. S. (1989). Does violence beget violence?: A critical examination of the literature. *Psychological Bulletin, 106,* 3–28.

Chapter 4

Kleck, R. E., & Strenta, A. (1980). Perceptions of the impact of negatively valued physical characteristics on social interaction. *Journal of Personality and Social Psychology, 39,* 861–873.

Levinger, G. (1983). Development and change. In H. Kelley, E. Berscheid, A. Christensen, J. Harvey, J. Huston, G. Levinger, et al. (Eds.), *Close relationships*. San Francisco: Freeman.

Chapter 5

Cohen, S., Kamarck, T., & Mermelstein, R. (1983). A global measure of perceived stress. *Journal of Health and Social Behavior, 24*(4), 385–396.

Cohen, S., & Williamson, G. (1988). Perceived stress in a probability sample of the United States. In S. Spacapan & S. Oskamp (Eds.), *Social psychology of health* (pp. 31–67). Thousand Oaks, CA: Sage.

Milgram, S. (1963). Behavioral study of obedience. *Journal of Abnormal and Social Psychology, 67,* 371–378.

Chapter 6

Christensen, A. (2011). *Communication During Conflict Questionnaire.* Unpublished questionnaire.

Chapter 11

Christensen, A., Sullaway, M., & King, C. C. (1983). Systematic error in behavioral reports of dyadic interaction: Egocentric bias and content effects. *Behavioral Assessment, 5,* 129–140.

Chapter 14

Goodman, G., & Esterly, G. (1988). *The talk book: The intimate science of communication in close relationships.* Emmaus, PA: Rodale Press.

Chapter 15

Barling, J., O'Leary, K. D., Jouriles, E. N., Vivian, D., & MacEven, K. E. (1987). Factor similarity of the Conflict Tactics Scale across samples, spouses, and sites: Issues and implications. *Journal of Family Violence, 2,* 37–54.

Breiding, M. J., Black, M. C., & Ryan, G. W. (2008). Prevalence and risk factors of intimate partner violence in eighteen U.S. states/territories, 2005. *American Journal of Preventive Medicine, 34,* 112–118.

Doss, B. D., Simpson, L. E., & Christensen, A. (2004). Why do couples seek marital therapy? *Professional Psychology, 35,* 608–614.

Gagnon, J. H., Michael, R. T., Laumann, E. O., & Kolata, G. (1994). *Sex in America: A definitive survey.* Boston: Little, Brown.

Jacobson, N. S., & Gottman, J. (1998). *When men batter women: New insights into ending abusive relationships.* New York: Simon & Schuster.

Lawson, A. (1988). *Adultery.* New York: Basic Books.

Simpson, L. E., Atkins, D. C., Gattis, K. S., & Christensen, A. (2008). Low-level relationship aggression and couple therapy outcomes. *Journal of Family Psychology, 22,* 102–111.

Simpson, L. E., Doss, B. D., Wheeler, J., & Christensen, A. (2007). Relationship violence among couples seeking therapy: Common couple violence or battering? *Journal of Marital and Family Therapy, 33,* 270–283.

Straus, M. A., & Gelles, R. J. (1986). Societal change and change in family violence from 1975 to 1985 as revealed in two national surveys. *Journal of Marriage and the Family, 48,* 465–479.

Chapter 16

Christensen, A. Principal Investigator. *Acceptance and change in marital therapy* (National Institute of Mental Health grant). 9/1/97–2/29/04.

Christensen, A. Principal Investigator. *Acceptance and change in marital therapy* (National Institute of Mental Health grant). 12/1/03–11/30/07.

Christensen, A. Co-Principal Investigator. *Empirically-based couple interventions on the web: Serving the underserved* (Subcontract to the University of Miami that is part of a National Institute of Child Health and Human Development grant to Brian Doss, Principal Investigator). 9/30/2009–7/31/2014.

Christensen, A., Atkins, D. C., Baucom, B., & Yi, J. (2010). Marital status and satisfaction five years following a randomized clinical trial comparing traditional versus integrative behavioral couple therapy. *Journal of Consulting and Clinical Psychology, 78,* 225–235.

Christensen, A., & Heavey, C. L. (1999). Interventions for couples. *Annual Review of Psychology, 50,* 165–190.

Doss, D. B. Principal Investigator. *Empirically-based couple interventions on the web: Serving the underserved* (National Institute of Child Health and Human Development grant). 9/30/2009–7/31/2014.

Hooley, J. M., & Teasdale, J. D. (1989). Predictors of relapse in unipolar depressives: Expressed emotion, marital distress, and perceived criticism. *Journal of Abnormal Psychology, 98,* 229–235.

Jacobson, N. S. Principal Investigator. *Acceptance and change in marital therapy* (National Institute of Mental Health grant). 9/1/97–2/29/04.

Whisman, M. A. (1999). Marital dissatisfaction and psychiatric disorders: Results from the National Comorbidity Study. *Journal of Abnormal Psychology, 108,* 701–706.

Index

Abandonment, sensitivity to, 65–68, 73–74, 80, 83, 95–96, 109, 313
Abuse. *See also* Violence in relationship
discouraging, 296–298
emotional, psychological, and verbal, 133, 287, 293–298, 307–308
physical, 68, 132–133, 140, 287–288, 291–293, 307
Acceptance
before change, 131–132
combined with change, 130–131
definition, 125–126, 127
description of, 14–15, 126–131, 138–140
development of, 15, 122, 142, 154, 158, 180
example of, 125–131, 137
experience as promoting, 15, 131, 140–142
plan for your relationship, 140–141
spontaneous change and, 14, 131–132, 140, 158, 198, 202
trust and, 141–142
versus change, 127–129
versus submission, 126
what should not be accepted, 132–135
what should be accepted, 135–137
Accusation
hindsight awareness and, 231–236, 244, 269
of lack of love, 148, 163, 274
overreaction and, 6, 102, 110–115, 157, 192
toxic cures and, 105–117, 122
truth in, 36–37, 183
of unconscious motive, 154–157
Action–reaction conflict, 81–83

Active listening, advice about, 249–254
Advice. *See also* Communication tips
"apple pie" type, 240–241, 258
"express your feelings," 244–249
listen to what partner says, 249–254
negotiate compromise, 254–258
overview of, 239–240
when good advice is bad, 241–242
Affair. *See* Infidelity
Agent, description of, 127–129
Agreement regarding differences, changing, 137
Alcoholism. *See* Special problems in relationship
Alienation after argument, 116–117
Alliances with others, 109–111
Ambivalence, 55–58, 205
Anatomy of argument, 103, 144, 157. *See also* Problem story
Anger
expressing, 6, 8–9, 161–162
"I" statements and, 247–248
pattern of chronic in relationship, 159–160
Anticipating communication pattern, 114, 167–169, 189–190
Apology, 170, 174, 241, 272, 304–305
Approval, sensitivity to, 73, 76–77, 82–83, 211
Argument. *See also* Communication problems; Communication pattern; Problem story; Toxic cures; Violence in relationship
alienation after, 6, 9, 113, 116–117, anatomy of, 103, 144, 157
beginning of, defining, 112–113

337

About the Authors

Andrew Christensen, PhD, is Professor of Psychology at the University of California, Los Angeles. Dr. Christensen has spent more than 30 years studying intimate relationships and working with couples in therapy. He has conducted extensive research on the impact of couple therapy, including the approach on which this book is based, which he developed with the late Neil S. Jacobson. Dr. Christensen and his wife, who live in Los Angeles, have two grown children.

Brian D. Doss, PhD, is Associate Professor of Psychology at the University of Miami, where he teaches and conducts research on couple therapy and romantic relationships. Dr. Doss lives in Miami with his wife and two children.

Neil S. Jacobson, PhD, was Professor of Psychology at the University of Washington until his death in 1999.